Anglo-Saxon Studies 38

MEDICAL TEXTS IN ANGLO-SAXON LITERARY CULTURE

Anglo-Saxon Studies

ISSN 1475-2468

GENERAL EDITORS
John Hines
Catherine Cubitt

'Anglo-Saxon Studies' aims to provide a forum for the best scholarship on the Anglo-Saxon peoples in the period from the end of Roman Britain to the Norman Conquest, including comparative studies involving adjacent populations and periods; both new research and major re-assessments of central topics are welcomed.

Books in the series may be based in any one of the principal disciplines of archaeology, art history, history, language and literature, and inter- or multi-disciplinary studies are encouraged.

Proposals or enquiries may be sent directly to the editors or the publisher at the addresses given below; all submissions will receive prompt and informed consideration.

Professor John Hines, School of History, Archaeology and Religion, Cardiff University, John Percival Building, Colum Drive, Cardiff, Wales, CF10 3EU, UK

Professor Catherine Cubitt, School of History, Faculty of Arts and Humanities, University of East Anglia, Norwich, England, NR4 7TJ, UK

Boydell & Brewer, PO Box 9, Woodbridge, Suffolk, England, IP12 3DF, UK

Previously published volumes in the series are listed at the back of this book

MEDICAL TEXTS
IN ANGLO-SAXON
LITERARY CULTURE

Emily Kesling

D. S. BREWER

© Emily Kesling 2020

All Rights Reserved. Except as permitted under current legislation no part of this work may be photocopied, stored in a retrieval system, published, performed in public, adapted, broadcast, transmitted, recorded or reproduced in any form or by any means, without the prior permission of the copyright owner

The right of Emily Kesling to be identified as the author of this work has been asserted in accordance with sections 77 and 78 of the Copyright, Designs and Patents Act 1988

First published 2020
Paperback edition 2023

D. S. Brewer, Cambridge

ISBN 978-1-84384-549-2 hardback
ISBN 978-1-84384-683-3 paperback

D. S. Brewer is an imprint of Boydell & Brewer Ltd
PO Box 9, Woodbridge, Suffolk IP12 3DF, UK
and of Boydell & Brewer Inc.
668 Mt Hope Avenue, Rochester, NY 14620–2731, USA
website: www.boydellandbrewer.com

A CIP catalogue record for this book is available
from the British Library

The publisher has no responsibility for the continued existence or accuracy of URLs for external or third-party internet websites referred to in this book, and does not guarantee that any content on such websites is, or will remain, accurate or appropriate

Yûzen to
Shite yama wo miru
Kawazu kana!

Ah, the frog
Who looks at the mountain
With utter calm!

--Issa
(trans. J. Hoyt)

Contents

List of Tables	viii
Acknowledgements	ix
Abbreviations	x
Introduction	1
1 *Bald's Leechbook*: A Medical Compendium	23
2 Elves, the Demonic, and *Leechbook III*	57
3 The *Lacnunga* and Insular *Grammatica*	95
4 The *Old English Herbarium* and the Monastic Reform	130
5 Medicine in Anglo-Saxon England	153
Appendices: Extended Quotations	187
A. *Bald's Leechbook* and its Latin Source Material	187
B. Parallel Passages in the *Lacnunga* and MS CCCC 41	194
Bibliography	199
Index	229

Tables

Table 1: Herbs used against Elves   69
Table 2: Herbs used against Demons   70
Table 3: Herbs used in only Elf-Related Remedies   70

Acknowledgements

I have been working on this project for several years and in that time have accrued many debts. In particular, I am grateful to Francis Leneghan and Heather O'Donoghue who have been unceasingly generous in their support and encouragement from the beginning of my graduate studies. I would also like to thank Andy Orchard and Debby Banham for their meticulous comments and suggestions on an early version of this work, as well as the anonymous reviewer.

I am likewise very thankful for the wider community of medievalists at the University of Oxford, where I completed the greater part of this book. My years there were formative ones, and I feel exceedingly blessed to have spent this time surrounded by so many enthusiastic and dedicated scholars. In particular, I would like to thank Mark Atherton, Simon Horobin, and Sarah Foot for their help and advice, as well as David Langslow for sharing his unpublished work on the *Latin Alexander*. More recently, I am indebted to the support of the University of Oslo, where I completed the final part of my work on this project, and its warm and welcoming scholarly community.

I would also like to thank my friends who have read and commented on parts of this book, among them Sheri Chriqui, Susanna Bennett, and my Aunt Kathy. Finally, and most importantly, I would like to thank my mother, Sarah Norton, who has always supported me – even in the most esoteric endeavours – and my husband Fabio who is my co-adventurer and the best in all ways.

Abbreviations

ASE	*Anglo-Saxon England*
ASPR	*The Anglo-Saxon Poetic Records*, ed. George Philip Krapp and Elliot Van Kirk Dobbie. 6 vols. Columbia University Press: New York, 1932–53
BL	British Library
BLB	*Bald's Leechbook* in *Leechdoms, Wortcunning, and Starcraft of Early England, Being a Collection of Documents Illustrating the History of Science in this Country Before the Norman Conquest*, ed. and trans. Oswald Cockayne. 3 vols. Rolls Series. London, 1864–66. Reprinted as part of the Cambridge Library Collection. Cambridge University Press: Cambridge, 2012. Volume II, Books I and II
CCCC	Corpus Christi College, Cambridge
DOE	*Dictionary of Old English: A to H*, ed. Angus Cameron, Ashley Crandell Amos, Antonette diPaolo Healey, *et al.* Dictionary of Old English Project: Toronto. Consulted at <www.doe.utoronto.ca>
EETS o.s.	Early English Text Society – original series
EETS s.s.	Early English Text Society – supplementary series
G&L	Helmut Gneuss and Michael Lapidge. *Anglo-Saxon Manuscripts: a Bibliographical Handlist of Manuscripts and Manuscript Fragments Written or Owned in England up to 1100*. University of Toronto Press: Toronto and London, 2014
JEGP	*The Journal of English and Germanic Philology*
Ker	Neil R. Ker, *Catalogue of Manuscripts Containing Anglo-Saxon*. Clarendon Press: Oxford, 1957
LAC	*Lacnunga* from *Anglo-Saxon Remedies, Charms, and Prayers from British Library MS Harley 585: the Lacnunga*, ed. and trans. with Introduction, Appendices and Commentary by Edward Pettit. Edwin Mellen Press: Lewiston, 2001
LBIII	*Leechbook III* in *Leechdoms, Wortcunning, and Starcraft of Early England, Being a Collection of Documents Illustrating the History of Science in this Country Before the Norman Conquest*, ed. and trans. Oswald Cockayne. 3 vols. Rolls Series. London, 1864–66. Reprinted as part of the Cambridge Library Collection.

Abbreviations

	Cambridge University Press: Cambridge, 2012. Volume II, Book III
MÆ	*Medium Ævum*
MDQ	*Medicina de Quadrupedibus* from *The Old English Herbarium and Medicina de Quadrupedibus*, ed. Hubert Jan De Vriend. EETS o.s. 286. Oxford University Press: London, 1984
MED	*Middle English Dictionary*, ed. Hans Kurath. University of Michigan Press: Ann Arbor, 1952–2001. Consulted at <http://quod.lib.umich.edu/m/med/>. Accessed on 10 August 2016
OEH	*Old English Herbarium* from *The Old English Herbarium and Medicina de Quadrupedibus*, ed. Hubert Jan De Vriend. EETS o.s. 286. Oxford University Press: London, 1984
PL	*Patrologia Latina*, ed. Jacques Paul Migne. 221 vols. Presses Universitaires de France: Paris, 1844–65

Introduction

The Old English medical collections were first edited for the Rolls Series by Oswald Cockayne in the 1860s as part of a three-volume publication with the engaging title *Leechdoms, Wortcunning, and Starcraft of Early England*. The major part of these volumes is dedicated to printing four collections of medical material in Old English. These texts are still largely known by the names drawn from Cockayne's edition: *Bald's Leechbook*, *Leechbook III*, the *Lacnunga*, and the *Old English Herbarium* and *Medicina de Quadrupedibus* (known together as the *Old English Pharmacopeia*). In their various manuscript copies, these collections span across five manuscripts and more than 500 folia and represent the earliest complete collections of medicine in a Western vernacular.

As texts whose aims are principally functional, these collections can be considered part of *Fachliteratur* or technical literature and as such have generally been of most interest to scholars of the history of medicine, codicology, or cultural history and folklore. When these texts have drawn the attention of scholars of literature or history, they have tended to be perceived as evidence of the poor quality of medical knowledge in the period or as a testimony to lingering paganism or popular belief and practice. Evaluations that suggest these works to be of only questionable orthodoxy and outside mainstream ecclesiastical practice are visible even in twenty-first-century publications. For instance, in the most recent edition of one of these texts the editor suggests it was compiled by someone who was 'not a model of orthodox piety', perhaps a lay person, who 'had access to both popular and learned traditions of charms and superstitious practices'.[1] Although assessments of this type have been widespread, this book will contend instead that all four collections mentioned above were almost certainly compiled in major ecclesiastical centres. Rather than being texts which by-and-large depict native pre-Christian tradition or popular yet heterodox Christian practice, these texts reflect the learned environments in which they were compiled and copied.

The four extant collections of medical material mentioned above by name of course do not represent the entirety of vernacular medical writing from the Anglo-Saxon period. Aside from the undoubtedly substantial body of works lost to time, there are also numerous remedies (or

---

[1] *Anglo-Saxon Remedies, Charms, and Prayers from British Library MS Harley 585: The Lacnunga*, ed. and trans. by E. Pettit (Lewiston, 2001), liii, liiii.

Introduction

sometimes groups of remedies) found in otherwise non-medical manuscripts, as well as smaller portions of what may have once been complete collections. For instance, a leaf belonging to the Bibliothèque Centrale in Louvain may be the final folio of an originally complete but no longer extant collection of medical material in Old English. Multiple remedies were also once found in a British Library manuscript, Cotton Otho B. xi, whose several folia of remedies now only survive in Lawrence Nowell's sixteenth-century transcript.[2] Another work deserving of mention here is the so-called *Peri Didaxeon*. This text is found only in MS Harley 6258b, a manuscript of the twelfth century that also contains the latest extant version of the *Old English Pharmacopeia*. This work appears more closely related to texts arriving in England in the eleventh century than the earlier tradition of Anglo-Saxon medicine.[3] As such, this work offers an important testimony to medicine in post-conquest England, but is beyond the scope of this study. The four named works mentioned above are the only complete vernacular medical collections dating from the Anglo-Saxon period, and, as coherent works, I suggest they offer the best possibility for a contextualized study of medical material in the period.

Although this book will suggest that each of the collections of medical material extant in Old English is drawn from a distinctly learned milieu, this does not mean that the four texts should be taken as a unified corpus. While the most probable location and date for the original compilation of each collection will be a topic of discussion throughout this book, in all cases the dates and origins of the texts will remain to varying degrees uncertain. Nevertheless, there is no reason to believe that any of the four extant medical collections were compiled at the same time or in the same milieu.

It has been common in the world of Old English scholarship for the four extant medical texts to be treated as a more-or-less homogeneous body of evidence from which remedies can be excerpted at will for whatever discussion is at hand. This type of approach can be seen in studies which isolate a single group of remedies related by a particular subject or

---

[2] For discussion of these fragments, see A. Meaney, 'Variant Versions of the Old English Medical Remedies and the Compilation of Bald's Leechbook', *ASE* 13 (1984), 235–68; C. B. Voth, 'An Analysis of the Tenth-Century Anglo-Saxon Manuscript London, British Library, Royal 12. D. xvii', unpublished PhD dissertation (Cambridge, 2015), pp. 115–25.

[3] For a discussion of *Peri didaxeon* in a broader context of new medical texts arriving in the eleventh century to England, see D. Banham, 'England Joins the Medical Mainstream: New Texts in Eleventh-Century Manuscripts', in *Anglo-Saxon England and the Continent*, ed. H. Sauer and J. Story (Tempe, 2011), pp. 341–52; D. Banham, 'A Millennium in Medicine? New Medical Texts and Ideas in England in the Eleventh-Century', in *Anglo-Saxons: Studies presented to Cyril Roy Hart*, ed. S. Keynes and A. P. Smyth (Dublin, 2006), pp. 230–42. A new edition is available in an unpublished dissertation: D. Maion, 'Traduzione e Commento del Peri Didaxeon', unpublished PhD dissertation (Università degli Studi Roma Te, 1998).

style; this has been done most frequently with the Old English 'metrical charms' and with remedies related to elves but also in studies of particular ailments. There is much to be gained in these types of studies, and it is perhaps the only way to approach certain subjects, but there is also much lost when remedies are removed from their larger context within a particular collection.

Instead of taking this type of thematic approach, I have chosen to organise this book around the four extant collections, with one chapter dedicated to each collection. Each of these texts reflects the availability of different types of material as well as the local interests of their compilers. It is also my contention that some of these collections can be best appreciated in the context of specific literary or historical developments, which include the period of vernacular translation associated with King Alfred, the ascendency of the hermeneutic style in the tenth century, and the Benedictine reform movement. Nevertheless, across varied periods, styles, and interests these collections continuously demonstrate their connections to intellectual culture and monasticism rather than lay practice.

One danger with the approach taken here is that it could run the risk of underemphasising important commonalities between the collections. Certain commonalities between these texts are clear to anyone familiar with the medical corpus. In many instances these collections were drawing upon the same sources, both in the vernacular and in Latin; indeed, in some cases, the same English translation of a Latin remedy is found in multiple collections. Beyond this, *Bald's Leechbook*, the *Lacnunga*, and *Leechbook III* can also be seen as occurring in broadly the same tradition. Each of these works collects entries from a variety of disparate texts and appears to aspire (successfully or otherwise) to the same organisational style of presenting together remedies for particular parts of the body or similar conditions (unlike, however, the *Old English Pharmacopeia*, which is organised by the herb and animal products used in its recipes). On an even more general level, all four collections share a predominately pharmaceutical outlook, that is, they rely primarily on the use of herbal, and in some cases animal-based or mineral, treatments.[4] It is not my aim to ignore or diminish these important similarities. Instead, I hope to demonstrate that, while these texts occur in broadly the same tradition, consideration of each of the Old English medical collections in its own right can contribute in different ways to a richer understanding of the literary production of the Anglo-Saxon period.

---

[4] The fact that these texts were primarily pharmaceutical does not mean that surgery was not practised in Anglo-Saxon England; it may have simply been learned through experience rather than through written sources. For a discussion of this issue, see D. Banham and C. Voth, 'The Diagnosis and Treatment of Wounds in the Old English Medical Collections: Anglo-Saxon Surgery?',

Introduction

The other risk taken by my organisation is that it may tend to overemphasise the planned and intentional aspect of these texts. It is the nature of manuscript culture for texts to be somewhat fluid; each scribe can unwittingly create errors, produce emendations, or otherwise affect the text. This is particularly true of medical compendia, where adding new recipes (whether known from other sources or from personal experience) appears a logical and obvious thing to do. Faith Wallis has argued that, unlike texts with canonical status, in the case of medical texts, 'the more important the text was for the early medieval reader, the more it was used, and hence the more it was subject to dismemberment, rearrangement, abbreviation, interpolation and so forth'.[5] The best evidence of later additions or changes in the Old English medical collections can be seen in *Bald's Leechbook*. Although this collection was meticulously organised, remedies listed in particular chapters often do not correspond directly to the tabulation of remedies given in the table of contents. This clearly suggests that remedies were added, removed, or moved in subsequent copies of the collection.[6] Some remedies were also added to the end of the *Lacnunga*, apparently by someone other than the original compiler as they occur in a different hand.[7] This is a reminder that, rather than existing as static monuments, these collections were part of the living tradition of Anglo-Saxon medicine. While this is important to acknowledge, I do not believe that it contradicts the fundamental nature of these collections as independent (if evolving) works created in different times and places and to different purposes.

The Four Collections

The chapters of this book have been arranged broadly to reflect date, with the two earliest collections *Bald's Leechbook* and *Leechbook III* being treated before the *Lacnunga* and the *Old English Pharmacopeia*, both of which date from the end of the Anglo-Saxon period.

---

in *Wounds and Wound Repair in Medieval Culture*, ed. L. Tracy and K. DeVries (Leiden, 2015), pp. 153–74. For a more general discussion of the non-textual aspects of medical training in the Anglo-Saxon period, see A. Van Arsdall, 'Medical Training in Anglo-Saxon Engalnd: An Evaluation of the Evidence', in *Form and Content of Instruction in Anglo-Saxon England in the Light of Contemporary Manuscript Evidence: Papers Presented at the International Conference, Udine, 6–8 April 2006*, ed. P. Lendinara, L. Lazzari, and M. A. D'Aronco (Turnhout, Belgium, 2007), pp. 415–34.

[5] F. Wallis, 'The Experience of the Book: Manuscripts, Texts, and the Role of Epistemology in Early Medieval Medicine', in *Knowledge and the Scholarly Medical Traditions*, ed. D. Bates (Cambridge, 1995), pp. 101–26, at 104.

[6] Voth, 'An Analysis', p. 134.

[7] *LAC*, vol. I, pp. 134–35, n. 10.

Introduction

The first chapter considers the text widely known as *Bald's Leechbook*. This title refers to the first two books of the three found in British Library MS Royal 12 D. xvii.[8] This work boasts the most complex organisational structure of all the texts and the highest proportion of translated Latin-based cures (excluding the *Pharmacopeia*). *Bald's Leechbook* contains an impressively wide-ranging collection of remedies, as well as sections of careful and sustained discussion drawn from Late Antique medical compendia. As these selections are drawn from a defined set of source texts and are found in no other extant vernacular collection, I argue that it is likely they were translated expressly for this collection. These passages, which provide theoretical details about bodily organs and certain ailments, may reveal an educational ambition on the part of the compiler of this text. I will suggest that these characteristics, moreover, may have spurred its recopying during the period of vernacular flourishing associated with King Alfred's court, as this movement appears to have prized the educational and encyclopaedic in its vernacular texts.

A collection known as *Leechbook III* follows immediately after *Bald's Leechbook* in the same manuscript. Although Cockayne's edition printed all three books as part of a single collection, this text is now widely recognised as an independent work. This collection is frequently prized for its 'Germanic' content and indeed contains the highest proportion of remedies to treat ailments related to *ælfe* ('elves') and other disease-agents such as the *mæra* ('the mare') and *nihtgengan* ('night-goers'). As will be seen, however, even the remedies for these very remedies contain a variety of learned material. In the second chapter I revisit the question of the relationship between demonic possession and elf-related illness and explore how liturgical material was used in the creation of these remedies, sometimes in subtle and complex ways such as in the remedy for *ælf-sogoþa*.

The third chapter will turn to the collection widely known as the *Lacnunga* ('remedies') found in British Library MS Harley 585.[9] This work was less clearly organised with the intention of forming a discrete medical collection as it contains a wider variety of materials than found in the other collections. It has drawn the attention of scholars primarily for its 'magical' content and its comparatively high proportion of metrical charms. However, when examined in a broader context much of the 'magical' material of the *Lacnunga* reveals an ultimately learned interest of the compiler in the alphabet, enumeration, and the power of words. I show that whoever assembled the *Lacnunga* must have had on hand a large selection of Hiberno-Latin texts (or materials otherwise influenced by Irish tradition) and an unusually large number of long metrical pieces in Old English. These elements have frequently been taken as signs of

---

[8] Ker no. 264; G&L no. 479.
[9] Ker no. 231; G&L no. 421.

superstition and ignorance, but instead reveal a milieu where learned and sometimes esoteric material was available to the compiler.

The fourth chapter addresses the *Old English Herbarium* and the *Medicina de Quadrupedibus*, which stand apart from the other collections as each being the work of a single translator. This is also the only collection to exist in multiple manuscript copies.[10] I will suggest that the principles underlying the translation of the *Old English Herbarium* were practicality and ease of use. However, the creation of this text would have required high quality exemplar texts, some possibly even in multiple copies. Such an endeavour of compilation and translation almost certainly took place at a major centre of learning, and likely one with active connections to the continent. These factors, coupled with a probable date for the collection in the late tenth century, position the translation of this text within the tenth-century Benedictine reform movement and may even indicate that medicine and medical learning was important to leaders of the reform movement, such as Æthelwold.

Taken together the production of these texts conforms to the positive portrayal of medicine found in literary and ecclesiastical sources of the period, something explored in the final chapter. Although the classical authors had differing opinions on the value and appropriateness of medicine (especially within a monastic setting), Anglo-Saxon sources portray a fundamentally positive view of medicine and doctors – a feeling apparently guided by the patristic vision of Christ the good physician. The texts of the medical corpus are often portrayed as liminal works sitting on the outer limits of theological acceptability, yet this conclusion is not supported by study of penitentials and homiletic texts from the period, in which prohibitions against forbidden practices such as *drycræft* or *galdru* occur almost exclusively in the context of popular folk tradition and heathen practice. I will suggest there is no reason for assuming that such prohibitions were meant to include the learned textual traditions found within the medical corpus.

Enthusiasm for uncovering popular practices, paganism, and oral traditions in these texts has frequently left their learned and literary elements unexamined. This is not to suggest that early belief systems or residual popular practice do not colour some of the remedies in these collections, but that many aspects of these texts can only be understood in the context of learned traditions. Each of the medical texts extant from Anglo-Saxon England reflects the ideas and approaches of different compilers and

---

[10] The *Old English Pharmacopeia* (which refers to the composite collection made up of the *Old English Herbarium* and the *Medicina de Quadrupedibus*, respectively) is found in four manuscripts: British Library MS Cotton Vitellius CIII (Ker no. 219; G&L no. 402), Bodleian Library MS Hatton 76 (Ker no. 328; G&L no. 632, 633), British Library MS Harley 585 (in which it precedes the *Lacnunga*), and British Library MS Harley 6358b, which dates to the twelfth century.

the different intellectual milieux where they were created. However, in its own way, each collection interacts purposefully with intellectual and monastic culture. Rather than simply being the domain of history of medicine or folklore, these texts also belong to the wider tradition of Anglo-Saxon literary culture.

This book engages with and builds upon a rich history of scholarship on these four texts. Since the time of Cockayne's editions, these collections have been the subject of on-going interest and inquiry to different generations of scholars, although only the *Old English Pharmacopeia* and the *Lacnunga* have since been republished in new editions.[11] The significance of Cockayne's editions for the subsequent study of medical collections cannot be overstated. Cockayne was a skilful philologist and his editions are generally reliable.[12] However, the facing-page translations he provided have been the subject of some criticism, mostly for their antiquating and Germanising style, popular in the nineteenth century. This is highlighted in particular by Ann Van Arsdall in her new translation of the *Old English Herbarium*, who provides examples taken from Cockayne's prose such as 'in case that any man with difficulty can pass water, take ooze of this same wort with vinegar, give it him to drink; wonderously it healeth'.[13] Such a translation, she suggests, transforms 'the Anglo-Saxon text from a medical reference' written in a reasonably plain style into fanciful literary arcana'.[14] Yet despite this outdated style, the editions produced by Cockayne had a significant role in making widely available for the first time the major works of the Old English medical corpus.

---

[11] A critical edition of the *Old English Herbarium* was published in 1984 by Hubert Jan De Vriend; this is referenced as *OEH*. A new translation of this text is also available: A. Van Arsdall, *Medieval Herbal Remedies: The Old English Herbarium and Anglo-Saxon Medicine* (London, 2002). The most recent critical edition of the *Lacnunga* was published in 2001 by Edward Pettit. However, an earlier edition had been published in 1952: J. H. G. Grattan and C. Singer, *Anglo-Saxon Magic and Medicine, illustrated specially from the semi-pagan text 'Lacnunga'* (Oxford, 1952). I rely on Pettit's edition, which is referenced as *LAC* throughout.

[12] Cockayne's general accuracy has been acknowledged by all editors of new editions of these collections: C. Wright, *Bald's Leechbook: British Museum Royal Manuscript 12 D. xvii*, Early English Manuscripts in Facsimile 5 (Copenhagen, 1955), pp. 27–28; Van Arsdall, *Medieval Herbal Remedies*, p. 63; *LAC*, p. xxxv. De Vriend makes no comment on the quality of Cockayne's edition of the *Herbarium*, but suggests that his purpose in creating a new edition was not to supersede Cockayne's version but instead to provide facing-page Latin text and an edition of Manuscript O (*OEH*, preface). As Voth points out, however, in some cases Cockayne's edition provides an edited version of the text without noting manuscript readings in his critical apparatus: Voth, 'An Analysis', p. 18.

[13] Van Arsdall, *Medieval Herbal Remedies*, p. 63. For a discussion of this translation style in its historical context, see S. Bassnett, *Translation Studies*, revised edition (London, 1980), pp. 68–73.

[14] Van Arsdall, *Medieval Herbal Remedies*, p. 57.

Introduction

Beyond simply providing reliable editions, Cockayne also took the first steps towards understanding the Latin sources underlying many of the Old English cures found in the medical collections. Wherever Cockayne was able to identify a classical source for a passage, he makes note of it in the margins alongside his edition of the Old English text. However, Cockayne appears to have drawn on a reasonably small selection of classical medical works, so in some cases this sourcing is inaccurate. Additionally, he believed that Anglo-Saxon translators would have been drawing directly on Greek medical sources, whereas later scholars have generally agreed that Greek sources would only have been known through Latin translations.[15] The next scholar to make a major contribution to understanding the Latin medical sources used in the compilation of these collections was M. L. Cameron, whose work culminated in the publication of his book *Anglo-Saxon Medicine* in 1993.[16] Aided by Cockayne's marginal notation, Cameron identified numerous sources for passages in the Old English texts, with a particular emphasis on *Bald's Leechbook*. The most recent work in this area has been undertaken by Conan Doyle, whose 2017 PhD provided an appendix compiling the previous source work done by Cockayne, Cameron, and others on *Bald's Leechbook* and extending it with his own research.[17] However, the question of which Latin medical sources were available in Anglo-Saxon England and how, when, and why these were translated into Old English is still an area in need of much further research.

The advancing research on the Latin background of the Old English medical collection has increased scholarly appreciation for the sophisticated nature of these collections. Some early commentators, by contrast, emphasised what they perceived to be the foolish and ineffective nature of Old English medicine. This viewpoint is most strongly voiced by Charles

---

[15] T. O. Cockayne, *Leechdoms, Wortcunning, and Starcraft of Early England: Being a Collection of Documents, for the most Part Never before Printed, Illustrating the History of Science in this Country before the Norman Conquest*, 3 vol. (London, 1864), vol. II, p. xxix (hereafter cited as Cockayne); cf. M. L. Cameron, 'Bald's *Leechbook*: Its Sources and Their Use in its Compilation', *ASE* 12 (1983), 153–82, at 154.

[16] M. L. Cameron, *Anglo-Saxon Medicine* (Cambridge, 1993). Previous articles published by Cameron on related topics include: M. L. Cameron, 'The Sources of Medical Knowledge in Anglo-Saxon England', *ASE* 11 (1982), 135–55; Cameron, 'Bald's *Leechbook*: Its Sources and Their Use in its Compilation'; M. L. Cameron, 'Anglo-Saxon Medicine and Magic', *ASE* 17 (1988), 191–215; M. L. Cameron, 'Bald's *Leechbook* and Cultural Interactions in Anglo-Saxon England', *ASE* 19 (1990), 5–12. Marilyn Deegan also made a significant contribution to the study of Latin sources of *Bald's Leechbook* in her unpublished doctoral dissertation: M. Deegan, 'A Critical Edition of MS B.L., Royal 12. D. xvii: Bald's "Leechbook"', unpublished PhD dissertation (Manchester, 1988).

[17] C. Doyle, 'Anglo-Saxon Medicine and Disease: A Semantic Approach', unpublished PhD dissertation (University of Cambridge, 2017), vol. II: Appendix.

Introduction

Singer, whose incendiary comments are often quoted in accounts of the mid-twentieth-century scholarship of these texts. Singer writes, for instance, that '[the Anglo-Saxon leech] had no understanding of even the rudiments of the science of classical antiquity', and that Anglo-Saxon medical texts should be considered as 'good examples of the darkest and deliquescent stage of an outdated culture'.[18] However, Charles Talbot, a contemporary of Singer, espoused a different view, praising the sophistication of *Bald's Leechbook* as containing 'the teaching of Greek writers as transmitted by Latin translations' and 'embod[ying] some of the best medical literature available to the West at that time'.[19] More recent scholarship has continued to combat Singer's portrayal, showing the intelligent way Anglo-Saxon compilers and translators dealt with their classical sources. This has been emphasised in particular by work done on the *Old English Herbarium* by Linda Voigts, Maria D'Aronco, and Ann Van Arsdall.[20] Cameron's work on *Bald's Leechbook* has also served to expose the complex organisational structure underlying this collection and Doyle has emphasised the degree to which Latin technical vocabulary was understood by Anglo-Saxon translators.[21] The use of classical sources in *Leechbook III* and the *Lacnunga* has received the least attention, but these collections also demonstrate in some cases a sophisticated use of Latin material.

A related area of debate has been the efficacy and usability of the medical collections. Cockayne himself saw Anglo-Saxon medicine as necessarily lower than classical medicine in terms of sophistication and effectiveness, yet he did not deny that some cures may have had efficacy, writing in the preface to the first volume of his *Leechdoms*: 'perhaps herbs are more really effectual than we shall easily believe.'[22] However, Singer

---

[18] These quotations come from Singer's introduction to the 1961 reprint of Cockayne's editions: *Leechdoms, Wortcunning, and Starcraft of Early England*, ed. T. O. Cockayne with a new introduction by C. Singer (London, 1961), vol. I, pp. xix, lvii.

[19] C. H. Talbot, *Medicine in Medieval England* (London, 1967), pp. 18–19.

[20] See L. Voigts, 'Anglo-Saxon Plant Remedies and the Anglo-Saxons', *Isis* 70 (1979), 250–68; M. A. D'Aronco, 'The Transmission of Medical Knowledge in Anglo-Saxon England: The Voices of the Manuscripts', in *Form and Content of Instruction in Anglo-Saxon England in the Light of Contemporary Manuscript Evidence*, pp. 35–58; M. A. D'Aronco, 'Anglo-Saxon Plant Pharmacy and Latin Medical Tradition', in *From Earth to Art. The Many Aspects of the Plant-World in Anglo-Saxon England* (Amsterdam, 2003), pp. 133–51; M. A. D'Aronco, 'L'erbario anglosassone, un'ipotesi sulla data della traduzione', *Romanobarbarica* 13 (1994–95), 325–65; Van Arsdall, *Medieval Herbal Remedies*; A. Van Arsdall, 'Challenging the "Eye of Newt" Image of Medieval Medicine', in *The Medieval Hospital and Medical Practice*, ed. B. Bowers (Aldershot, 2007), pp. 195–206; A. Van Arsdall, 'Rehabilitating Medieval Medicine', in *Misconceptions about the Middle Ages*, ed. B. Grigsby and S. Harris (New York, 2008), pp. 135–41.

[21] Cameron, 'Bald's *Leechbook*: Its Sources and Their Use in its Compilation'; Cameron, *Anglo-Saxon Medicine*, pp. 74–99.

[22] Cockayne, vol. I, p. liii.

Introduction

(and his student Bonser) questioned whether such texts were made to ever be used and suggested that the *Herbarium* in particular contained 'sterile formulae' which were copied without being used or even properly understood.[23] The general scholarly consensus no longer supports this conclusion, and the texts of the medical corpus are now widely considered to have been intended as useful works.[24] Nevertheless, the question of efficacy of individual remedies is much more fraught. The fundamental argument of Cameron's *Anglo-Saxon Medicine* is that, far from being based solely on superstition, many remedies in Old English are in fact 'rational' and would in all likelihood have had some degree of efficacy. Positioning himself against Singer and Bonser, Cameron writes:

> 'Did ancient and medieval physicians use ingredients and methods which were likely to have had beneficial effects on the patients whose ailments they treated?' [...] I think the answer is 'Yes, and their prescriptions were about as good as anything prescribed before the mid-twentieth century.'[25]

Cameron based his analysis of the efficacy of individual remedies on his background as a biologist. Since the publication of *Anglo-Saxon Medicine* in 1993, some of the conclusions made by Cameron have been questioned; in particular, a remedy from *Bald's Leechbook* involving garlic, ox gall, and other ingredients (which Cameron describes as 'an outstanding example of a remedy likely to have been helpful') has been the topic of ongoing debate.[26] One of the challenges in addressing the efficacy of individual

---

[23] W. Bonser, *The Medical Background of Anglo-Saxon England: A Study in History, Psychology and Folklore* (London, 1963), p. 35. See also C. Singer, *From Magic to Science: Essays on the Scientific Twilight* (New York, 1958), p. 24.

[24] A counterpoint to this trend is found in F. E. Glaze, 'The Perforated Wall: The Ownership and Circulation of Medical Books in Medieval Europe, ca. 800–1200', unpublished PhD dissertation (Duke, 1999), pp. 5–9, 143–57. Glaze positions herself between these two viewpoints, suggesting that some medical texts were not studied or copied primarily for practical purposes but instead for their linguistic qualities.

[25] Cameron, *Anglo-Saxon Medicine*, p. 117.

[26] See B. Brennessel, M. D. C. Drout and R. Gravel, 'A Reassessment of the Efficacy of Anglo-Saxon Medicine', *Anglo-Saxon England* 34 (2005), 183–95; E. Rayner, 'AncientBiotics - A Medieval Remedy for Modern Day Superbugs?' (University of Nottingham), consulted at <http://www.nottingham.ac.uk/news/pressreleases/2015/march/ancientbiotics---a-medieval-remedy-for-modern-day-superbugs.aspx> (Accessed 27 June 2016). Cf. Cameron, *Anglo-Saxon Medicine*, p. 119. For a more general discussion of the potential of the Old English medical collections for providing insights into new medicinal uses of drugs, see F. Watkins *et al.*, 'Anglo-Saxon Pharmacopoeia Revisited: A Potential Treasure in Drug Discovery', *Drug Discovery Today* 16 (2011), 1069–75; F. Watkins *et al.*, 'Antimicrobial Assays of Three Native British Plants Used in Anglo-Saxon Medicine for Wound Healing Formulations in 10th Century England', *Journal of Ethnopharmacology* 144 (2012), 408–15.

Introduction

remedies lies in correctly identifying the modern equivalents of medieval herbs, an area in which current research is being undertaken by Debby Banham.[27] In some cases this type of identification can be extremely difficult as even within the Anglo-Saxon period the same name was sometimes applied to multiple plants.[28] Although important work is being done in this area, questions of efficacy are unlikely ever to be completely resolved and this is not an area that I engage in this book.

Another discussion relevant to understanding how 'mainstream' these texts might have been has concentrated on their status as licit or illicit within the Anglo-Saxon Church. Whereas the discussion of Latin sources, translation, and efficacy has largely centred around *Bald's Leechbook* and the *Old English Herbarium*, the question of theological acceptability has more frequently revolved around the *Lacnunga*. Amongst the medical corpus, the *Lacnunga* is widely held to contain the largest number of 'charms', and, as that term suggests, it is these remedies that have been at the centre of the debate over acceptability. In 1909, Felix Grendon's 'The Anglo-Saxon Charms' included a list of the laws prohibiting the practice of magic and the use of 'charms' (*galdru*).[29] Grendon suggests that the 'uncompromising tone' of these injunctions should be taken in contrast to earlier more liberal positions held before Christianity was fully 'entrenched in the soil of Europe'; it was during this earlier, less-regulated period that many heathen charms were essentially Christianised, he argues.[30] The idea that a number of remedies within the medical collections were forbidden within the Anglo-Saxon Church is also evident in Grattan and Singer's 1952 edition of the *Lacnunga*. The authors suggest that the *Lacnunga* was com-

---

[27] D. Banham, 'Investigating the Anglo-Saxon *Materia Medica*: Archaeobotany, Manuscript Art, Latin and Old English', in *The Archaeology of Medicine: Papers Given at a Session of the Annual Conference of the Theoretical Archaeology Group held at the University of Birmingham on 20 December 1998*, ed. R. Arnott (Oxford, 2002), pp. 95–99.

[28] See, for example, Maria D'Aronco's discussion of the herb *elehtre* which is clearly identified with lupin in the *Old English Herbarium* but seems to have signified a different plant (probably squirting cucumber) earlier in the period: M. A. D'Aronco, 'A Problematic Plant Name: *Elehtre*. A Reconsideration', in *Herbs and Healers from the Ancient Mediterranean through the Medieval West: Essays in Honor of John M. Riddle*, ed. A. Van Arsdall and T. Graham (Farnham, 2012), pp. 187–216. For further discussion, see J. Riddle, *Dioscorides on Pharmacy and Medicine* (Austin, 1985), pp. xxii–xxv.

[29] F. Grendon, 'The Anglo-Saxon Charms', *The Journal of American Folklore* 22 (1909), 105–237, at 140–42.

[30] Grendon, 'The Anglo-Saxon Charms', pp. 143–50. Grendon gives several examples of how these practices would have been Christianised: 'Christian ritual was boldly introduced in the charms to replace Heathen rites. Making the sign of the cross naturally became a favorite observance in magical remedies [...]. To give a flavor of Christianity to the herbal hodge-podges which had long been brewed according to Heathen recipes, the exorcist added holy water or a little frankincense.'

piled in stages, with one stratum of remedies being added by a 'leech who was only very superficially Christianised and was quite familiar with the persistent Paganism of local folk. He was not a resident in a monastery.'[31] As can be seen from this observation, the debate over the acceptability of these cures also intersects with the broader question of how 'popular' we should consider the remedies of the medical collections, in particular those relating to elves or dwarves.

The perception that many of the remedies found within the *Lacnunga* (and elsewhere in the corpus) were essentially unorthodox has since been challenged, in particular in the work of Karen Jolly.[32] Jolly argues that the remedies commonly referred to as charms have in fact been thoroughly Christianised in their textual manifestations and exhibit a Christian worldview. Similarly, Lea Olsan has highlighted the necessary involvement of clergy in many medical remedies, and new work by Ciaran Arthur has questioned the usefulness of the term 'charm' in relationship to these texts and as a translation of the term 'galdor', emphasising the close connections between such texts and ecclesiastical ritual.[33] This is still an open area of discussion, however, with some critics such as Edward Pettit and Stephanie Hollis still asserting the essentially pagan (and likely officially forbidden) nature of some entries.[34]

This book continues a trend in scholarship towards recognising the skilful and learned nature of these collections. While some portions of these texts may well represent popular practice or preserve folkloric motifs, a more significant portion reveals literate interests in Latin tradition and intellectual culture.

The Latin Tradition and the Medical Corpus

The works of the Old English medical corpus are the earliest examples of vernacular medical texts extant from the Early Middle Ages and as such are a unique phenomenon. They are also unusual for their inclusion

---

[31] J. H. G. Grattan and C. Singer, *Anglo-Saxon Magic and Medicine: Illustrated specially from the Semi-Pagan Text 'Lacnunga'* (Oxford, 1952), p. 19.

[32] K. Jolly, 'Anglo-Saxon Charms in the Context of a Christian World View', *Journal of Medieval History* 11 (1985), 279–93; K. Jolly, *Popular Religion in Late Saxon England: Elf Charms in Context* (Chapel Hill, 1996). See also V. Flint, *The Rise of Magic in Early Medieval Europe* (Oxford, 1991); C. Arthur, 'Ex Ecclesia: Salvific Power Beyond Sacred Space in Anglo-Saxon Charms', *Incantatio* 3 (2013), 9–32.

[33] L. Olsan, 'Latin Charms of Medieval England: Verbal Healing in a Christian Oral Tradition', *Oral Tradition* 7 (1992), 116–42; C. Arthur, *'Charms', Liturgies, and Secret Rites in Early Medieval England* (Woodbridge, 2018).

[34] S. Hollis and M. Wright, *Old English Prose of Secular Learning* (Cambridge, 1992), pp. 225–29; *LAC*, pp. xlviii–li.

Introduction

alongside standard ailments widely acknowledged in Western texts of remedies for *ælfe* ('elves'), *dweorh* ('dwarf'), and other otherwise unattested ailments such as *þeor*. However, while the Old English collections exist as distinctively English works and each answer to local concerns and interests, at the same time they draw upon and participate in a wider pan-European medical tradition.

All four of the extant works of the medical corpus draw to varying degrees on Latinate medical tradition. A list of works whose passages have found their way into these Anglo-Saxon collections would include the Late Antique encyclopaedic works of authors such as Oribasius and Alexander of Tralles, the Gaulish author Marcellus's mixture of classical medicine with incantations, derivative works based on Pliny and Dioscorides, Galen's *Ad Glauconem de methodo medendi* and the pseudo-Galenic *Liber Tertius*, as well as herbal works including the popular *Pseudo-Apuleius Herbal*.[35] These texts represent some of the most popular medical texts available in the Early Middle Ages. In particular, these texts correspond closely to the medical texts being used and copied in Carolingian monasteries and it is probable that many of these collections may have come to Anglo-Saxon England through Carolingian channels.[36] While more details on how or when these various texts (whether complete or in excerpted form) arrived in England are largely unknown, through these types of Latin texts Anglo-Saxon translators and compilers had access to the shared medical heritage of the West. The rest of this introduction will be dedicated to introducing the most important classical (and post-classical) influences on the Old English medical collections.

---

[35] Background on these texts is available elsewhere. The most thorough treatment is found in Doyle, 'Anglo-Saxon Medicine and Disease', pp. 57–73. For the works of Pliny, Dioscorides and Pseudo-Dioscorides, Oribasius, Alexander of Tralles, the *Liber tertius*, and the *Passionarius Galeni*, see also below. The texts of the Herbarium Complex are treated in Chapter 4, pp. 131–34. Treatments of other authors are also found in Glaze, 'The Perforated Wall', pp. 24–39; Cameron, *Anglo-Saxon Medicine*, pp. 65–73.

[36] In his survey of medicine in France during the reign of Charles the Bald, Contreni offers a list of the most frequently cited medical authors that overlaps closely with those used in the Anglo-Saxon medical corpus: 'Hippocrates, Galen, Oribasius, Dioscorides, Soranus, Alexander of Tralles, Theodorus Priscianus, Pliny, Quintus Serenus, Cassius Felix, and Marcellus Empiricus': J. Contreni, 'Masters and Medicine in Northern France During the Reign of Charles the Bald', in *Charles the Bald: Court and Kingdom*, ed. M. Gibson and J. Nelson (Oxford, 1981), pp. 262–82, at 269. For the transmission of medical text to Anglo-Saxon England through Carolingian monasteries, see D'Aronco, 'L'erbario anglosassone', pp. 353–55 and Chapter 4, pp. 148–50.

Introduction

Pliny the Elder

Pliny, in his *Naturalis historia*, advocates the use of simple, naturally derived medicines. Although cures are easily available through natural remedies, he laments that these simple cures have been forgotten and replaced with complicated mixtures peddled by foreign doctors:

> ulcerique parvo medicina a Rubro mari inputatur, cum remedia vera cotidie pauperrimus quisque cenet. nam si ex horto petantur, aut herba vel frutex quaeratur, nulla artium vilior fiat. ita est profecto, magnitudine populi R. periit ritus, vincendoque victi sumus. paremus externis, et una artium imperatoribus quoque imperaverunt.[37]

> [For even a small sore, medicine is imported from the Red Sea, when true remedies are consumed daily by even the poorest people. For if [remedies] were to be sought from the garden, or a plant or bush, no art would be cheaper than medicine. Thus it is certain, that through their greatness the Roman people have abandoned their customs, and having been conquerors we ourselves have been conquered. In one art we are the subject of foreigners and they control their rulers.]

In keeping with this general perspective, the medical remedies Pliny records are often very simple in their ingredients and preparation.

Pliny the Elder's medical philosophy and writings formed the basis for much of medicine practised in the Early Middle Ages. It seems unlikely that Pliny's great work the *Naturalis historia* was ever translated in its entirety into Old English, yet at least some books of the Latin text were available in Anglo-Saxon England as sections are cited by Bede as well as other authors including Aldhelm, Alcuin, Abbo, and Byrhtferth. Lapidge records four manuscripts from Anglo-Saxon England that contained some of the *Naturalis historia* and draws the conclusion that Bede's library likely contained about half of its books.[38] In its complete form, Pliny's large work contains 37 volumes addressing the very broad subject of the *rerum natura, hoc est vita* ('the nature of things, that is life').[39] In his preface, Pliny claims that he drew upon some 2,000 sources for this endeavour. Regardless of the accuracy of this boast, it is clear that he drew upon many sources for

---

[37] Pliny the Elder, *Natural History: With an English Translation in Ten Volumes*, ed. H. Rackham, Loeb Classical Library, I (Cambridge, 1975), XXIV, 5. Henceforth referred to as *Naturalis historia* (citations are given by chapter number and paragraph number).

[38] M. Lapidge, *The Anglo-Saxon Library* (Oxford, 2006), p. 325; M. Chibnall, 'Pliny's *Natural History* and the Middle Ages', in *Empire and Aftermath: Silver Latin II*, ed. T. Dorey (London, 1975), pp. 57–78, at 61.

[39] *Naturalis historia*, preface, 13.

Introduction

his remedies, both of Roman and Greek origin.[40] Pliny plainly intended this achievement as a reference text and appended a list of contents to its preface. A large share of this work was therapeutic, with Books 20 to 32 dealing extensively with medical material. The books range between various topics; some of them appear to be organised by drug origin (for example, Book 24 deals mostly with drugs obtained from foreign trees), but others are arranged by disease.

Pliny's remedies are particularly dominant in the *Old English Pharmacopeia*, as its two main sources (the *Pseudo-Apuleius Herbal* and the *Liber medicinae ex animalibus*) owe much of their content to Pliny.[41] However, remedies derived from Pliny are also found in *Bald's Leechbook*, the *Lacnunga*, and *Leechbook III*.[42] In general, this material was probably not taken directly from Pliny's great work, the *Naturalis historia*, but from derivative works compiled in the Late Antique period. In the fourth century, the medical material found in Pliny's *Naturalis historia* was extracted and compiled into a shorter collection now generally known as the *Medicina Plinii*; this work in turn was the basis for the *Physica Plinii*, a later work that drew mainly upon the *Medicina Plinii* but also used other sources.[43] Some books of *Naturalis historia* would have been available in Anglo-Saxon England, but the translators of medical material were more likely relying on one or both of these derivative collections. The testimony of *Bald's Leechbook* suggests the availability either of a no longer extant, expanded version of the *Physica Plinii* or the presence as well of the more complete *Medicina Plinii*.[44] Through these derivative sources Anglo-Saxon translators had access to a wide variety of Plinian remedies.

Dioscorides

A second major influence on the Old English medical collections, and early medieval medicine more generally, was the Greek author Dioscorides. Unlike his contemporary Pliny, who was trying to record all things per-

---

[40] M. Beagon, *Roman Nature: The Thought of Pliny the Elder* (Oxford, 1992), p. 204.
[41] De Vriend, pp. lvii–lviii, lxvi.
[42] J. Adams and M. Deegan, 'Bald's *Leechbook* and the *Physica Plinii*', *ASE* 21 (1992), 87–114. This work has been updated in Doyle, 'Anglo-Saxon Medicine and Disease', pp. 9–11. For examples of how these remedies are integrated within the collection, see Doyle, 'Anglo-Saxon Medicine and Disease', Volume II: Appendix.
[43] Adams and Deegan, 'Bald's *Leechbook* and the *Physica Plinii*', p. 89; Cameron, *Anglo-Saxon Medicine*, p. 69.
[44] Adams and Deegan, 'Bald's *Leechbook* and the *Physica Plinii*', p. 110. Adams and Deegan argue that 'the compiler was either using a fuller version of the *Medicina Pliniii* than that which is extant, or a version of the *Phyisca* which was closer to the original *Medicina Plinii* in various respects.'

Introduction

taining to the natural world, Dioscorides's aim was to systematically and conclusively cover the subject of pharmacy.[45] Like the *Naturalis historia*, Dioscorides's Περὶ ὕλης ἰατρικῆς ('On Medical Materials') is a massive work that comprises, in its full form, information on over 600 medical substances and around 2,000 recipes.[46] However, Dioscorides's influence in the Middle Ages came not only from his Περὶ ὕλης ἰατρικῆς, which was probably fully translated into Latin by the sixth century and is known under the title *De materia medica*, but also from derivative works.

As the foremost ancient author on pharmacy, his work was the *fons et origo* for other medieval herbals, and, due to the magnitude of Dioscorides's work, it was often abridged and used in new smaller herbal collections.[47] There is no indication that the Anglo-Saxon translators had access to the full *De materia medica*, but two derivative collections were clearly known, as they supply most of the remedies found in the last third of the *Old English Herbarium*.[48] These two works, the *Curae herbarum* and the *Liber medicinae ex herbis femininis*, are now most often attributed to 'Pseudo-Dioscorides' because they differ from Dioscorides's original work in significant ways. The *Ex herbis femininis* in particular enjoyed great popularity in the Early Middle Ages.[49] Dioscorides's *De materia medica* very much constitutes the core source for this text, but the sixth-century author was keen to amend or modify the remedies as well as to reduce its size to only 71 chapters. These factors led Riddle to label this a 'largely new work', one which

---

[45] P. Dioscorides, *De materia medica*, trans. L. Beck (Hildesheim, 2011), p. xv. In her introduction, Beck notes that Dioscorides's observations on pharmacy may well have been written in the same decade as the *Naturalis historia*.

[46] Dioscorides, *De materia medica*, p. xviii; Riddle, *Dioscorides on Pharmacy and Medicine*, p. xviii. Riddle remarks on the size of Dioscorides's endeavour: 'when one considers that the entire Hippocratic corpus listed only about 130 medicinal substances – and the Hippocratic works were by far the largest in volume of the extant medical writings before Dioscorides – then the scale of Dioscorides' work becomes clearer.'

[47] J. Riddle, 'Pseudo-Dioscorides' *Ex herbis femininis* and Early Medieval Medical Botany', *Journal of the History of Biology* 14 (1981), 43–81, at 43; J. Stannard, 'The Herbal as a Medical Document', in *Herbs and Herbalism in the Middle Ages and Renaissance* (Aldershot, 1999), pp. 212–20, at 215.

[48] Philip Rusche has argued that the Greek text of the *De materia medica* may have been known at the school of Theodore at Canterbury in the late seventh century. However, if this is the case, there is no evidence that it was known in the later period or to the compilers of any of the Old English collections. See P. Rusche, 'Dioscorides' *De materia medica* and Late Old English Herbal Glossaries', in *From Earth to Art: The Many Aspects of the Plant-World in Anglo-Saxon England; proceedings of the First ASPNS Symposium, University of Glasgow, 5–7 April 2000*, ed. C. P. Biggam (Amsterdam, 2003), pp. 181–94, at 191–92.

[49] Riddle, 'Pseudo-Dioscorides' *Ex herbis femininis*', pp. 43–44. The Old Latin full version of this text has survived in three complete or nearly complete manuscripts dating from the ninth and the tenth centuries; the shorter *Ex herbis femininis* is found in some 29 manuscripts, 13 of which date from the twelfth century or earlier.

Introduction

'reflects a higher level of medical-botanical lore than currently attributed to the era, an uncommon linguistic skill in Greek and Latin, and some degree of originality, perhaps as much as can be expected in any herbal, whatever the time.'[50] The name *Ex herbis femininis* pertains to the idea that this tract contains information on female herbs, according to the classical system in which plants were sometimes categorised by gender.[51] The title of this treatise may in fact be related to its association with the *Pseudo-Apuleius Herbal*, which is occasionally referred to as being a reference for masculine herbs.[52] The *Curae herbarum* is a similar work, sharing about a third of its chapters with the *Ex herbis femininis*, and both deriving from a lost Latin translation of Dioscorides's work.[53]

De materia medica is noteworthy on several accounts, not only for its volume but perhaps even more so for its thoroughness and organisation. Like the *Pseudo-Apuleius Herbal*, Dioscorides's compendium is organised by herb (or substance), with entries generally following a specific pattern. Lily Beck outlines this general structure as: morphology, habitat, relative qualities, method of preparation, general properties and specific therapeutic applications, adulteration, compounding, and directions for storage.[54] Not every drug contains all of these pieces of information in its entry, but the details included typically follow this structure. Dioscorides is the first author to reference at length the idea of 'properties' (in Greek, δυνάμεις) of different medical substances.[55] According to this theory, every substance has properties that refer to its effect on a patient. A drug can be, for example, warming, cooling, staunching, binding, or softening. This theory of therapeutics would come to full fruition in the works of Galen in the second century. Although the Anglo-Saxons had access to Dioscorides's work only through derivative collections, these collections maintained his basic structure within herbal entries and his philosophy of the properties of drugs.

---

[50] Riddle, 'Pseudo-Dioscorides' *Ex herbis femininis*', p. 43.
[51] Riddle, 'Pseudo-Dioscorides' *Ex herbis femininis*', p. 47. Male plants were those generally considered to be harder, drier, and less fruitful than female plants, which were softer and more moist.
[52] Riddle, 'Pseudo-Dioscorides' *Ex herbis femininis*', p. 47.
[53] A. Bracciotti, 'Osservazioni sulla forma del latino *lauer* nell'edizione Wellmann di (pseudo-) Dioscoride e nelle edizioni di alcuni erbari latini', *Filologia antica e moderna* 26 (2004), 45–55, at 46.
[54] Dioscorides, *De materia medica*, p. xxiii.
[55] Dioscorides, *De materia medica*, p. xxiii. Pliny mentions properties in passing but never treats them systematically.

Introduction

Byzantine and Galenic Medicine

Although practical, pharmaceutical medicine was the most widely translated medical material in Anglo-Saxon England, at least as evidenced by surviving sources, more theoretical humoral medicine was also known. This type of medicine is most evident in certain passages of *Bald's Leechbook*, which draw on a variety of Late Antique sources heavily influenced by Galen's medical theory.[56] Galen, born in Pergamon in the second century, is best known for his humoral theory. He believed that there were four major humours: blood, yellow bile, black bile, and phlegm, which correspond to the four elements: fire, earth, air, and water.[57] Galen's theories on anatomy, based in part on the dissection of animals, were also influential. He was an exceedingly prolific author, yet due in part to the extreme length and verbosity of his works, they were most often known in the Middle Ages through later authors, in particular in the works of Byzantine physicians Oribasius and Alexander of Tralles, who helpfully excerpted and abridged Galen's work.[58]

Oribasius was born in the Greek city of Pergamon near the beginning of the fourth century.[59] He is most famous for having been the personal physician of the Roman Emperor Julian, known as 'the Apostate'. In the 350s, Oribasius completed his great work *Medical Collections* (Ἰατδιχαὶ Συναγωγαί), in 70 books.[60] Later in his life, he produced two abridgements of this massive work: the *Synopsis to Eustathius* and the *Synopsis to Eunapius*, also known respectively as the *Synopsis* and the *Europistes*.[61] The greater part of the *Medical Collections* had been lost by the seventh century, and it is mostly through these shorter works that Oribasius was known in the medieval West. These two collections were translated into Latin twice in the Late Antique period; originally scholars referred to these two translations as the 'old' and 'new' translations, yet more recently they have been shown to both date from around the same period – probably from the late sixth or early seventh century. The corresponding passages

---

[56] For a discussion of the character of these passages in *Bald's Leecbook*, see pp. 37–42. For an overview of the question of how much humoral theory would have been transmitted and understood in Anglo-Saxon England, see Doyle, 'Anglo-Saxon Medicine and Disease', Chapter 5. See also L. Ayoub, 'Old English *wæta* and the Medical Theory of the Humours', *JEGP* 94 (1995), 332–46.

[57] O. Temkin, *Galenism: Rise and Decline of a Medical Philosophy* (London, 1973), p. 17.

[58] For a discussion of Byzantine influences on medieval Western medicine, see Glaze, 'The Perforated Wall', pp. 32–36.

[59] M. Grant, *Dieting for an Emperor: A Translation of Books 1 and 4 of Oribasius' Medical Compilations with an Introduction and Commentary* (Leiden, 1997), p. 1.

[60] Cameron, *Anglo-Saxon Medicine*, p. 67.

[61] Grant, *Dieting for an Emperor*, p. 4; Oribasius, *Œuvers d'Oribase*, ed. U. C. Bussemaker, C. Daremberg, A. Molinier, 6 vols. (Paris, 1856–76), VI, p. ii.

in *Bald's Leechbook* appear to be taken from both translations, suggesting the availability of multiple copies of the text in Anglo-Saxon England.[62]

The second author mentioned above, Alexander of Tralles, was born two centuries after Oribasius, probably near the beginning of the sixth century, in a region that is now modern Turkey.[63] Like Oribasius, Alexander's works were originally written in Greek, his most famous being the *Therapeutica* (Θεραπευτικά), which gives advice on the diagnosis and treatment of many diseases, the majority of which deal with internal problems. Its chapters are ordered generally from the head downwards (an organisation resembling *Bald's Leechbook*). The exact date is uncertain but at some point, probably close to the creation of the Greek text, a shorter Latin translation was made, covering about 80% of its content. This 'Latin Alexander' included both the *Therapeutica* and a tract by Alexander on fevers.[64] It is likely that this is the form in which the Anglo-Saxons would have encountered Alexander's writings.

The medical texts of both Oribasius and Alexander are encyclopaedic works. Neither author is typically praised by modern medical historians for their originality or ingenuity. However, both are important conduits of classical medical learning – Oribasius especially was often content to simply compile what he viewed as the best works on a certain subject without heavily editing them.[65] The primary sources for each author were the texts of the Greek Hippocratic corpus, and, most significantly, those of the famous Roman physician Galen.[66] The works of Alexander of Tralles and Oribasius were significant in exposing the Anglo-Saxons to Greek medical theory (albeit in a derivative form).

In addition to these two major authorities, there is another group of texts worth mentioning because of their frequent use in *Bald's Leechbook*. These include Galen's *Ad Glauconem de methodo medendi*, the pseudo-Galenic *Liber tertius*, and the *Aurelius-Esculapius* complex.[67] These texts are best known in the form in which they were edited and compiled in the mid-eleventh century by the Salernitan author and physician, Gariopuntus.

---

[62] Cameron, *Anglo-Saxon Medicine*, p. 24.
[63] D. Langslow, *The Latin Alexander Trallianus: The Text and Transmission of a Late Latin Medical Book*, Society for the Promotion of Roman Studies, monograph 10 (London, 2006), p. 2.
[64] Langslow, *The Latin Alexander Trallianus*, pp. 6, 8. The earliest manuscript copy of the Latin Alexander dates c. 800 AD.
[65] *Œuvers d'Oribase*, VI, p. iv.
[66] Langslow, *The Latin Alexander Trallianus*, p. 6; *Œuvers d'Oribase*, VI, p. iv.
[67] F. Glaze, 'Galen Refashioned: Gariopontus in the Later Middle Ages and Renaissance', in *Textual Healing: Essays on Medieval and Early Modern Medicine*, ed. E. Furdell (Leiden, 2005), pp. 53–75, at 53–54. The *Ad Glauconem de methodo* is a loose translation of Galen's original (Cameron, *Anglo-Saxon Medicine*, p. 71; Glaze, 'The Perforated Wall', p. 39). For more information on this text, see also: P. Kibre and I. Kelter, 'Galen's "Methodus medendi" in the Middle Ages', *History and Philosophy of the Life Sciences* 9 (1987), 17–36.

Introduction

This compilation is known as the *Passionarius*, or the *Liber nosematon*.[68] The Anglo-Saxons would not have had the texts in their post-Salernitan form, as this medical movement postdates the Anglo-Saxon period, but it is clear from the extended quotations in the *Leechbook* that some of the individual treatises and possibly an early form of composite text were consulted. The most frequently used is the *Liber tertius*, an anonymous early Byzantine work.[69] However, other sections appear to be taken either from the *Ad Glauconem de methodo medendi* or from an early version of the *Passionarius*.[70] Alongside the *Latin Alexander*, the *Europistes* and *Synopsis* of Oribasius, these treatises represent some of the most popular medicine in the Early Middle Ages and provide *Bald's Leechbook* with many of its more theoretical passages.

Medical Texts and Anglo-Saxon Libraries

When considering the corpus of Latin medicine translated into Old English, it is difficult to prove that a particular text was known, entire, to an Anglo-Saxon audience. However, the texts mentioned above must have been sufficiently available to allow them to be drawn upon at considerable length by Anglo-Saxon translators and compilers. It is thus worth taking a moment to consider this testimony against the manuscript record from Anglo-Saxon England, in which only a few Latin medical texts survive; those that do include: some books of the *Naturalis historia*, the *Herbarium Complex* texts (including the *Ex herbis femininis*), Galen's *Ad Glauconem de methodo medendi*, and a text by the same author on fevers.[71] Of course extant manuscripts represent only a percentage of those existing in Anglo-Saxon libraries. This is clearly recognised in works such as Michael Lapidge's catalogue of classical and patristic authors known in Anglo-Saxon England which includes works cited directly by major Anglo-Saxon authors, as well as those found in booklists from the period. Yet in the case of medical collections, the only texts to be included in this catalogue are those still surviving in manuscript form. This exception likely reflects both the difficulties sometimes encountered with identifying medical quotations as well as the treatment of medical texts in the booklists, which is not helpful in identifying particular texts. However, this should not be

---

[68] Glaze, 'Galen Refashioned', pp. 53–54.
[69] For more background on this text, see K. Fischer, 'Der pseudogalenische *Liber tertius*', in *Galenismo e medicina tardoantica: fonti greche, latine e arabe: atti del Seminario internazionale di Siena, Certosa di Pontignano, 9–10 settembre 2002*, ed. I. Garofalo and A. Roselli (Naples, 2003), pp. 101–32.
[70] The difficulty of sometimes distinguishing passages from these sources is discussed by Cameron: 'Bald's *Leechbook*: Its Sources and Their Use in its Compilation', pp. 163–66.
[71] Lapidge, *The Anglo-Saxon Library*, pp. 303, 325, 340.

Introduction

taken to suggest that the only medical texts known were those still extant in manuscript copies.

In the collection of known booklists from Anglo-Saxon England, medical texts are decisively mentioned four times, and less conclusively in two additional instances. The only author or text to be identified by name is Pliny (which presumably indicates either books of the *Naturalis historia* or the *Physica Plinii*). In other instances, manuscripts are simply identified as *liber medicinalis, medicinalis,* or *lece boc*.[72] It is difficult to know if these titles indicated collections in Latin or Old English and the individual texts specified here are impossible to identify; nevertheless such lists testify to the fact that medical texts were reasonably standard features of Anglo-Saxon libraries.

The booklists may also sometimes reveal something about how these manuscripts were used. In a list of books in the possession of monks of Bury St Edmunds, a 'Sigar preost' is recorded as having two books: *þe lece boc ond blake had boc*.[73] The *lece boc* appears to refer to a medical text of some sort, yet it seems possible that the *blake had* book might also refer to a collection of medical cures specifically relating to leprosy.[74] If this were the case, it would seem to be evidence of a member of the monastic community specialising in medicine. A further point of interest is an erased entry in this same list which Lapidge reads as *þe [lece]*.[75] This too may well be a medical text of some sort, in which case this list of 15 books may have contained three independent medical works. This might reflect a level of specialisation within the monastic centre; intriguingly, Debby Banham has suggested that there might have been some form of 'medical school' at Bury in the late eleventh century under abbot Baldwin, which could possibly reflect a continuation of this earlier tradition at the monastery.[76]

The evidence of booklists, as well as the Latin source material underlying the vernacular remedies of the Old English medical corpus, suggests that current catalogues do not fully convey the variety and number of

---

[72] M. Lapidge, 'Surviving Booklists from Anglo-Saxon England', in *Learning and Literature in Anglo-Saxon England: Studies Presented to Peter Clemoes on the Occasion of his Sixty-Fifth Birthday*, ed. M. Lapidge and H. Gneuss (Cambridge, 1985), pp. 33–89, at lists I, IV, VIII, and XII.
[73] Lapidge, 'Booklists', list XII.
[74] Lapidge, 'Booklists', pp. 75–76. Lapidge suggests several possible meanings for this designation. It is possible that 'had boc' could stand in for 'hand boc' with a missing suspension-mark, or that 'blake' could refer to the colour of the binding. Most interesting, however, is the suggestion that it could be a form of *blæco* (meaning pallor or leprosy) plus *had* and meaning 'a condition of leprosy'. If this were the case, a 'blake had boc' would probably designate a collection of treatments for leprosy.
[75] Lapidge, 'Booklists', list XII.
[76] D. Banham, 'Medicine at Bury in the Time of Abbot Baldwin', in *Bury St Edmunds and the Norman Conquest*, ed. T. Licence (Woodbridge, 2014), pp. 226–46, at 244–45.

Introduction

Latin medical texts available to an Anglo-Saxon audience. The variety of texts employed in the translated passages of the Old English medical corpus indicates that classical and Late Antique medical learning was important in some Anglo-Saxon intellectual circles, and the inclusion of these translated texts (and in some cases new acts of translation) testifies to the importance of the wider European tradition to the compilers of the Old English medical collections.

Although medical material has been treated as marginal in the study of Anglo-Saxon literature and intellectual history, this does not appear to accurately reflect its status in the period. It is clear that medical texts held an important place in Anglo-Saxon libraries, and medical remedies are a frequent choice for marginal editions in texts of all sorts. Medical texts were also among the genres of text most chosen for translation, even if translation in this field would have required special expertise. It is my hope that this book will help to further illuminate the place of medical writings in wider Anglo-Saxon literary and intellectual culture.

1

Bald's Leechbook: A Medical Compendium

The British Library manuscript Royal 12 D. xvii contains three books of medical material. Cockayne referred to the collections in this manuscript as a *Leech Book*, which he then further divided into three volumes. However, he recognised the third book as having a different 'somewhat more monkish character', and it is now widely agreed that these three volumes actually represent two separate collections of medical material.[1] The first two books of the Royal manuscript are commonly referred to as *Bald's Leechbook*: the best known and likely oldest of the Old English medical collections, which, as such, represents the earliest complete medical collection in a Western vernacular. The final book is identified by scholars as *Leechbook III* (a name taken from Cockayne's original idea of a *Leechbook* in three parts) and will be the focus of Chapter 2.[2]

The name *Bald's Leechbook* is taken from a verse colophon that occurs at the end of the second book. This colophon, which serves to divide the two books of *Bald's Leechbook* from *Leechbook III*, is written in Latin hexameters:[3]

> Bald habet hunc librum cild quem conscribere iussit;
> Hic precor assidue cunctis in nomine Xristi.
> Quo nullus tollat hunc librum perfidus a me.
> Nec ui nec furto nec quodam famine falso.
> Cur quia nulla mihi tam cara est optima gaza.
> Quam cari libri quos Xristi gratia comit.[4]

---

[1] See Cockayne, vol. II, p. xx; Wright, *Bald's Leechbook*, p. 14.
[2] *Bald's Leechbook* and *Leechbook III* have each been edited as an unpublished PhD dissertation. An edition of *Bald's Leechbook* is found in M. Deegan, 'A Critical Edition of MS B.L., Royal 12. D. xvii'; a less thorough treatment of the third book is found in B. Olds, 'The Anglo-Saxon Leechbook III: A Critical Edition and Translation', unpublished PhD dissertation (Denver, 1984). I have made reference to both of these editions. However, I have worked primarily from Cockayne's editions of these two collections, with reference to the published facsimile (Wright, *Bald's Leechbook*) and in some cases the British Library manuscript.
[3] Royal 12 D.xvii is Ker no. 264; G&L no. 479. For discussion of *Leechbook III*'s status as a separate collection, see Wright, *Bald's Leechbook*, p. 14. See also Chapter 2, pp. 57–59.
[4] BL, Royal MS 12 D. xvii, f. 109r; *hund* emended in line 1 to *hunc*, following Wright, *Bald's Leechbook*, p. 13; expansions also following this edition. Throughout this book expansions will be rendered silently; the symbol *wynn* is

[Bald owns this book, which he commanded Cild to write/copy. I earnestly ask this of everyone in the name of Christ, that no perfidious person take this book from me either by force, or by stealth, or by any false speech. Why? Because the highest treasure is not more dear to me than those dear books which the grace of Christ adorns/brings together.]

The colophon has attracted some attention because it associates the collection with an author (this is the only one of the four Old English medical texts to be associated, however tenuously, with a named author). The names themselves are unusual and it seems most likely that they are shortened versions of longer names. Both 'Bald' (or 'Beald') and 'Cild' appear much more often as a component in Anglo-Saxon names rather than as a name themselves.[5] The shortened versions are probably given to meet the requirements of the hexameter verse.

As has been noted frequently in the scholarship surrounding this collection, the colophon does not make it clear if Cild is the author of the text or merely a scribe; similarly Bald could be interpreted as the author or simply the owner.[6] The difficulty lies in the verb *conscribere* which could mean to write in the authorial sense or could mean to produce a copy or even to compile a collection. There may be a play on this last meaning in the final line of the colophon where *comit* could be understood to mean 'adorn' or 'ornament' but can also carry the meaning of bringing together or compiling. This second sense might be appropriate here, as, aside from being the only collection associated with a named author, *Bald's Leechbook* would have required considerable effort to compile and stands apart from the other extant Old English medical collections for its complexity of organisation.

The two books of the collection are each headed by a table of contents and contain chapters demarcated by roman numerals.[7] Both books are generally organised to follow the body in a head-to-foot organisation, with the first chapter of Book I beginning: *on þissum ærestan læcecræftum gewritene sint læcedomas wið eallum heafdes untrymnessum* ('in these first

---

normalised as *w* and the Tironian note as *ond*. Translations are my own unless otherwise noted.

[5] PASE lists the colophon as the only instance of the name 'Bald'; 'Cild' occurs elsewhere only as the name of an eleventh-century moneyer: 'bald', 'cild', *Prosopography of Anglo-Saxon England*, <http://www.pase.ac.uk> (Accessed, 26 Sept 2017). Cecily Clark suggests the possibility of shortening two-part names and Colman lists both names as potentially hypocoristic (short names) or bynames (nicknames): C. Clark, 'Onomastics', in *The Cambridge History of the English Language, Volume 1: The Beginning to 1066*, ed. R. M. Hogg (Cambridge, 1992), pp. 452–89; F. Colman, *The Grammar of Names in Anglo-Saxon England: The Linguistics of Culture of the Old English Onomasticon* (Oxford, 2014), p. 253.

[6] Wright, *Bald's Leechbook*, p. 13.

[7] For a recent and thorough description of the manuscript, see Voth, 'An Analysis', pp. 23–38.

remedies are written treatments for all sicknesses of the head').[8] This organisation (also known as *a capite ad calcem*) is not unusual amongst Late Antique and early medieval medical collections. This system continues throughout Book I from head diseases, down through problems like knee and thigh pain, to remedies for cold feet in Chapter 30. In the second half of Book I, the organisation is less clear, but similar diseases are grouped together, with Chapters 31–44 generally dealing with skin conditions, 45–53 dealing with sicknesses from various worms, and 54–65 mostly relating to fever or paralysis. The final chapters, 66–88, have no discernible organisation and address a large variety of ailments, ranging from the bite of a rabid dog to hair thinning.

On the surface, the structure of Book II appears relatively similar to Book I. Typically, scholars have described the two books as treating external and internal ailments respectively.[9] The second book does not move as clearly down the body, but instead describes different internal organs (and their ailments) in turn. Thus, the first 16 chapters relate to the *maga* (considered to be the digesting part of the stomach),[10] chapters 17–24 to the liver, 25–35 to the *wamb* (the belly or intestines), 36–45 to the spleen, 46–50 to sore of the side, and 51 to lung disease. The structural complexity in these sections is higher than in most sections of Book I. Most sections on the different organs begin with a description of the organ, its location, and its most typical ailments before several additional chapters with remedies for different sorts of afflictions relating to that organ. The sections of Book II on internal ailments are followed by a few chapters on making *spiwedrencas* ('emetic drinks') and *leohte drencas* ('light drinks'),[11] after which occur a variety of remedies for various ailments without clear organisation. It is probable that in some cases these end chapters may be later additions to the original collection, especially as there is other evidence

---

[8] *BLB*, I 1.1. References to *Bald's Leechbook* are given first by book in roman numerals, followed by the chapters in Arabic numerals; these follow the numeration in Cockayne's edition. If there are further subdivisions within a chapter in Cockayne's edition, these are designated by the number following the full stop.

[9] See, for instance, Wright, *Bald's Leechbook*, p. 14; R. S. Nokes, 'The Several Compilers of *Bald's Leechbook*', *ASE* 33 (2004), 51–76, at 55–56; Meaney, 'Variant Versions', p. 251.

[10] There are two organs associated with the stomach in the Old English medical collections, the *maga* and the *wamb*. The meaning of these two terms is dealt with in detail by Doyle: 'Anglo-Saxon Medicine and Disease', pp. 90–107. The difference between the two terms in the medical corpus appears to correspond at least partially to the Latin distinction between *stomachus* and *venter*, which they frequently gloss. *Stomachus* refers more specifically to the digesting organ and *venter* refers to the whole abdomen area, i.e. the belly. In the Old English medical corpus *wamb* is used most frequently to refer to the intestines or bowel.

[11] Cockayne translates *leohte drencas* as light drinks. Deegan notes that in some cases these occur with *unspiwol* ('non-emetic') and *stille* ('calm') and suggest that these drinks might have been used to soothe an upset stomach (Deegan, 'A Critical Edition of MS B.L., Royal 12. D.XVII', vol. II, p. 322).

of emendations and additions being made to the original exemplar of the text.[12] However, as these remedies are included in the table of contents at the beginning of each book and are written in the same hand as the body of the text, such additions presumably preceded the Royal manuscript.

Latin Sources and the Creation of the Text

The 'Latinity' of *Bald's Leechbook* is widely recognised in scholarship surrounding the text. Especially amongst scholars of medicine, the collection is generally deemed the 'best' of the Old English medical corpus, largely because Latinate content has traditionally been held in higher esteem than other types of content. However, few studies have discussed the nature of this Latinity or the relevance of this work to other types of translations produced in Anglo-Saxon England. As will be explored later in this chapter, the Royal manuscript itself was almost certainly produced in Winchester during the period when many of the extant 'Alfredian' translations were being copied. This does not mean that the original composition of the collection necessarily took place in this same centre, but suggests that the recopying of the manuscript formed part of this larger literary movement.

Unlike the other texts associated with this movement, however, *Bald's Leechbook* is not generally considered to be a unified work undertaken by a single author or even group of authors. Indeed, the degree to which *Bald's Leechbook* can be considered a work of translation has been a subject of some discussion and reassessment in recent decades. Cameron's early work on the Latin sources of the text was guided by the underlying assumption that the compiler of the collection was also in fact the translator of its remedies, which he or she drew from Latin sources to hand. Relying on this principle, Cameron identified 'a small number of works which were unquestionably known at first hand to the compiler' and proposed that only Old English remedies which differ significantly from their Latin counterparts were encountered at second hand by the compiler.[13] This assumption was later challenged by Audrey Meaney's work on remedies occurring in multiple versions and across different collections in the wider corpus of Old English medicine. Meaney compares 52 occasions where individual remedies (or

---

[12] Christine Voth discusses this issue at length: Voth, 'An Analysis', pp. 129–68.

[13] Cameron, 'Bald's *Leechbook*: Its Sources and their Use in its Compilation', pp. 154–55. He includes in the list of those known at first hand: Oribasius's *Synopsis* and *Euporistes*, the *Practica Alexandri*, *De Medicamentis* by Marcellus, the *Physica Plinii*, and possibly the *Medicina Plinii*. In the second category of works known at second hand he includes: *Epitome altera* by Vindicianus, the *Herbarium Complex* texts, Galen's *Ad Glauconem Liber I*, *Ad Glauconem Liber II*, and *Liber tertius*, the *Passionarius Galeni*, the *Petrocellus*, the *Liber Aurelii* and *Liber Esculapii*. For more information on these works, see the introduction.

occasionally passages including several remedies) are shared between two or more sources.[14] Her analysis of these comparisons indicates that although material was shared between Anglo-Saxon collections, no single extant collection was the direct ancestor of another. She suggests instead that a body of remedies was translated at an early date into Old English and that these texts 'circulat[ed] more or less independently' and in 'little groups' rather than in intentionally collated collections.[15]

These findings undermined the traditional view of the creator of *Bald's Leechbook* as the independent translator of the content of his or her text, causing Cameron to revise his prior position on the collection. Speaking of the similarities between the remedies of the Nowell transcript and *Bald's Leechbook*, he writes that:

> we cannot claim that [the compiler of *Bald's Leechbook*] had copies of the works of Pliny and Marcellus and Oribasius before him as he worked. What we can say is that, if he did not have them, someone before him had access to them, so that Anglo-Saxons had in their libraries the works (or extracts from them) which we find used as sources for these entries in the *Leechbook*. Bald himself may have had them too, but the evidence does not permit us to say so.[16]

Cameron here asserts that although we can judge that certain medical texts were known in Anglo-Saxon England, it is not possible to say which might have been used by the compiler of *Bald's Leechbook* specifically. This perspective, which has been more widely adopted, suggests that the major achievement of the creator of this collection lies not in translating medical material into Old English, but in collecting and organising already circulating translated items. This stance takes into account commonalities between various texts and remedies shared across the corpus. However, as will be seen, such a view is likely an overcorrection and does not adequately account for the intellectual and literary project involved in the creation of *Bald's Leechbook*. Although it is clear that many remedies within *Bald's Leechbook* must have been circulating in an already translated form, this does not mean that novel translation played no part in the creation of the collection. A close analysis of the text suggests that those involved in the creation of the collection were in fact responsible for trans-

---

[14] See Meaney, 'Variant Versions'. Meaney considers not only the four major Old English medical collections but also remedies that occur on single leaves of manuscripts dedicated to other uses, as well as the transcript made by Lawrence Nowell in 1562 of MS Cotton Otho B. xi, which contained over 50 remedies but was damaged beyond legibility in the Cotton fire of 1731. A new transcription and translation of this text is now available in Voth, 'An Analysis', pp. 182–90.

[15] Meaney, 'Variant Versions', pp. 250–51.

[16] Cameron, *Anglo-Saxon Medicine*, p. 88.

lating a portion of its content, and that, furthermore, it may be possible to determine specifically which texts this translator had to hand. A new understanding of how this collection may have been created could serve to cement the place of *Bald's Leechbook* alongside other complex works of translation from the period, not least the so-called Alfredian translations.

Books I and II: Separate Works or a Single Text?

One of the main tasks of the redactor of *Bald's Leechbook* was almost certainly the compilation of remedies. As Meaney has established, some of the remedies in *Bald's Leechbook* are shared with other Old English collections or manuscript leaves. In some instances it seems likely that these were single remedies, yet they would have often travelled in small groups, which were then sorted and rearranged according to the complex classification system of the collection. Richard Nokes suggests that various remedies were written out on small slips of parchment that were then organised and copied into the chapters of the text.[17] Such a system, or another similar to it, would have been necessary to achieve the complex organisational system found in the text.

It is clear that additions were made to the collection following its original compilation. This can be seen in the fact that the organisational system begins to break down in the last few chapters of each book and that the table of contents often varies from the chapters themselves. In both books the table of contents normally gives a tally of how many remedies for an ailment are found within a chapter, but in many cases this differs (sometimes significantly) from the number of remedies actually present in the chapter. Voth has analysed these deviations in detail and suggests that they demonstrate extensive scribal interaction with the text following the creation of the original exemplar.[18] If this is the case, remedies were inserted carefully to preserve the original organisational scheme established by the compiler, which is itself a testimony to the remarkable organisational structure of the original compilation.

Differences between the two books of *Bald's Leechbook* have fostered some speculation over their origin and compilation. Nokes has put forward the suggestion that there was no single individual masterminding *Bald's Leechbook*, but at least two principal writers with discernibly different styles. He posits a 'Writer A', who 'wrote most of book I and seems to have influenced Writer B, who wrote the greater part of book II'.[19] Nokes sup-

---

[17] Nokes, 'The Several Compilers of Bald's *Leechbook*', p. 51.
[18] Voth provides a useful table detailing the remedy tallies reported in the table of contents and those found in the chapter itself: Voth, 'An Analysis', p. 137.
[19] Nokes, 'The Several Compilers of Bald's *Leechbook*', p. 57.

ports this theory with a rhetorical analysis of the text, but his conclusions are undermined by the fact that he focuses on the Old English text alone and does not examine its Latin source material. His analysis focuses on the transitional phrases at the beginning and end of remedies, which he saw as being independent from the source texts. However, these transitional phrases are in fact often borrowed directly from their Latin source. For instance, he observes a preference for beginning a remedy with *wiþ* and *gif* in Book I compared to *be* (or other more elaborate phrases) in Book II, yet frequently these introductory phrases have distinct Latin counterparts. Generally, *wiþ* ('against/for [a condition]') functions as a translation of the Latin *ad* ('against/for [a condition]'), formulas frequent in the *Physica Plinii* or Marcellus's *De medicamentis*. Likewise, the Old English *be* ('about') is generally correlative with the Latin *de* ('about/concerning'), which is also used frequently in the *Liber tertius*.[20] Although there are some cases where the Old English introduction might vary from its Latin counterpart, these occasions are fewer than those where they align, and often those instances isolated by Nokes as expressing the stylistic proclivities of the Anglo-Saxon writer are in fact closely following a source text.[21]

Although *Bald's Leechbook* exists in two separate books with different focuses, there is reason for viewing them as two separate collections, either in origin, or in compiler. The two books are both of a mixed dialectal character, but in her recent analysis of the language of the collection Voth suggests a basic linguistic similarity between the books (and a clear distinction between these books and *Leechbook III*).[22] This finding is further supported by the complementary nature of the two books. Both books follow a similar organisational system, even if some sections of Book II are particularly complex, and there is very little overlap in content between the books. It seems unlikely that if Book I were produced independently it would overlook a number of basic conditions that arise in Book II. I would suggest that if Book I was originally independent, or fashioned out of an existing collection, then the creator of Book II must have exercised strong editorial oversight over the refashioning of Book I. It is uncertain, but not

---

[20] This is notable throughout the collection (cf. Doyle's appendix, where Latin sources are listed alongside their corresponding Old English remedies: Doyle, 'Anglo-Saxon Medicine and Disease', Volume II: Appendix).

[21] For example, Nokes attempts to distinguish a second voice in the text by pointing to the chapter beginning *Her sint tacn aheardodre lifre* ('here are the signs of a hardened liver'), noting that this is 'much more conversational than we usually see in the *Leechbook*'. Yet although this type of introduction differs from most chapters which often begin with the simpler *wiþ*, the content of this chapter is in fact derived largely from the Latin text of Alexander of Tralles, where the opening formula *signa si* occurs frequently, e.g. *signa si in cirta epatis flegmon fuerit* ('signs if there should be inflammation around the liver') (*Alexandri Practica cum optimis declarationibus Jacobi de partibus et Simonis Januensis* (Venice, 1522), ch. 58).

[22] Voth, 'An Analysis', pp. 46–47.

improbable, that this master compiler was either the Bald or Cild of the colophon.

The differences between the two books of this collection may be best explained as reflecting differences in source content rather than the rhetorical penchants of different compilers. Of course it is possible (perhaps even probable) that *Bald's Leechbook* was in some way a group project, yet there is no compelling reason to believe that there are two or more main voices at work in the text. Instead of dividing the collection by books, it is more useful to consider different chapter-types: those made up of groups of short, practical remedies, and those passages which tend to be longer, more complex, and often causally oriented. More passages of this second sort appear in Book II, whereas Book I is more dominated by the first type, but examples of each type of passage are found in both books. All the remedies from *Bald's Leechbook* identified by Meaney as being shared between two or more sources, 49 in all, are remedies or passages of this shorter, more practical sort. I suggest that rather than seeing the two books of *Bald's Leechbook* as the work of two different Anglo-Saxon authors, we should consider its two books as comprising a single unified text, combining short, useful remedies with longer more theoretical sections.

Short Remedies: Translation Styles

Those pieces termed 'short remedies' generally demonstrate less stylistic consistency in translation method than the longer, more theoretical passages found in *Bald's Leechbook*. This inconsistency is reasonable, however, given that many of these remedies are found in other Old English sources. If many of these shorter remedies were not translated by the author of this collection but instead by a variety of anonymous Anglo-Saxon predecessors, a unity of style could hardly be expected. Remedies of a similar type and also displaying inconsistency in form and translation method are also found in the *Lacnunga* and *Leechbook III*. It is difficult to know what percentage of the shorter remedies found in *Bald's Leechbook* would have been drawn from pre-existing collections or flyleaves and which may be original to the collection. Given that so many works from Anglo-Saxon England are no longer extant, the simple fact that a remedy is now evidenced only in a single collection does not demonstrate it was original to that text. I am inclined to believe that a very large proportion of the shorter remedies were of this already pre-translated sort, which were collected by a skilled compiler who organised them into this impressive collection. This would account for discrepancies of form found amongst these remedies.

As mentioned above, certain chapters in *Bald's Leechbook* contain a large number of these shorter remedies. These are arranged by ailment (or bodily area) without regard for source. An example passage can help to demonstrate the typical form of these chapters. This section is taken from the second chapter of Book I, which deals with eye-related ailments. Within the text, it is titled *Læcedomas wiþ eagne miste* ('Remedies against eye mistiness/cloudiness'); remedies are numbered for clarity.

> (1) Eft grene cellendre gegniden ond wiþ wifes meoluc gemenged alege ofer þa eagan. (2) Eft haran geallan genime ond smire mid. (3) Eft cwice winewinclan gebærnde to ahsan ond þa ahsan gemenge wið dorena hunig. (4) Eft ryslas ealra ea fisca on sunnan gemylte ond wið hunig gemengde smire mid. (5) Wið eagna miste eft betonican seaw gebeatenre mid hire wyrttruman ond awrungenre ond gearwan seaw ond celeþonian emmicel ealra meng togædere do on eage. (6) Eft finoles wyrttruman gecnuadne gemeng wið huniges seaw seoð þonne æt leohtum fyre listelice oþ huniges þicnesse. gedo þonne on ærene ampullan ond þonne þearf sie smire mid þis todrifþ þa eahmistas þeah þe hie þicce synd.[23]

> [(1) Again, rubbed fresh *cellendre* and mixed with woman's milk, lay over the eyes. (2) Again, take hare's gall and anoint [the eyes] with it. (3) Again, living *winewincle* burned to ash and the ashes mixed with honey of bumblebees. (4) Again, the fat of all river fish melted in the sun and mixed with honey, anoint with [it]. (5) Against eye mistiness, again, the juice of *betonica* beaten with its roots and wrung and juice of *gearwe* and *celeþonie* in equal amounts; mix together, apply on the eye. (6) Again, mix pounded root of *finol* with the juice of honey [pure honey?], then boil carefully over a light fire to the thickness of honey; put it in a brass ampulla and then when there is need, anoint with it. This drives away the eye-mists though they might be thick.]

The remedies given above are translated from a variety of sources. The first two remedies appear to come from the *Physica Plinii*, with the third paralleling a remedy from the *Naturalis historia*, the fourth and sixth from Marcellus's *De medicamentis*, and the fifth having no yet discovered source. It is unknown exactly which versions of these texts would have been known in Anglo-Saxon England, but in the case of the remedies from the *Physica Plinii* and *De medicamentis* similarities with the Old English suggest a close relationship. I have listed below the published versions of these texts for comparison (with the number in front corresponding to the remedy numbers given in the Old English passage above). Due to our lack of knowledge of the precise nature of the Latin sources available to the Old English authors, the following discussion is necessarily somewhat provisional.[24]

---

[23] *BLB*, I 2.5–2.9.

[24] Quotations given are from primary sources. However, identifying sources of these texts has been the on-going project of several scholars. In my writing of this chapter, I was extremely indebted to M. L. Cameron's work. More recently, Conan Doyle has published an appendix of *Bald's Leechbook* which compiles

1) Physica Plinii 13.9: Item coriandrum viridem trito admixto lacte mulieris inunguis et super tumentes oculos inpones.[25] [*For the same, you smear green coriandrus with mixed, rubbed (sifted?) woman's milk and put it over swollen eyes.*]

2) Physica Plinii 18.3: Item de fel leporinum subinde inungue, et caliginem tollit. [*Likewise anoint frequently with hare's gall, and it removes the cloudiness.*]

4) De medicamentis 138.9: Adipes omnium fluuialium piscium in sole liquefactae adiunctoque melle inunctioni adhibitae mirifice oculis caligantibus prosunt.[26] [*The fats of all river fish, melted in the sun, and with honey added, the ointment applied, are wonderfully helpful for clouded eyes.*]

6) De medicamentis 136.5: Feniculi radicis contusae suco tantundem mellis optimi despumati utinam Attici misceto eaque lento igne ad mellis crassitudinem discoquito repositaque in pyxide etiam aerea habeto. Cum erit opus, cum aqua cisterina aut muliebri lacte inungueto; quamuis crassas caligines cito discuties. [*You shall mix the same amount of the best skimmed honey, ideally Attic, with the juice of the pounded roots of* feniculum *and carefully cook the same with a light fire until the honey thickens and have it kept in a small brass box. When there should be a need, anoint with well water or with woman's milk, however thick the darkness you will remove it quickly.*]

A quick overview of these four examples shows that the technique of translation appears to differ somewhat from one to the other. The rendering of the Latin word order stays similar throughout while the loyalty to the source text varies, with no apparent consistency within the remedies taken from individual texts. Although we must allow for the possibility that the Old English versions were translated from Latin originals differing in some ways from those given above, comparison of the texts nonetheless is suggestive of different approaches to translation. Remedies 2 and 4, seemingly based on the *Physica Plinii* and *De medicamentis* respectively, are those which appear to render the source text most closely, and in each case the main difference is that the closing assurance of the remedy's efficacy has been omitted. It is fairly typical for Old English remedies to skip this unnecessary comment on the effect of a remedy, although this is done in

---

and extends the work done by Cameron and others: 'Anglo-Saxon Medicine and Disease', Volume II: Appendix.

[25] Citations from the *Physica Plinii* are taken from Pliny the Elder, *Physica Plinii Bambergensis*, ed. A. Önnersfors (Hildesheim, 1975). Due to the degree of uncertainty in identifying the modern equivalent of medieval herbs, I have left all herb names in the Old English or Latin in my translations. For a discussion of this problem, see the introduction.

[26] Citations are given from Marcellus, *Marcelli de Medicamentis Liber*, ed. M. Niedermann (Leipzig, 1916).

by no means every instance.[27] As can be seen, even though the last remedy given appears to be otherwise the most significantly altered, it has kept the declaration of result found in the source text.

The first and final remedies given above appear to differ more markedly from their source texts among these examples, although some of these changes could have existed in the Latin source text used by each translator. The Old English version of the first entry for eye disease seems to make better sense than the Latin version; the Old English may possibly render the intended meaning of the Latin but at the loss of the literal grammatical meaning of the source text. In the Latin, *trito* ('rubbed') and *admixto* ('mixed') are adjectives in the ablative agreeing with *lacte* ('milk'). The Anglo-Saxon translator appears to have altered the passage so that, more logically, it is the herb that is 'rubbed' and then mixed with the milk. Additionally, the detail describing the eyes as swollen has apparently been removed. Similarly, Remedy 6 also seems to deal rather freely with its source. The Old English version omits the instruction that ideally one use Attic honey (classically honey from Athens was viewed as the purest and of the highest quality), as well as the statement at the end that the herbal mixture should be combined with well water or woman's milk before being used on the eyes.

It is difficult to know if this type of substantial variation between the Old English text and the Latin source material marks a deliberate change by a translator or the accumulation of small errors made in copying over time. In a system like the one described by Meaney, where, once translated, remedies became a common commodity, it is predictable that as translated remedies were recopied, certain changes are more likely to occur. For instance, although this chapter in *Bald's Leechbook* is for eye mistiness (or cloudiness), the second remedy listed above forms part of a Latin chapter called *ad acie oculorum* ('for keenness of the eyes'). Although ostensibly related, this is of a different purpose than a remedy for clouded sight (generally *caligines oculorum*). Since the Latin remedy begins with *item*, translated by *eft* and meaning *likewise*, or *again*, it was probably disassociated from its original purpose, especially through multiple instances of recopying or reordering. It is easy to see how this sort of confusion could occur.

In discussing style, it can be helpful to compare the remedies of *Bald's Leechbook* with the variant versions found in other sources. In some instances, remedies are very close in form to the remedies found in another collection. For instance, the remedies in the Nowell transcription are in many cases very similar to some found in *Bald's Leechbook* and Meaney has suggested that they may go back to a common ancestor.[28] But in other collections,

---

[27] For other instances where the assurance of efficacy is omitted in *Bald's Leechbook*, cf. *BLB*, I 2.1 and *Physica Plinii* 17.1 and 17.8; *BLB*, I 2.3 and *Physica Plinii* 17.8; *BLB*, I 2.4 and *Physica Plinii* 17.11; *BLB*, I 2.8 and *De medicamentis* 138.9; *BLB*, I 2.11 and *Physica Plinii* 17.9; *BLB*, I 4.3 and *De medicamentis* 15.5 and 15.83.

[28] For a more in-depth examination of the correspondences between the remedies

the remedies appear to be shared at a greater distance with perhaps more intermediary steps between. It is useful to compare entries translated from the Herbarium Complex texts with the independent version found in the *Old English Herbarium*. These should not be considered shared remedies with *Bald's Leechbook* in the sense that the *Old English Herbarium* appears in all accounts to be an independent translation project. However, these parallel remedies provide an opportunity for considering and contrasting the treatment of sources in these two different collections.

The treatment of the sources found in the short remedies collected in *Bald's Leechbook* stands in contrast to the methods of the *Old English Herbarium*. As will be seen in Chapter 4, the translation of the *Herbarium* was a single large-scale project of translation and demonstrates a general unity of style and purpose; minor changes to the source text were made by the translator to make Latin *Herbarium* more useful for his or her (likely monastic) audience, yet the translation as a whole is very faithful to its source text. This faithfulness and consistency stands in marked contrast to many of the remedies found in *Bald's Leechbook*, which, as mentioned above, were likely translated by a variety of individuals in different times and circumstances. Listed below is a remedy found in both collections with its Latin source:

Latin (OEH, 1.8):
Ad dentium vitia. Vettonica ex vino veteri aut aceto ad tertias decoque, gargarizet, dentium dolorem discutiet.

[*For diseases of the teeth, let him gargle* vettonica *reduced down to a third in aged wine or vinegar. It dissipates the pain of the teeth.*]

Old English Herbarium MS V: 1.8
Wiþ toðece genim þa ylcan wyrte betonican ond wyl on ealdan wine oþþe on ecede to þriddan dæle, hit hælþ wundurlice þæra toða sar ond geswell.

[*For toothache, take this same herb* betonica *and boil in aged wine or vinegar to the third part, it wonderfully heals pain of the teeth and swelling.*]

Bald's Leechbook I 6.2
Wið toþ wærce. betonican seoð on wine oþ þriddan dæl swile þonne geond þone muð lange hwile.

---

of the Nowell transcript and *Bald's Leechbook*, as well as a discussion of their possible relation, see Meaney, 'Variant Versions', pp. 245–50, 265–68. See also Voth, 'An Analysis', pp. 117–25.

[For toothache, boil betonica *in wine to the third part, swish it then throughout the mouth for a long while.]*

Given the level of variation within these remedies, single examples cannot be comprehensive, but certain aspects of the translation here, if not universal, appear to be fairly typical of the short remedies in *Bald's Leechbook*. In particular, the fact that the *Leechbook* version omits the assurance of efficacy is similar to those remedies seen in the previous section and appears to be a fairly standard variation; it is certainly more common in this work than in the *Herbarium*. In general, the *Herbarium* remedies tend to be more faithful to the Latin, but this example is interesting because each Old English version omits an instruction that the other includes. The version in *Bald's Leechbook* simplifies the instruction that the herb be boiled in either wine or vinegar, mentioning only wine, whereas the *Herbarium* version completely omits the direction that the herb be gargled, an instruction that is emphasised and expanded in the *Bald's Leechbook* remedy. Perhaps the *Herbarium* author thought this instruction was redundant in a remedy for tooth pain.

We can also compare a set of remedies from the Herbarium Complex found not only in *Bald's Leechbook* and the *Old English Herbarium* but also in the *Lacnunga*:

Latin (*OEH*, 1.9):
Ad lateris dolorem. Vettonicae dragmas iii cum vino veteri quiatos iii et piperis grana xxvii, contritum et calefactum ieiunus bibat.

[For pain of the side, three drams of vettonica *with three cups of aged wine and 27 grains of pepper; let [him] drink this ground together and warm while fasting.]*

Old English Herbarium MS V: 1.9
Wiþ sidan sare genim þære ylcan wyrtc þreora trymessa wæge; seoð on ealdum wine ond gnid þærto xxvii piporcornu, gedrinc his þonne on niht nistig þreo full fulle.

[For pain of the side, take three shillings weight of this same herb, simmer in old wine and grind with 27 peppercorns; then drink it after a night of fasting, three bowls full.]

Bald's Leechbook I 21
Eft betonican swilc swa þry penegas gewegen. ond pipores seofon ond xx. corna to Somne getrifulad. geot ealdes wines þry bollan fulle to. ond gewlece sele nihtnestigum drincan.

[*Again, in the same way, three pennyweight of* betonica, *and seven and twenty corns of pepper triturated together, add old wine, and give to drink three bowls full, warmed, after a night of fasting.*]

Lacnunga 116:
Wyrc godne drenc wið sidece: wyl betonican ond pollegan in aldum wine; do in XXVII piporcorn gegrundenra; syle him on nihtnyhstig godne scenc fulne wearmes, ond gereste gode hwile æfter ðæm drence on ða saran sidan.[29]

[*Make a good drink for side-pain: boil* betonica *and* pollegie *in old wine; put in twenty-seven ground peppercorns; give him a good full cup of the warm drink, fasting for a night, and let him rest for a good while after the drink on the painful side.*]

In this instance the remedy from *Bald's Leechbook* is more precise than the *Herbarium*'s version. In this triad, the *Leechbook* remedy is the only one to retain the specification of how much wine is to be added. Additionally, this version uses the rare, technical term *getrifulian* (from the Latin *tribulare*) to describe the condition of the peppercorns, a very close rendering of the Latin term used. In general, the tone and diction of this remedy are more technical than those found in the previous remedies listed above. This is a typical example of the diversity possible among the short remedies of *Bald's Leechbook*. In this instance, the most elaborate departures from the Latin remedy are found in the *Lacnunga* version. Rather than being incomplete, this remedy expands upon the original, adding an ingredient *pollegie* as well as the instruction that the patient rest on his side after partaking of the remedy. These sorts of additions likely indicate a further distance from the original translation than the version found in *Bald's Leechbook*.

In these examples we can see three translated remedies, each with a different style. In this case, the version from *Bald's Leechbook* is uncharacteristically technical, the *Lacnunga*'s apparently amended and expanded, and the *Herbarium* version straightforward and generally faithful. These remedies provide a practical example of how a single Latin source could give birth to a variety of Old English cures. The level of variation found in the *Lacnunga* remedy also demonstrates how remedies could become so changed over time as to be almost unrecognisable. Audrey Meaney records examples where the same Latin remedy could appear twice in a collection, after the variants apparently rendered the two different enough to have been not recognised as sharing the same original identity.[30] In comparison, the *Herbarium* stands out for its consistency and the practical

---

[29] Translations from the *Lacnunga* are Pettit's unless otherwise noted, but herb names (translated in Pettit's edition) have been rendered in Old English for consistency in this book.

[30] Meaney, 'Variant Versions', pp. 249–50.

nature of its translation. A combination of different translators as well as the process of change over time through recopying is likely responsible for the level of variation found in *Bald's Leechbook*'s short remedies.

Long Passages: Structure

In the examples given thus far, the remedies examined have all been brief, self-contained units. Occasionally a couple of these remedies might be taken together from a source text, but more frequently the individual remedies in a passage come from a variety of different sources. The long passages of *Bald's Leechbook* are structured differently. Indeed, the use of the term 'passage' rather than remedy is expressive of this distinction, for these chapters or sections are made up of longer extracts from source texts, each often containing several remedies. As above, any analysis of these passages is provisional due to our lack of exact knowledge of the form of source texts available, but I would suggest such an examination can still be revealing of general tendencies in the translation of these texts. As an illustration of how these long passages often appear, I have provided an outline of the structure of the first 16 chapters of Book II, the section related to the internal organ the *maga* ('stomach').

> Chapter 1: a long extract that appears to be taken from the Latin Alexander of Tralles, informing the reader about the signs of a diseased *maga* and its location next to the heart and spine.
>
> Chapter 2: remedies for swollen and sore *maga* from Alexander of Tralles.
>
> Chapters 3–7: chapters taken from a variety of chapters in the *Liber tertius*. These treat a number of conditions associated in that text with the *stomachus* (the Latin equivalent for the *maga*).
>
> Chapters 8–16: chapters with content mostly taken from the *Liber tertius*, and from Alexander of Tralles.

The organisation of the following sections on the liver, *wamb*, and spleen follow a similar structure, with an introductory section followed by a number of chapters providing cures and other information. This type of careful, sustained, and at least partly theoretical discussion of particular organs or ailments is not found in the other medical collections extant from Anglo-Saxon England.

The distinction between this sort of structure and that found in the chapters containing shorter remedies is obvious. Additionally, differences in the source texts used are also noticeable. Although not conforming to a strict rule, the shorter passages tend to draw on a different group of sources from the longer passages. The majority of the short remedies come from Plinian sources (including the *Physica Plinii* and occasionally the *Medicina Plinii*),

Marcellus's *De medicamentis*, or the various treatises making up the Latin Herbarium Complex. Some of these sources are the same as those which lie behind the *Old English Herbarium*, and the theory of medicine found therein generally has its genesis in Pliny the Elder and Dioscorides.[31] The longer passages, on the other hand, are rarely taken from this sort of herbalist source. Indeed, the nature of the texts mentioned above would make it difficult to elicit a single, long passage that was not made up of numerous separate remedies. Instead, in the long passages the translator draws on a collection of sources of a different nature, with the greater part taken from the medical works of Alexander of Tralles and Oribasius, as well as the *Liber tertius*, an early Byzantine work which also forms part of a compilation later known as the *Passionarius*. Although there are no long sections taken from the Latin Oribasius texts in these chapters on the *maga*, they are sources used frequently in other similar sections.

To understand the structure of one of these chapters, it is useful to look at an example passage. It is difficult to convey structure with a small excerpt, so the entirety of Chapter 21 of Book II is provided in the appendix alongside the corresponding chapters from Latin sources that make up its contents.[32] This extended selection will be used as a starting point for discussing both the structure and translation methods found in these longer passages. The chapter given deals with hardness (or dryness) of the liver. In Galenic tradition the liver was seen as the centre in which food was converted into blood.[33] The particular disease described relates to inflammation of the liver resulting in mal-digestion of food. The beginning reads as follows:

> Her sint tacn aheardodre lifre ge on þam læppum ond healocum ond filmenum. Sio aheardung is on twa wisan gerad. Oþer biþ on fruman ær þon þe ænig oþer earfeþe on lifre becume. oþeru æfter oþrum earfeþum þære lifre cymð. sio biþ butan sare. ond þonne se man mete þigð þonne awyrpð he eft ond onwendeþ his hiw ond hæfð ungewealdene wambe ond þa micgean. ond þonne þu ðine handa setst ufan on þa lifre þonne beoð swa hefige swa stan ond ne biþ sar. gif þæt lange swa biþ þonne gehæfþ hit on uneþelicne wæterbollan.

---

[31] See the introduction for discussion of these authors, pp. 14–17.

[32] For other examples of these 'long passages', see *BLB*, I 35, 18; II 17, 21, 22, 30, 36. Sections of Chapter 22 of Book II are discussed alongside their Latin source in D. Banham and C. Doyle, 'An Instrument of Confusion: The Mystery of the Anglo-Saxon Syringe', in *Recipes for Disaster*, ed. J. Rampling, D. Banham, and N. Jardine (Cambridge, 2010), pp. 27–38.

[33] M. Grant, *Galen on Food and Diet* (London, 2000), p. 8; A. Debru, 'Physiology', in *The Cambridge Companion to Galen*, ed. R. J. Hankinson (Cambridge, 2008), pp. 263–82, at 265–66. For more background on the medical theories associated with Galen, see Temkin, *Galenism*; J. Longrigg, *Greek Rational Medicine: Philosophy and Medicine from Alcmaeon to the Alexandrians* (London, 1993).

[Here are the signs of a hardened liver either in the lobes or the crevices or the membranes. The hardening occurs in two manners: one is from the beginning before there is any other condition in the liver, the second comes after other pains of the liver; it is without soreness and when the person eats food, then throws it up again and he changes his colour and has lack of control over his stomach and urine, and when you set your hand over the liver it is as heavy as a stone and it is not sore. If it is like that for a long time, then it becomes a dropsy that is difficult to cure.]

As can be seen more clearly in the appendix, in Chapter 21 several independent paragraphs from Latin sources have been combined into a single cohesive piece of Old English. Often, the long passages are arranged in *Bald's Leechbook* into chapters formed from a single source, yet it is almost as common for a chapter to be made up of long sections from several sources (as is the case in Chapter 21).[34] However, when they contain material from more than one Latin source, these excerpts are still comparatively longer in relation to the individual remedies encountered earlier. The organisation of this chapter suggests that the translator went through both the Latin Alexander and *Liber tertius* extracting whatever material he or she deemed related to the topic.

The content of the Old English paragraph given above is drawn from the *Liber tertius*, but the translator has taken two Latin chapters dealing with two specific ailments, *scleria* and *scirrosis* (terms coming from Greek both generally meaning 'hardness'), and combined them into this single passage. Doyle notes that even though these Greek pathological terms do not appear to have had one-to-one equivalents in Old English, the translator is able to differentiate between the ailments by referring to different manners (*gerad*) of hardening with different symptoms.[35] The use of this free technique shows the confidence of the translator, who had enough expertise to sort through Latin texts and collect remedies for ailments he or she judged to be fundamentally the same, even if they were labelled differently in the Latin sources.

---

[34] Other examples of chapters drawn from two or more Latin sources in Book II include Chapter 16, Chapter 17, Chapter 22, Chapter 31, and Chapter 36. For details on these parallels, see Doyle, 'Anglo-Saxon Medicine and Disease', Volume II: Appendix.

[35] For a discussion of these two terms, see Doyle, 'Anglo-Saxon Medicine and Disease', pp. 200–02. More chapters from the discussion of liver hardness in the *Liber tertius* were the source for Chapter 22 of Book II (or possibly similar passages in the *Passionarius* texts). For a discussion of this, see Banham and Doyle, 'An Instrument of Confusion', pp. 31–37.

Long Passages: Style

When Chapter 21 is compared to its Latin source material there is an obvious difference with regard to length, as the Old English chapter has been condensed from a significantly larger amount of Latin material. Five chapters dealing with liver hardness, taken from two different works, have been combined into a single cohesive chapter in the Old English. More than this, however, the translator has apparently sifted through the Latin material, condensing and synthesising his or her sources. The appendix makes clear which parts of the Latin content were incorporated (however loosely) into the Old English by putting these sections in bold. In many of the Latin chapters the content has been cut by around a third, and by more than half in the case of Chapter 58 from the Latin Alexander. It is always possible this could reflect a heavily abridged source text. However, in general, most of the omitted material appears to have been skipped because of its repetitive nature. For instance, the translator often omits the beginning sections of chapters where the disease is being introduced. These sections would have been necessary as an introduction to individual chapters, but are unnecessary when those chapters become incorporated into a single more-comprehensive Old English chapter. The sentence missing from the end of Chapter 59 from the Latin Alexander is also repetitive, restating what has come before it, and was probably omitted for a similar reason.

In other instances, however, it can be harder to understand why certain sections may have been omitted. For instance, in the Old English rendering of the Latin Alexander Chapter 57 (found in the appendix) a partial sentence and one whole sentence appear to have been omitted. The Old English connects the two sentences that discuss places in the liver where there could be inflammation, omitting the intermediate statement on when fever might arise. It is possible that the translator found the Latin text's description of the absence of a symptom (that is, that there will not be fever if the patient suffers from liver inflammation) unimportant.

In a few instances, omissions in the text may reflect a difference of opinion between the Anglo-Saxon translator and the source texts. For instance, there are passages such as in Book I Chapter 35 where ingredients listed in the Latin version of a remedy are expanded in the Old English. In this instance the closest Latin parallel for a poultice of *hordeo calido* ('warm barley'), but the Old English has *weax hlafe ond of wearmum bere. ond of swelcum þingum* ('wax cake and warm barley and such things').[36] Changes like this seem to be a knowing departure from the source text.

---

[36] *Passionarius*, V 34; *BLB*, I 35. Citations from this text are taken from *Galeni Pergameni Passionarius, a doctis medicis multum desideratus: Egritudines a capite ad pedes usque* (Lyon, 1526) (references are by book and chapter). With many others, I wait in anticipation for Professor Eliza Glaze's edition of the *Passionarius* texts to be completed.

In other instances motivations are less clear, such as in Chapter 17 of Book II where the Anglo-Saxon version differs significantly from the Latin description of the liver as both creating blood (*inde sanguinem fit*) and as containing the *anima* or spirit.[37] The Old English version does not say that the liver creates blood, simply that it collects it (*blod gesomnaþ*), and also skips all reference to the *anima* as dwelling in the liver. Omissions such as this might possibly hint at differences in opinion between Anglo-Saxon tradition and the Latin sources. The idea that the *mod* or mind was located in the chest – not the liver – is a well-recognised Anglo-Saxon concept and may be the reason for this change.[38] In general, however, the majority of omissions appear to be less a matter of medical opinion and more one of making a clearer, more direct text.

Another stylistic feature of these long passages is a tendency to simplify overly complex Latin syntax. The translator does this in a number of ways, one of which is to render passive Latin constructions into active ones. In the chapter given in the appendix, for example, passive constructions occur 27 times in the Latin chapters and only twice in the Old English chapter.[39] Old English prose does not rely as heavily on passive constructions as Latin, so this is not an unusual approach for making a readable text. Sometimes the translator also helps to clarify slightly opaque Latin sentences by providing a subject.[40] Likewise, the abundant use of impersonal constructions in these Latin passages is reduced, and the translator also generally renders the complex hypotactic Latin sentence structures used both in the *Liber tertius* and Latin Alexander into paratactic Old English sentences, most often using *ond*. Together these traits combine to make a readable and clear style in these longer passages. This could be contrasted with the style used in the *Medicina de Quadrupedibus*, for instance, which tends to try to imitate Latin syntax.[41]

This translator also has another notable trait, visible in some of the sections discussed above. Near the middle of the Latin Alexander Chapter 57, the translator has skipped a section of the text, one full sentence and two half sentences. However, this transition is handled with noteworthy

---

[37] Cf. *BLB*, II 17 and *Theodori Prisciani Euporiston Libri III cum Physicorum Fragmento et additamentis Pseudo-Theodoris, accedunt Vindiciani Afri quas feruntur Reliquiae*, ed. V. Rose (Leipzig, 1874), *Epitome altera* XVIIII.

[38] See L. Lockett, *Anglo-Saxon Psychologies in the Vernacular and Latin Traditions* (Toronto, 2011), pp. 55–62; M. Godden, 'Anglo-Saxons on the Mind', in *Learning and Literature in Anglo-Saxon England*, pp. 271–98.

[39] For more examples, cf. BLB, I 35 and *Passionarius*, V 34; BLB, II 4 and *Liber tertius*, 18.1; BLB, II 7 and *Liber tertius*, 21.1, 22.1.

[40] See for instance the last sentence in the Latin Alexander 57 in the appendix where the subject is not identified but in the Old English we are told that it is the doctor, specifically, who should be able to understand the signs of the disease.

[41] See pp. 133–34.

skill, as the two bookending sentences are combined seamlessly into a single, cogent Old English sentence. In Book II Chapter 17, the translator does something very similar, omitting the middle of a Latin sentence, and re-stitching it into a comprehensible whole.[42] This method, of re-crafting Latin sentences or clauses around omitted material into a new sentence in Old English, is common in the translation of these longer passages.[43] In general, I would argue that this type of translation exhibits a higher level of skill than that deployed in most of the short remedies. The translator of these passages clearly felt enough confidence with this (often very difficult) Latin source material to be able to manoeuvre with ease, restructuring and in some instances transforming it.

Continuity Between Books One and Two

Thus far, the discussion of the longer passages has focused primarily on the sections from Book II related to the bodily organs. Now it will turn to Book I. As previously mentioned, scholars have generally noted differences between the two books of *Bald's Leechbook*, with some even arguing for separate authorship. In the previous discussion, I have proposed a different theory which defines two distinct types of passages within the text: short self-contained remedies which vary in their style, but tend to be basically literal in their translation, and longer passages which differ more elaborately from their source text, and are often severely condensed – simplifying and synthesising sometimes repetitive and pedantic Latin authors. Although more common in Book II, this second type of passage is also found in several places in Book I.

The greater majority of Book I is made up of the short-type remedies, yet in a few instances a style similar or identical to the long passages of Book II can be seen. An example is Chapter 18 of Book I, relating to a condition called *micla geoxa*, roughly translated as 'great spasm'. The majority of the passage appears to have been translated from an Oribasius chapter

---

[42] In this instance, the Latin appears to be taken from the *Epitome altera*, XVIIII: *tunc que sordidissima et iudicio suo reprobata sunt, exonerantur in ventrem, intestines repletantur. accipit iecor sordidissima ex cibo et illa calore suo tam diu decoquendo liquescit.* ('then the things which are most dirty, and condemned by its judgement, are unloaded into the stomach; the intestines are filled up. The liver receives the very dirty things from food and melts them by cooking them down in its own heat for quite a long time.') The Old English reads: *þonne þara metta meltung biþ ond þynnes þa becumaþ on þa lifer þonne wendaþ hie hiora hiw ond cerrað on blod. ond þa unsefernessa þe þær beoþ hio awyrpþ ut.* ('then there is a melting of the foods, and fluid is produced in the liver; then they change their character, and turn into blood; it [the liver] rejects the impurities which are there.')
[43] For examples from Book I, compare: *BLB*, I 2.30 and *Oribase* V 33; *BLB*, I 36 and the *Epitome altera*, XX.

on *singultus* (spasm or hiccup).⁴⁴ However, as in the example chapter given above from Book II, this passage has been dramatically altered by its Anglo-Saxon translator. For the sake of comparison, this passage has also been included in the appendix. As in Chapter 21, the Latin text has been dramatically shortened (reduced by about a third), with omissions handled in a very similar way to the longer passages discussed before. The original source text by Oribasius is less verbose than previous examples taken from the Latin Alexander, using fewer passive or impersonal constructions. However, the Old English again restructures and clarifies syntax at the same time as synthesising the content. The omissions of Latin text are handled with skill: omitting a section on pepper and other causes of hiccups, our translator binds together an early mention in the Latin passage of vomiting with a later elaboration on the same remedy. This treatment is comparable to the style examined above.

Similar stylistic techniques are at work in other places in Book I. Instances of this sort of translation appear to be found not only in stand-alone chapters but also sometimes in passages interspersed among lists of shorter remedies. For instance, a passage taken from Oribasius occurs near the beginning of Chapter 2, a chapter on eye diseases, which contains a variety of different cures from different sources. I have not reproduced this entire passage as it can be found in Cameron's *Anglo-Saxon Medicine*.⁴⁵ However, an example reveals similar methods to those seen above. The Latin source reads:

> in aqua frigida [...] longius videre possunt in visum. Non enim inpedit ad legendum visio; additus enim ex hoc virtus. In suspitionem sit vinus multus et dulces et cibos qui in superiora ventris multum manet et indigestis [...]⁴⁶

> ['[If immersed] in cold water, they are able to see things further away. Nor does it impair the vision for reading, for from this [treatment] the strength is increased. Let much wine be distrusted, and sweet things, and foods which in the upper stomach (*venter*) frequently remain without digesting'.]

---

⁴⁴ The last few lines of text are not from Oribasius's works. In Cockayne's edition he indicates that the entire chapter was taken either from Alexander of Tralles or Paulus of Ægina. However, the last few lines are not found in either of these sources (indeed, the whole chapter is missing from the Latin Alexander, and only the first section is found in the Greek version). After comparing these texts, I have found that the chapter in Oribasius's *Synopses* is much closer to the Old English passage than those found in the other two authors and seems more likely to have been the source text. However, I have not been able to locate the origin of the final lines.
⁴⁵ Cameron, *Anglo-Saxon Medicine*, pp. 84–85.
⁴⁶ Oribasius, *Synopses*, V. 33. Citations for this source are taken from *Œuvers d'Oribase*, ed. Bussemaker, VI, p. ii (references are by volume and chapter number).

The Old English shortens this, omitting references to the remedy actually enhancing one's vision and dropping the reference to reading:

> Wiþ eagna miste monige men þy læs hiora eagan þa adle þrowian lociað on ceald wæter. ond þonne magon fyr geseon ne wyrt þæt þa seon. ac micel win gedrinc ond oþre geswette drincan ond mettas […][47]

> [Against cloudiness of the eyes, many people, lest their eyes should suffer from this ailment, look into cold water and then they can see far, nor does that herb harm the vision, but drinking much wine, and other sweet drinks, and foods […].]

The manner of translation here is characteristic of earlier examples where the translator binds two sentences together around the omitted content. Another example is found in Chapter 4, where two sections from the *Liber tertius* on diseases of the neck and jaw have been added following a series of remedies from Marcellus and other sources.[48] These are of a similar style to the long passages elsewhere and may have apparently been added as a supplement to this section. I would suggest these sections were translated by the same person responsible for translating the long passages in Book II.

To bring together this discussion, certain passages in *Bald's Leechbook*, which I designate as the 'long passages', appear to show a stability of translation style across the two books. The most plausible explanation for this occurrence is that while there was already a significant body of cures translated into Old English, an individual translator decided to supplement this collection by translating more theoretical passages from the Latin texts available in his or her library. Although it is conceivable that this might have occurred at any time in the early history of Anglo-Saxon medicine, it may well have happened in tandem with the original creation and compilation of *Bald's Leechbook*, as these longer passages are shared with no other text. In this case, the creation of this text should be viewed as an important intellectual achievement. For perhaps the first time in the vernacular the practical cures of Pliny and Dioscorides were supplemented with Galenic and Late Antique material from sources such as the Latin Alexander and the *Liber tertius*. This resulted in a text that functioned not just as a practical guide for doctors but also as a type of compendium, a vernacular encyclopaedia of medical learning.

---

[47] *BLB*, I 2.1.
[48] *BLB*, I 4.4 and *Liber tertius*, 75.1–2; cf. Doyle, 'Anglo-Saxon Medicine and Disease', Volume II: Appendix, ch. 4.

Situating Bald's Leechbook

It is difficult to securely tie the compilation of *Bald's Leechbook* to a specific location. The majority of scholars have placed the creation of the original collection in Winchester. However, some voices have questioned this association. In particular, Christine Voth has recently argued that the language of the collection reveals an underlying Anglian dialect and suggests that it is more reasonable to assume a West Mercian centre.[49] She records the two principal dialectal components as Anglian and West Saxon. However, Voth acknowledges the 'mixed' nature of dialectical features found in the manuscript and refers to the text as a '*Mischsprache*, a mixture of linguistic and orthographic forms from a variety of sources'.[50] This must be at least partly a result of the fact that the collection was partially compiled from pre-translated remedies. Dating this original exemplar collection is also difficult. Even if it originated in an Anglian centre, as Voth suggests, this tells us little about the date of the collection. The extant manuscript is dated by Ker to the middle of the tenth century.[51] The additions and emendations made to the text suggest that there was time for substantial interaction following the drafting of the exemplar, yet a more precise date is elusive. However, notwithstanding the difficulty of dating or locating the original exemplar of the collection, there are several reasons for linking the existing manuscript copy with the period of Alfredian translation.

The nature of 'Alfredian translation' has long proved contentious in Anglo-Saxon literary studies. In the twentieth century, the King of Wessex was typically regarded as the personal translator of a number of works in Old English, although which texts specifically belonged to this royal corpus was a point of contention. Boethius's *Consolation of Philosophy*, Augustine's *Soliloquies*, Gregory's *Pastoral Care*, and sometimes the first 50 psalms are the works that have most commonly been considered to have been either translated by Alfred himself or under his direct oversight.[52] However, in the last decades, largely due to the work of Malcolm Godden, the question of the king's personal authorship of any of these works has come under scrutiny. The Old English versions of the *Boethius*, *Soliloquies*, *Pastoral Care*, and *Dialogues* all contain prefaces explicitly claiming royal authorship, while other works do not contain royal prefaces but make ref-

---

[49] Voth, 'An Analysis', pp. 43–50, 158–59.
[50] Voth, 'An Analysis', p. 46.
[51] Ker no. 264; G&L no. 479.
[52] Cf. D. Whitelock, 'The Prose of Alfred's Reign', in *Continuations and Beginnings*, ed. E. G. Stanley (London, 1966), pp. 67–103, at 71; M. Alexander, *Old English Literature* (London, 1983), p. 153; *King Alfred's Old English Prose Translation of the First Fifty Psalms*, ed. P. O'Neill (Cambridge, 2001), introduction; J. Bately, *The Literary Prose of King Alfred's Reign: Translation or Transformation* (London, 1980), pp. 14–15; D. Pratt, *The Political Thought of Alfred the Great* (Cambridge, 2009), p. 118.

erence to Alfred internally in their translation. Yet Godden suggests that the invocation of the king in these prefaces should not be taken literally but is better understood as a conventional literary trope.[53] In response to these concerns, scholarship has generally shifted from viewing Alfred as a translator to the broader focus of a period of cultural renaissance and the flourishing of vernacular writing (especially prose) during his reign and in the decades following.

Yet despite the recent revival of interest in Alfredian texts, the place of *Bald's Leechbook* within this context has been largely ignored. This exclusion is at least partially due to the fact that, unlike some of the other texts, *Bald's Leechbook* was never thought to be a translation in the king's own hand. However, as the debate within the field of Alfredian scholarship moves away from a focus on personal royal authorship toward a looser understanding of a vernacular revival centred in Wessex, the peripheral status of *Bald's Leechbook* needs to be revaluated.

As with the *Orosius* and *Soliloquies*, *Bald's Leechbook* situates itself in an Alfredian context by direct textual reference to King Alfred. This comes at the end of Chapter 64 of Book II, a chapter offering numerous remedies, mostly for internal disorders. The description of this chapter in the table of contents summarises its contents thus:

> Læcedom semonian wiþ innoþes forhæfdnesse ond gutomon. wið milte wærce ond stice ond spican wiþ utsihtan ond dracontian wiþ fule horas on men. ond alwan wiþ untrymnessum ond galbanes wiþ nearwum breastum. ond balzaman smiring wiþ eallum untrumnessum ond petraoleum to drincanne an feald wiþ innan tydernesse ond utan to smerwanne. ond tyriaca is god drenc wiþ innoþ tydernessum. ond se hwita stan wið eallum uncuþum brocum.[54]

[A remedy: *semonia* for constipation of the innards, *gutomon* for spleen pain and stabbing pain, and *spica* for diarrhea; and *dracontia* for vile phlegm in persons; *alwe* for infirmities; and *galbanes* for narrow chests [possibly asthma, angina]; and balsam ointment for all infirmities; and *petraoleum* to drink unmixed for inner tenderness, and to be applied

---

[53] For this argument, see M. Godden, 'Did King Alfred Write Anything?', *MÆ* 76 (2007), 1–23; as well as M. Godden, 'The Alfredian Project and its Aftermath: Rethinking the Literary History of the Ninth and Tenth Centuries', Sir Israel Gollancz Memorial Lecture, *Proceedings of the British Academy* 162 (2008), 93–122, at 99. See also, 'Authorship and Date', in *The Old English Boethius: An Edition of the Old English Versions of Boethius's De Consolatione Philosophiae*, ed. S. Irvine and M. Godden, (Oxford, 2009), pp. 140–51. Responses to Godden's article include J. Bately, 'Did King Alfred Actually Translate Anything: The Integrity of the Alfredian Canon Revisited', *MÆ* 78 (2009), 189–215, and D. Pratt, 'Persuasion and Invention at the Court of King Alfred the Great', in *Lay Intellecutals in the Carolingian World*, ed. J. Nelson (Cambridge, 2007), pp. 162–91.

[54] *BLB*, I 64 (table of contents). *An feald* read according to Voth's edition. For background and analysis of these ingredients, see Voth, 'An Analysis', pp. 164–65.

externally; and *tyriaca* is a good drink against intestinal tenderness, and the white stone for unknown diseases.]

Unfortunately, in the body of the text, the beginning of this passage is on a missing quire, yet the second half of the prescription is intact. After giving instructions for treating the ailments listed above, the chapter ends with the inscription: *þis eal het þus secgean ælfrede cynige domne helias patriarcha on gerusalem* ('all this Lord Elias, the Patriarch in Jerusalem, commanded to be said to King Alfred').[55] This suggests that the recipes listed above, and perhaps others, were sent from Jerusalem in the late ninth century to the court of Alfred. The plausibility of this statement is supported by Asser's account of letters and gifts being sent to Alfred by the patriarch in Jerusalem: *Nam etiam de Hierosolyma ab Elia patriarcha epistolas et dona illi directas vidimus et legimus* ('For we have even seen and read the letters and gifts sent directly [to Alfred] from Elias the Patriarch in Jerusalem').[56] Audrey Meaney has also demonstrated that the drugs mentioned are products that would have been available in Syria and the surrounding regions.[57] There is no strong reason, therefore, to suspect the report of this passage to be false. Christine Voth has suggested these remedies are written in a West Saxon dialect (as would be expected if the remedies are genuine), although she considers these remedies to be a later addition to the collection, which she believes to be originally Anglian.[58] It is certainly possible that this section could have been added to an already extant collection. Nevertheless, such an addition would still underline that a purposeful adaptation of this collection was being made during the period associated with Alfredian translation and very possibly close to the court circle of the king, the place where the record of this communication would have been available.

This view is supported by the fact that the Royal manuscript was almost certainly produced in Winchester. In his catalogue entry for the manuscript, Ker notes that the main hand of the text is identical to the third hand of the Parker Chronicle, that responsible for the years 925–55. This manuscript houses the oldest extant version of the *Anglo-Saxon Chronicle* and laws and

---

[55] *BLB*, II 64.
[56] *Asser's Life of King Alfred: Together with the Annals of Saint Neots Erroneously Ascribed to Asser*, ed. W. Stevenson (Oxford, 1904), ch. 91.
[57] A. Meaney, 'Alfred, the Patriarch and the White Stone', *AUMLA: Journal of Australian Universities Language and Literature Association* 49 (1978), 65–89, at 66–70. See also Cockayne, vol. II, introduction, pp. xx–xxvii; Cameron, *Anglo-Saxon Medicine*, p. 73.
[58] Voth writes: 'The chapter's location at the end of the second book, the singular subject in the table of contents and its unusual form and style are indicative of an addition to the text rather than part of the original compilation': 'An Analysis', p. 160.

is generally assumed to have been copied at Winchester.[59] It is logical that this scribe would have still been located there when he produced the Royal manuscript. This seems even more likely considering the similarity of this hand to the two previous hands found in the chronicle: these similarities are so great that Malcolm Parkes has argued that they were all produced as part of the same scriptorium and represent 'different states in the evolution of what was, in the first instance, a local style'.[60] This same 'scriptorium' is associated with other Alfredian works, as the second hand of the chronicle – responsible for the entries immediately preceding those copied by the *Leechbook* scribe – is also the main hand of the Tollemache manuscript, which contains the oldest extant copy of the Old English *Orosius*.[61] The two hands are similar enough that Alistair Campbell believed the two manuscripts to be the product of a single scribe, although this is not generally accepted.[62] Voth catalogues some differences between the two hands but concurs that similarities in script and punctuation indicate that the two scribes were 'trained in the same centre'.[63] The hand responsible for the *Orosius* is very close in date to that found in the *Leechbook*, with the former being dated by Ker to the first half of the tenth century (s. x^1) and the latter to the middle (s. x med).[64] All evidence therefore appears to indicate that the Royal manuscript and the Tollemache *Orosius* were produced in the same place at nearly the same time, and it seems not too far a leap to suggest that their scribes either knew one another or, alternatively, that the scribe of the *Leechbook* could have been the earlier scribe's replacement.

Of course, neither the extant copy of *Bald's Leechbook* nor of the *Orosius* are thought to be the original manuscript copies of these works. Thus, the simple fact that both extant manuscripts were copied in Winchester does not mean that the originals were compiled there. As has been discussed, the mixed dialectical features of *Bald's Leechbook* suggest that portions of the book might have originally been composed in different centres. Dialectical features themselves do not necessarily preclude an association with the period of Alfredian translation, as the figure of Wærferth, bishop of Worcester, has been associated with the translation of Gregory's *Dialogues*, a project undertaken perhaps even at King Alfred's request, and the importance of Mercian scholars in the translation project begun

---

[59] The Parker Chronicle is CCCC 173 (Ker no. 39; G&L no. 52).
[60] M. Parkes, 'The Paleography of the Parker Manuscript of the Chronicle, Laws and Sedulius, and Historiography at Winchester in the Late Ninth and Tenth Centuries', *ASE* 5 (1976), 149–71, at 159.
[61] The Tollemache *Orosius* is London, BL, MS Add. 47967 (Ker no. 133; G&L no. 300).
[62] *The Tollemache Orosius (British Museum Additional Manuscript 47967)*, ed. A. Campbell (Copenhagen, 1953), p. 16, cited in Voth, 'An Analysis', p. 23; see also Wright, *Bald's Leechbook*, pp. 19–21.
[63] Voth, 'An Analysis', pp. 54–55.
[64] Ker, p. 332. Wright also dates the text to c. 950 (*Bald's Leechbook* p. 23).

at Winchester is generally acknowledged.[65] Overall, the evidence linking the Royal manuscript with the West Saxon capital and the presence of the remedies referencing King Alfred (included both within the body of the text and in the table of contents) strongly suggests that, even if the original collection may not have been compiled in Winchester, at the very least this was where a new and revised copy was made.

As is well known, the late-ninth and early-tenth century saw the translation of a number of famous Latin works into Old English. The surviving corpus includes the translation of practical works such as the *Prose Psalms* and the *Pastoral Care*, philosophical and theological works like the *Boethius* and *Soliloquies*, as well as historical and geographical works such as the *Orosius* and the *Anglo-Saxon Chronicle*. The location of the extant copy of *Bald's Leechbook* in Winchester suggests the relevance of this collection to the literary translation projects being undertaken in Wessex during this period, and a work on medicine and medical theory would fit well within a corpus of works that apparently aimed for range and diversity of subject.

The Leechbook *in the Context of Other Alfredian Texts*

Even within the collection of works traditionally considered to be 'Alfredian' there appears a variety of styles. It is generally acknowledged that the *Dialogues* and the *Pastoral Care* follow their Latin source more closely than do the Old English *Orosius*, *Boethius*, or *Soliloquies*. Now that these texts are generally assumed to be independent works, undertaken by different translators, they can be used to convey the varieties of translations that were being undertaken in Wessex in the late-ninth and early-tenth centuries.[66] Comparison with other texts associated with the Alfredian programme helps us to situate *Bald's Leechbook* within the context of Old English prose of this period.

---

[65] Wærferth's involvement in the translation is mentioned in *Asser's Life of King Alfred*, ch. 77. For a discussion of Wærferth's role in the Alfredian translation, see M. Godden, 'Wærferth and King Alfred: The Fate of the Old English *Dialogues*', in *Alfred the Wise: Studies in Honour of Janet Bately on the Occasion of her Sixty-Fifth Birthday*, ed. J. Roberts and J. Nelson with M. Godden (Cambridge, 1997), pp. 35–51. The importance of Mercian learning to the Alfredian revival has been discussed by several scholars, including M. Brown, 'Mercian Manuscripts? The "Tiberius" Group and its Historical Context', in *Mercia: An Anglo-Saxon Kingdom in Europe*, ed. M. Brown and C. Farr (London, 2001), pp. 281–91; *Life of St. Chad: An Old English Homily*, ed. R. Vleeskruyer (Amsterdam, 1953), pp. 38–62. Other scholars have stressed the presence of Mercian 'helpers' at Alfred's court: J. Bately, 'Old English Prose Before and During the Reign of Alfred', *ASE* 17 (1988), 93–138, at 103; A. Lemke, *The Old English Translation of Bede's Historia Ecclesiastica Gentis Anglorum in its Historical and Cultural Context* (Göttingen, 2015), pp. 98, 104.

[66] However, the *Soliloquies* and *Boethius* are likely by a single author, see below.

As a translation which makes Latinate learning accessible in the vernacular, *Bald's Leechbook* appears to share the educational aims of several other Alfredian works. Like the medical text, the Old English *Boethius*, *Orosius*, and *Soliloquies* all attempt something more than simply translating an important Latin work into Old English. Each translation is filled with extra details beyond what is necessary for understanding the argument of the text. For instance, Godden and Irvine comment that: 'rewriting the [*De Consolatione Philosophiae*] was evidently an opportunity to embed and communicate a world of information about the contemporary and classical world.'[67] In some ways, these texts seem as concerned with communicating as much information as possible (whether about philosophy, or in the case of the *Orosius*, history) as with faithfully translating a Latin source. Although these works reflect on spiritual themes, they may reflect similar educational ambitions as held by the compiler of *Bald's Leechbook*. Just as the authors of the Old English *Boethius* or *Soliloquies* embellish their sources with outside information, so the translator of the *Leechbook* supplemented the existing body of cures available in Old English with new, more-complex passages taken from Latin texts.

The Old English versions of Boethius's *De Consolatione Philosophiae* and St Augustine's *Soliloquia* are the most free of the Alfredian translations. In both of these texts, the translator (generally considered to be a single author) makes significant departures from his or her source, often omitting long sections as well as adding large amounts of original material.[68] In *Bald's Leechbook*, by contrast, major alterations to content are more likely to be through selection and omission. In general, the translator of the long passages is less creative with his source content than the author of the Old English *Boethius* and the *Soliloquies*. He or she appears happy to condense, reword, and omit long passages of the source text but rarely adds more than minor details to its content, although this may of course also reflect the constraints of the medical genre. A closer comparison might instead be made between the style of *Bald's Leechbook* and the Old English *Orosius*. Lacking an explicit attribution to Alfred, this text has long occupied a contentious place within the Alfredian corpus. Yet, similarly to *Bald's Leechbook* (as well as the *Soliloquies*), it includes an internal reference to the king.[69] The Anglo-Saxon translator of the *Orosius* adapted and

---

[67] *The Old English Boethius*, p. 68.
[68] For a discussion of the authorship of the Old English *Boethius* and *Soliloquies*, see *The Old English Boethius*, p. 136. For a detailed overview of the differences between these Old English texts and their Latin sources, see N. Discenza, 'The Old English *Boethius*', in *A Companion to Alfred the Great*, ed. N. Discenza and P. Szarmach (Leiden, 2015), pp. 200–26; P. Szarmach, 'Augustine's *Soliloquia* in Old English', in *A Companion to Alfred the Great*, pp. 227–54.
[69] *The Old English Orosius*, ed. J. Bately, EETS s.s. 6 (Oxford, 1980), I. I l. 29–30, p. 13: *Ohthere sæde his hlaforde, ælfrede Cyninge, þæt he ealra Norðmonna norþmest*

amended his source, adding supplementary content not in the original Latin version. However, the most significant changes in the creation of this edition involve condensing the Latin original to around one half the length of the source text.[70] This tendency towards extreme abridgement and recasting mirrors the style of the *Leechbook* compiler. In both instances, the respective Anglo-Saxon authors apparently found sizable sections of their sources to be either repetitive or unnecessary. Although in both cases not as extreme as the transformations made in the *Boethius* or the *Soliloquies*, these works demonstrate a similar sense of the confidence and control felt by their translators, and the general sense of mastery exhibited in some of these other Alfredian texts.

Nonetheless, a major distinction between other Alfredian translations and the medical text is the fact that the former purport to be, although expanded, translations of a single text, whereas *Bald's Leechbook* is an independent vernacular creation made from passages taken from numerous texts. This distinction may be less significant than it at first appears, however. It is perhaps useful in the cases of the Old English *Boethius* and *Orosius*, where most expansions to the source seem to have come from glossed versions of the text rather than outside sources.[71] The method used in the creation of the Old English *Soliloquies*, on the other hand, is perhaps less different from that used by the compiler of *Bald's Leechbook*.

While the Old English *Soliloquies* is typically seen as a translation of Augustine's *Soliloquies*, it is in reality something closer to a pastiche. The first and second books of the *Soliloquies* are drawn primarily from Augustine's original, although the second book departs more dramatically from its source. However, the Anglo-Saxon 'translator' ventured to add a third book to what is in the Latin original an unfinished text in two books. This third book appears to be drawn from multiple sources, most notably the homilies of Gregory the Great and Augustine's *De videndo Deo*.[72] The author of the *Soliloquies* somewhat foreshadows this method in the preface to the text when he or she compares the task of translation to the building of a house:

---

    bude ('Ohthere said to his Lord, King Alfred, that he lived the furthest North of all Norwegians').

[70] M. Godden, 'The Old English Orosius and its Sources', *Anglia* 129 (2012), 297–320, at 318–19.

[71] For a discussion of this related to the Old English *Boethius*, see *The Old English Boethius*, pp. 54–55. For a similar discussion relating to the Old English *Orosius*, see Godden, 'The Old English Orosius and its Sources', pp. 301–05, and *The Old English Orosius*, pp. lv–lxxii.

[72] M. Gatch, 'King Alfred's Version of Augustine's *Soliloquia*: Some Suggestions on its Rationale and Unity', in *Studies in Earlier Old English Prose*, ed. P. Szarmach (Albany, 1986), pp. 17–46, at 35–36; Pratt, *The Political Thought of Alfred the Great*, pp. 318–22.

Gaderode me þonne kigclas, and stuþansceaftas [...] and bohtimbru and bolttimbru, and, to ælcum þara weorca þe ic wyrcan cuðe, þa wlitegostan treowo be þam dele ðe ic aberan meighte. Ne com ic naþer mid anre byrðene ham þe me ne lyste ealne þane wude ham brengan, gif ic hyne ealne aberan meighte; on ælcum treowo ic geseah hwæthwugu þæs þe ic æt ham beþorte.[73]

[I then gathered for myself sticks and posts ... and crossbars and beams and for each one of the structures which I knew how to build the finest timber in the quantities which I might carry. I never came away with one load without wishing to bring home whole forests, if I could have carried it all: in every tree I saw something for which I had a need at home.]

Similar metaphors such as blossoms being gathered into a bouquet, or nectar gathered by a bee, were used throughout the Middle Ages to refer to the reading and collecting of classical texts.[74] However, Godden has argued that the metaphor used in the *Soliloquies* is a particularly apt description for the Alfredian 'translations', for the author is not treating the texts of the Fathers as integral units but rather sources from which bits and pieces can be taken at will. Godden writes: 'the works of the Fathers cannot easily be equated to trees in the forest, they are rather the houses which the Fathers themselves had built, buildings from which Alfred is apparently taking materials in order to construct a different kind of house of his own.'[75] He relates this method to the looser 'translations' which are reworked to say and mean new things. On a more literal level, however, the closest parallel to the type of endeavour described in the preface is *Bald's Leechbook*, which does not claim to reproduce any single text but rather gathers 'timber' and 'crossbeams' from a large variety of sources.

Within the Alfredian corpus there appears to be an underlying desire to convey previously unavailable Latin content to a vernacular audience, albeit often in a revised, expanded, or condensed form. Malcolm Godden has argued that the purpose of Alfredian translations such as the *Boethius* and *Orosius* was largely encyclopaedic, intended to provide Anglo-Saxon readers with factual information about history, geography, and customs of the peoples of the world.[76] Whether or not the creation of the original collection was initiated as part of the Alfredian project, a work such

---

[73] *King Alfred's Version of St. Augustine's Soliloquies*, ed. T. Carnicelli (Cambridge, 1969), preface.

[74] For a discussion of these metaphors and the preface's choice of one in the *silva* [woods] tradition, see M. Irvine, *The Making of Textual Culture: 'Grammatica' and Literary Theory 350–1100* (Cambridge, 1994), pp. 435–37.

[75] M. Godden, *The Translations of Alfred and his Circle, and the Misappropriation of the Past* (Cambridge, 2004), p. 4.

[76] M. Godden, 'The Old English *Orosius* and its Context: Who Wrote It, for Whom, and Why?', *Quaestio Insularis* 12 (2011), 1–30; *The Old English Boethius*, p. 68.

as *Bald's Leechbook* might well have proved useful alongside these other vernacular works, as they could have been seen as sharing an educative and encyclopaedic purpose. This purpose is best seen in the addition of descriptive and theoretical material in the long passages of the text, passages not found in the other collections of medicine in Old English. If the text does not date from this time, then it may have been for these descriptive and educational passages in particular that the work was revised and recopied during this period.

The Library of Bald and the Making of Bald's Leechbook

The colophon found at the end of the second book in the Royal manuscript, and from which *Bald's Leechbook* has derived its name, has primarily attracted attention for its reference to two named figures and their possible roles in creating the text now known as *Bald's Leechbook*. However, its literary qualities have attracted much less notice. As mentioned at the beginning of the chapter, this short piece is written in Latin hexameter verse and reveals both skill and training on the part of its author. While meeting the requirements of hexameter verse, the lines also exhibit considerable alliteration (marked below by underlining):

> Bald habet hunc librum cild quem conscribere iussit;
> Hic precor assidue cunctis in nomine Xristi.
> Quo nullus tollat hunc librum perfidus a me.
> Nec ui nec furto nec quodam famine falso.
> Cur quia nulla mihi tam cara est optima gaza.
> Quam cari libri quos Xristi gratia comit.

> [Bald owns this book, which he commanded Cild to write/copy. I earnestly ask this of everyone in the name of Christ, that no perfidious person take this book from me either by force, or by stealth, or by any false speech. Why? Because the highest treasure is not more dear to me than those dear books which the grace of Christ adorns/brings together.]

Alliteration, while not essential to Latin verse, is a frequent element in Anglo-Latin poetry. The fourth line is particularly artful, exhibiting triple alliteration on 'n' and 'f' while presenting a thought-word-deed triad ('by force, by stealth, or by any false speech').[77] Certain cadences in this short text are also found elsewhere, most notably *conscribere iussit* occurs in

---

[77] I am very grateful to Prof. Andy Orchard for pointing out the artistry of this line to me. For more discussion of the literary qualities of this verse and its place within the genre of poetic colophons and framing texts from Anglo-Saxon England, see E. Kesling, 'The Artistry of Bald's Colophon' (forthcoming).

a series of colophons associated with Amand Abbey in Francia.⁷⁸ These similarities suggest that the author was drawing on literary models in the creation of this colophon, perhaps from the continent. It remains uncertain whether the author of this verse was involved in the creation of the medical text. However, these lines underline the fundamentally learned and literary nature of this text, which, while a vernacular creation, was considered worthy of a verse colophon in Latin. I would also suggest that whoever was responsible for translating the complex Latin medical material found in the long passages of *Bald's Leechbook* was surely confident enough to compose Latin verse and may also be the author of this poem.

I would like to conclude this chapter by considering again the library of the compiler of *Bald's Leechbook*. As mentioned above, in his early work on Anglo-Saxon medicine, Cameron began the process of collecting a list of those sources he believed to be known at first hand to the compiler of *Bald's Leechbook*, but some of his assumptions compromised the accuracy of these results and resulted in his later retraction of those conclusions. This has left the subject in need of revisiting.

As Cameron first demonstrated, *Bald's Leechbook* reproduces material from a large variety of Latin sources including Pliny's *Naturalis historia*, the later Plinian abridgment the *Physica Plinii* (and possibly the *Medicina Plinii*), Marcellus's *De medicamentis*, Oribasius's *Synopsis* and *Euporistes*, the Latin Alexander of Tralles, the *Epitome altera* by Vindicianus, the *Liber tertius* and possibly early versions of some of the other texts later called the *Passionarius*, as well as probably other yet unidentified sources. It seems unfeasible for this large selection of medical texts to have been available, entire, to an Anglo-Saxon audience, particularly in a single monastic house or secular library. As Cameron suggests, it is very possible that some sources would have been available only in selections.⁷⁹ For instance, the *Epitome altera* of Vindicianus is the source of some of the long quotations in Book II, but the fact that it is used only in a very few instances suggests that the complete work may not have been available, with perhaps only excerpts embedded within another collection.

However, some complete works do appear to have been in the hands of the compiler of *Bald's Leechbook*. As has been shown in this chapter, a particular group of sources – the Latin Alexander, the *Euporistes* and

---

⁷⁸ These are colophons associated with a monk, Lotharius. The closest match is: *Clauiger exiguus quondam Lotharius istum/ Librum, quem cernis, lector, conscribere iussit* ('Lotharius, the humble key-bearer, formerly ordered this book, which you behold, to be written/copied). This colophon is found in a ninth-century Amand collection of excerpts from the works of St Augustine (Paris, Bibliothèque Nationale, Lat. 2109). Two other colophons associated with Lotharius contain the phrases *scribere iussit* and *scriber iussit*: 'Appendix ad Milonem', ed. L. Traube, *Monumenta germaniae historica, Poetae Latini Carolini*, Volume III (Berlin, 1896), p. 675.

⁷⁹ Cameron, *Anglo-Saxon Medicine*, p. 88.

Synopsis of Oribasius, and the *Liber tertius* – are all quoted with frequency and at length in the longer passages of *Bald's Leechbook*. If it is indeed the case that these longer passages were added by the compiler, as seems likely, it seems very probable that he or she had this collection of texts to hand. Although we cannot know for certain the form these collections would have taken, the length of the segments borrowed and the frequency of their citation suggests that he had either extensive portions or the texts entire, rather than simply short extracts embedded in other works.[80] This conclusion is further evidenced by the head-to-toe order attempted not only in *Bald's Leechbook* but also in *Leechbook III* and the *Lacnunga*. It is probable that a Latin medical collection, organised in a head-to-foot order (such as the Latin Alexander), was responsible for influencing the organisational structure of these collections even if no extant text of this type has survived in the manuscript record.

Whatever library contained these texts must have possessed an unusually well-stocked collection of medical texts. This location may have been the Old Minster in Winchester, as has been suggested by several scholars. The *Old English Herbarium* was likely translated there in the tenth century, a fact which suggests that at least by this later date the library had an exceptionally good collection of medical texts.[81] However, this is not to preclude other possible centres where *Bald's Leechbook* could have been compiled, such as Worcester.[82] Irrespective of its place of compilation, this collection should be recognised as a complex and scholarly endeavour organised to make a comprehensive collection of Latin and native medical material available in the vernacular. Part of the plan for the collection also appears to have been to supplement the existing translation of Latin cures with more sustained and theoretical sections taken from Late Antique authors. This particular ambition does not appear to have been shared by the compilers of the other Old English medical compilations, and it is only by considering this collection individually, rather than simply as part of a larger corpus, that these characteristic qualities are brought to light.

Considering the text in this way – as an extensive project including both compilation and the translation of new materials – highlights its

---

[80] There are two manuscripts from the Carolingian monastery of St Gall written in an insular hand and containing large portions of Oribasius's texts (and in one case Galen's *Ad Glauconem de medendi methodo*). These are MS St Gall 761 and MS St Gall 759; both date to the ninth century. See W. M. Lindsay, *Notae Latinae: An Account of Abbreviation in Latin MSS. of the Early Minuscule Period (c. 700–850)* (Cambridge, 1915), p. 237; cf. Glaze, 'The Perforated Wall', p. 123. However, these manuscripts are not listed in G&L, which would suggest that in the authors' view they are not of Anglo-Saxon provenance.

[81] For an overview of the evidence for a Winchester location for this collection, see Chapter 4, pp. 147–52.

[82] For the suggestion of Worcester as a potential place of compilation, see Voth, 'An Analysis', pp. 125–26.

relevance to discussions about other large translation projects undertaken in the ninth and tenth centuries. Like texts such as the *Boethius* or *Orosius*, *Bald's Leechbook* converts and refashions complex scholarly Latin source material (in this case replete with complex medical vocabulary) into the Old English vernacular. Although its status as *Fachliteratur* has excluded *Bald's Leechbook* from many literary studies, the creation of this collection was a substantial intellectual and literary endeavour and the inclusion of this work is necessary for a full understanding of the broader literary landscape in the Anglo-Saxon period.

2

Elves, the Demonic, and *Leechbook III*

The only extant copy of *Leechbook III* occurs in the same manuscript as *Bald's Leechbook*, Royal 12 D. xvii. All three books were published together in their first edition by Cockayne, although he acknowledged the different (in his words, 'more monkish') character of the third book.[1] This third book shares a basic resemblance with the two books of *Bald's Leechbook*: they all contain medical remedies from Latin and native English sources, are prefaced by a table of contents, and more or less follow a head-to-toe organisational structure (although this structure is much weaker in *Leechbook III* than in *Bald's Leechbook*). It is easy to see these texts as three volumes of cures amounting to one very thorough reference text of remedies and information, and, indeed, whoever brought these collections together probably intended them to be used as such.

However, *Bald's Leechbook* and *Leechbook III* were most likely originally separate pieces. A colophon follows the two books of *Bald's Leechbook*, identifying them with the mysterious figures Bald and Cild and separating them from the third book, which follows on immediately from the colophon on the same page. This suggests that the scribe had two exemplars to hand as he or she worked. In keeping with this, Voth has pointed to dialectical differences between the two collections, and there are also a number of subtler differences between the collections.[2] *Leechbook III* lacks the thoroughness of *Bald's Leechbook*. In its two books (one directed towards external ailments and the other internal ailments), *Bald's Leechbook* contains remedies for a large number of conditions and in many cases lists multiple remedies for a single disease. The collection appears to have been designed as an encyclopaedic medical tool, a detailed reference text for a trained medical practitioner. The third book, on the other hand, is much less comprehensive. It is the shortest of the three books found in the Royal manuscript, spanning only 18 folia (in comparison to the 56 and 52 folia of Books I and II of *Bald's Leechbook* respectively).[3] The table of contents lists only 76 different chapters

---

[1] Cockayne, vol. II, p. xx.
[2] Voth, 'An Analysis', pp. 46–47.
[3] I have used Voth's foliation ('An Analysis', p. 26). In this count I have omitted the folia and quires missing from the manuscript. Citations from *Leechbook III* are given by chapter number; if there are further subdivisions within a chapter

and four are missing from the body of the text. Many of the illnesses treated are the same as in *Bald's Leechbook*. However, the entries for individual afflictions tend to be much less extensive, generally listing only one or two remedies (whereas *Bald's Leechbook* is more likely to list several, in some cases upwards of 20 remedies or more for a single affliction). Additionally, the third book appears less well organised, with remedies beginning at entry 30 occurring in little groups of related remedies but with no clear top-down structure. A final point of difference between the two collections is that the distinctive 'long remedies' described in Chapter 1, and characteristic of *Bald's Leechbook*, do not occur in *Leechbook III*, a fact which supports the conclusion that they were translated by the compiler of *Bald's Leechbook* as an intentional supplement to existing remedies. Together these various discrepancies support the widely accepted conclusion that these books should be considered as two separate collections.

Of all the surviving Anglo-Saxon medical collections, *Leechbook III* is frequently held to be the most reflective of native English medical practices. Cameron was the first to observe that *Leechbook III* contains the fewest remedies discernibly drawn from Latin sources. He also observed that 'the number of remedies containing only native ingredients is high and these ingredients are usually given native English names, not Anglicised Latin ones'.[4] Based on these observations, he argued that *Leechbook III* was probably the most indicative of traditional English medical practice prior to the influence of literacy and Mediterranean learning.

More than simply representing 'English' practice, however, *Leechbook III* is also often taken to be most reflective of Anglo-Saxon popular belief. Thus, Jolly describes *Leechbook III* as having 'more of the Christian-folk amalgamations' than *Bald's Leechbook*.[5] In a similar vein, Cameron also suggests that from *Leechbook III* 'we can learn something about the common folk background' of the people of Europe.[6] Jolly and Cameron are using the term 'folk' somewhat differently: Cameron means to signify herbs and remedies natively used in Britain prior to the influence of Latin medical texts and traditions, whereas Jolly is concerned with popular practices in England concurrent with the extant medical corpus. However, in both cases these observations likely stem in part from the fact that there is a higher number of cures in *Leechbook III* for ailments apparently associated with the traditional folk belief of Germanic-speaking cultures. These include elves (*ælfe* in Old English), the 'mare' (*mære*), and possibly a category of figures known as night walkers (*nihtgengan*).[7]

---

in Cockayne's edition, these are designated by the number following the full stop.

[4] Cameron, *Anglo-Saxon Medicine*, p. 36.
[5] Jolly, *Popular Religion*, p. 106.
[6] Cameron, *Anglo-Saxon Medicine*, p. 38.
[7] See DOE, s.v. 'ælf, ylfe (pl)'. Following Hall, I use the Old English term *ælf* and

The comparative abundance of these particular ailments is one of the factors that distinguish *Leechbook III* as an independent work, distinct from the other collections of Old English medicine. This unique profile of remedies is suggestive both of the material at hand for its compiler and possibly of his or her personal interests. Not only does *Leechbook III* contain the highest number of certain types of ailments (including those related to *ælfe*), its entries are also the most varied in terms of terminology and content. I will also argue that there are differences in how these types of ailments manifest between the collections, with the *Lacnunga* representing a different strand of tradition from the entries in *Leechbook III*.

This chapter will also address the 'popular' status of these types of remedies. Remedies against *ælfe* and related ailments are frequently brought into discussions of popular practice, unorthodox beliefs, and unsanctioned practices in Anglo-Saxon England. However, while these ailments (at least in their origin) may have reflected traditional folk beliefs in England, it does not follow that the entries found in the medical collections should be considered 'popular', at least when understood in the meaning that they do not contain learned elements. As will be seen in this chapter, even entries for the most seemingly 'Germanic' ailments engage carefully with learned material – the best example being the remedy for *ælf-sogoþa*, which will be considered at the end of the chapter. Frequently material used in these remedies is ecclesiastical in origin, offering a testimony to the intersection of ecclesiastical and medical forms of healing in the period, rather than the necessarily traditional or popular nature of these cures. Learned persons, in some cases certainly literate in Latin, must have been involved in the creation of these remedies in their extant form. It is possible that the remedies found in these collections may also represent common practices being used in Anglo-Saxon communities in the period when the collection was copied, but this is not known with any certainty.

Mære, Nihtgengan, *and* Ælfe

All three of the terms mentioned above, *mære*, *nihtgenga*, and *ælfe* are somewhat opaque afflictions in the medical texts. Excluding occurrences in glossaries, the word *mære* or *maran* occurs four times in the Old English corpus: twice in *Bald's Leechbook* (once in the table of contents and in one remedy), once in *Leechbook III*, and once in the Old English 'Journey Charm', found in the margins of Cambridge, Corpus Christi College 41.[8] The Epinal, Leiden,

---

ælfe (pl) rather than *ælf* and *ylfe* (pl.). For the linguistic background of this term, see A. Hall, *Elves in Anglo-Saxon England: Matters of Belief, Health, Gender and Identity* (Woodbridge, 2007), pp. 3–6.

[8] For all the attestation of *mære* and variants, see A. Hall, 'The Evidence for

and Corpus glossaries all record *mera* or *merae* as a gloss for Lat. *incuba*. Hall notes that the usage here is distinctively female, where one might expect the masculine *incubus*.[9] The general meaning of something that presses down or assaults someone in some way appears concordant with the description in *Bald's Leechbook*: *Gif mon mare ride* ('if one is ridden by a *mære*').[10] A more definite meaning of the word is elusive, although Hall suggests that associations between *maran* and *ælfe* were 'well established and widespread in the West Germanic-speaking world'.[11]

The term *nihtgenga* occurs four times in *Leechbook III*, in two separate remedies. The only other occurrence in the medical corpus is in the *Old English Herbarium*, where it is used to translate the Latin *nocturnas ambulationes*. The meaning in this second instance appears to be straightforward sleepwalking, as it is grouped with *egeslicum gesihðum ond swefnum* ('terrifying visions and dreams').[12] However, the context of one remedy in *Leechbook III* suggests a less run-of-the-mill meaning, where it occurs listed beside the devil and *ælf*-kind.[13] This usage appears more evocative of Grendel, the *sceadu-genga* ('shadow-walker'), than a typical sleepwalker.[14] However, as this term only occurs in these five places in the Old English corpus it is hard to offer a more precise definition.

Neither *nihtgengan* nor *maran* are common in the corpus of Old English medicine. Both appear in *Leechbook III*, but with less frequency than *ælfe*, although the fact that three of the six remedies dealing with these afflictions occur in *Leechbook III* (the shortest collection in the corpus) is perhaps slightly suggestive. It might also be noted that neither of these terms appears anywhere in the *Lacnunga*. However, a more important point of application for this chapter is that both of these terms are clearly associated within the medical texts with *ælfe*, or elves.

Of the four extant Old English medical collections, *Leechbook III* contains the largest proportion of elf-related remedies. In the two books of *Bald's Leechbook*, there are three remedies explicitly aimed at types of ailment containing some form of the term *ælf*.[15] There are a further two remedies also presumably for treating elf-diseases as they immediately follow treatments for elf-related ailments and do not name a new ailment. Four of

---

Maran, the Anglo-Saxon "Nightmares"', *Neophilologus* 91 (2007), 299–317, at 313–14.

[9] Hall, 'The Evidence for *Maran*', p. 302.
[10] *BLB*, I 64.
[11] Hall, *Elves*, p. 125.
[12] *OEH*, I. 1.
[13] *LBIII*, 61. *Wyrc sealfe wiþ ælfcynne ond nihtgengan ond þam mannum þe deofol mid hæmð* ('Make a salve for *ælf*-kind, *niht-gengan*, and those with whom the devil has intercourse').
[14] *Klaeber's Beowulf*, ed. R. D. Fulk, R. E. Bjork, J. D. Niles, 4th Edition (Toronto, 2008), l. 703.
[15] These remedies are *BLB*, I 64, II 5.

these five remedies occur in a single chapter of the first book. *Leechbook III* contains five remedies explicitly directed at ailments containing forms of the word *ælf*, and two additional remedies that follow on from such ailments beginning with the words *eft wiþ þon* ('again for this') and *wiþ þon ilcan* ('for the same').[16] Only two remedies in the *Lacnunga* involve the word *ælf* and none in the *Old English Pharmacopeia*.

From this we can see that of the four collections, *Leechbook III* contains the most remedies involving elves; *Bald's Leechbook* contains the second highest number. However, the difference between these collections becomes more pronounced when we consider that in these tabulations I have counted the two books of *Bald's Leechbook* as a single text, and that each of its two books individually cover more than double the folia of *Leechbook III*. The distinction may perhaps be further amplified as Hall and Nokes have both suggested that some of the elf-related diseases from *Bald's Leechbook* might represent a later addition to the text.[17] However, more significant than the fact that *Leechbook III* simply has 'the most' elf-related remedies is that the elf-diseases reflected therein are more clearly differentiated from one another than in the other collections and appear to reflect a more complex series of relationships, a fact that may reflect a compiler particularly concerned with diseases of this type. As these are some of the entries most frequently invoked in discussions of the popular or superstitious nature of the Old English medical collections, it is worth introducing the ailments treated in these passages in more detail.

Elves and Elf-Disease in Bald's Leechbook *and the* Lacnunga

Two remedies in *Bald's Leechbook* reference some form of elf-disease in their title. The first remedy reads *wiþ ælcre yfelre leodrunan ond wið ælfsidenne* ('against every evil *leod-rune* and against *ælf-siden*').[18] Interestingly, this

---

[16] *LBIII*, 62.

[17] A. Hall, 'Calling the Shots: The Old English Remedy *Gif hors ofscoten sie* and Anglo-Saxon "Elf-Shot"', *Neuphilologische Mitteilungen* 106 (2005), 195–209, at 196, n. 3; Nokes, 'The Several Compilers of Bald's *Leechbook*', pp. 66–68. Nokes suggests that both Chapter 64 of Book I and Chapter 65 of Book II (containing together all the elf-remedies in the collection) are later additions to the text. To me, this analysis relies too heavily on the assumption that the compiler of *Bald's Leechbook* had an inherent suspicion of 'supernatural' causes of disease. Nonetheless, it seems plausible that Chapter 65 might not have been original to the collection as the chapter is the last section of remedies and is followed by a somewhat incongruous piece on the properties of agate. Finally, as Hall points out, the remedy in Chapter 65 appears to be for the same ailment found in Book I 89 and 'it would have been characteristic of the compiler of Bald's *Læceboc* to have included such related remedies together if he meant to include them at all.'

[18] *BLB*, I 64.

remedy is close in form to one found in *Leechbook III, wið nihtgengan*.[19] The precise meaning of the term *ælf-siden* is unclear. Hall argues that *siden* is likely cognate with Old Norse *síða*, meaning 'to work magic'. Therefore he suggests that *ælf-siden* 'probably meant something along the lines of "the magic of *ælfe*"'.[20] *Leod-rune* is also mysterious. It does not occur elsewhere in the corpus of Old English in this form. Meaney has suggested that *rune* denotes some form of supernatural female.[21] However, Fell and Hall both follow Cockayne's earlier suggestion that the term implies singing and may mean something closer to 'rune lay'.[22] This interpretation would be concurrent with the suggestion that *ælf-siden* might represent some type of elf-magic. The other occurrence of the word *ælf* in *Bald's Leechbook* is in a remedy *wið ælfe ond wið uncuþum sidsan* ('against *ælfe* and against unknown *sidsa*'). As Hall suggests, it seems possible that this term *sidsa* (dat. *sidsan*) is related to *siden*.[23] In that case, it is notable that there appear to be both known and unknown forms of this *siden*. Together these two remedies are the only ones directly purporting to cure an exclusively elf-related affliction in *Bald's Leechbook*. In both cases these remedies appear to be directed against potentially similar ailments – something known as *siden* and associated with *ælfe*.

However, there is one more instance of *ælf* in *Bald's Leechbook*, which occurs in Book II, Chapter 65. In this case elves are mentioned only at the end of the remedy and not included in the title of the remedy or in the table of contents heading. The remedy begins with the title *Gif hors ofscoten sie* ('if a horse is *ofscoten*') and ends: *sy þæt ylfa þe him sie þis him mæg to bote*.[24] Hall suggests the translation: 'should it be ælfe's, which is on it [the horse], this will do as a remedy for it [the horse].' *Ofscoten* is often translated as 'shot' in this phrase and thus this remedy has often been taken as proof of the ailment 'elf-shot', that is, the idea that elves were seen to shoot their victims with darts (either real or metaphorical). This method of translation owes something to Cockayne's rendering of the title, which does not mention elves, as 'if a horse is elf shot'. Cockayne never meant this to imply dart-shooting elves, however, as in his glossary he clarifies that 'elf-shot' is to be understood 'in the Scottish phrase', that is, 'dangerously distended by greedy devouring of green food'.[25]

---

[19] Hall, *Elves*, p. 124; Meaney, 'Variant Versions', p. 239.
[20] Hall, *Elves*, p. 119; see also DOE, s.v. 'ælf-siden'.
[21] A. Meaney, 'Women, Witchcraft and Magic in Anglo-Saxon England', in *Medicine in Early Medieval England: Four Papers*, ed. D. G. Scragg and M. Deegan (Manchester, 1989), pp. 9–40, at 14–15.
[22] Hall, *Elves*, p. 124; C. Fell, 'Runes and Semantics', in *Old English Runes and their Continental Background*, ed. A. Bammesberger (Heidelberg, 1991), pp. 195–229, at 225–27.
[23] Hall, *Elves*, pp. 119–20. Cockayne instead suggests that we might translate this as 'against an elf and against a strange visitor': *BLB*, II 65.1.
[24] *BLB*, II 65.1.
[25] Cockayne, vol. II, p. 401.

In this remedy the involvement of elves appears of secondary importance (as can be seen in Hall's translation of the final phrase, given above). Although Hall posits that there is a collocation of *ælfe* with *sceotan* evidenced in Western Germanic languages, this remedy seems to imply that while a horse *can* become *ofscoten* through the agency of an *ælfe*, this affliction does not intrinsically need to be caused by them.[26] This reading would indicate that we ought not to view *gescot* as an affliction inherently related to elves, and that possibly we ought not to translate it as 'shot' at all. It is perhaps better, as Hall suggests, to understand the word having the more general sense of internal pains, which comes to be its meaning in later English.[27]

As mentioned above, the term *ælf* occurs twice in the *Lacnunga*. This collection contains only one remedy explicitly aimed at an elf-related disease. Entry 29 details instructions for the creation of a *halga drænc* ('holy drink') against *ælfsidene ond wið eallum feondes costungum* ('ælf-siden and against all the temptations of the Enemy'). The relationship between the devil (or demons) and elves will be discussed later. However, from its title, it appears that this recipe treats a similar type of ailment to that seen in *Bald's Leechbook* (the entire entry is given in Chapter 3).[28] It is difficult, of course, to know what symptoms might have been associated with this illness, and some of the ingredients prescribed in the remedies differ (the herbs in these cures will be discussed later in this chapter), but both collections testify to some type of affliction(s) known as *ælf-siden*.

The second, and final, instance where elves appear in the *Lacnunga* is in the metrical piece known as *Wið færstice*.[29] Like *Gif hors ofscoten sie*, this remedy does not name a specific elf-related ailment. Indeed, it arguably does not identify its use at all. The title *Wið færstice* ('for sudden stabbing-pain') comes from a short herbal remedy immediately preceding the poetic work. This remedy has generally been assumed to be related to the metrical composition; perhaps one sings the poem while preparing the herbal salve, though if this is so, this relationship is not made explicit. References to elves occur twice in the middle of the poetic piece:

Gif herinne sy   isenes dæl
hægtessan geweorc,   hit sceal gemyltan.
[...]
Gif hit wære esa gescot,   oððe hit wære/ *ylfa gescot*,
oððe hit wære hægtessan gescot,   nu ic wille ðin helpan.
Þis ðe to bote esa gescotes,   ðis ðe to bote *ylfa gescotes*,
ðis ðe to bote hægtessan gescotes;   ic ðin wille helpan.[30]

---

[26] Hall, *Elves*, pp. 102–03; Hall, 'Calling the Shots', pp. 201–03.
[27] Hall, 'Calling the Shots', p. 202.
[28] See Chapter 3, pp. 98–99.
[29] See Chapter 3, p. 113.
[30] *LAC*, vol. I, CXXVII b, ll. 16–17, 21–24. Emphasis mine; text and translation by Pettit. For the Old Norse collocation *æsir ok álfar*, see p. 73 n. 49.

[If there should be herein a sliver of iron
the work of a witch [or witches], it shall melt [(?)or heat shall melt (it)].
[...]
If it were shot of gods [or spirits], or if it were *shot of elves*,
or if it were shot of witch [or witches], now I will help you.
This is your cure for shot of gods [or spirits], this is your cure for *shot of elves*,
This is your cure for shot of witch [or witches]; I will help you.]

Here elves occur alongside other threatening forces, any of which apparently could have caused the ailment of the sufferer. This is clearly different from some of the other remedies mentioned and perhaps most similar to *Gif hors ofscoten sie* in considering *ælfe* as one of several possible causes of the ailment treated.

To briefly summarise, *Bald's Leechbook* contains one remedy in Book I against *ælfsiden* (with three untitled remedies immediately following), and a remedy in Book II against *ælfe* and *uncuþum sidsan* ('unknown *sidsa*'). Both of these remedies appear to relate to some type of power known as *siden* associated with elves. This same ailment appears in the title of a cure in the *Lacnunga*. Finally, two references (one in *Bald's Leechbook* and one in the *Lacnunga*) seem to associate *ælfe* with internal stabbing pains, but in this case it is not at all clear that elves are seen to be the exclusive cause of this ailment. If *Leechbook III* had not survived, *ælf-siden* would be the only named ailment from Anglo-Saxon sources linked explicitly to elves, and the only identifiable symptom of elvish trouble would be some type of internal pain. However, the folia of *Leechbook III* reveal a greater variety of medical terms related to elves.

Elves and Elf-Disease in Leechbook III

Five remedies directly employ some form of the term *ælfe* in *Leechbook III*. Each of these remedies uses the term in a different form, in some cases clearly indicating a separate ailment. Four of these remedies occur in close context in Chapters 61, 62, and 63; one mention occurs earlier in the collection in Chapter 41. The remedy found in Chapter 41 is the only one to use the term *ælf-siden*.[31] The fact that this remedy occurs separately from the other elf-related remedies, and that it is the only one to contain an elf-related term shared with the other Old English medical collections, could indicate that this remedy and the second grouping of elf remedies might derive from separate sources (although this is not to suggest that this source represents a clearly separate tradition, as Hall and Meaney

---

[31] *LBIII*, 41.

have both shown that there is a strong textual relationship between the earlier remedy against *ælf-siden* and a remedy from Entry 61, *wið ælfcynne*). The remedies in the later grouping, on the other hand, display a different (and more complex) understanding of elf-related afflictions than is found elsewhere in the Old English medical corpus.

Chapters 61, 62, and 63 of *Leechbook III* contain six remedies purported to be directed towards *ælfe* in some form. These include one for *ælf-cynne* (apparently, 'elven-race'), three remedies for *ælf-adl* ('elf-disease'), one for *ælf-sogoþa* ('elf-pains/hiccup(?)'), and one for *wæter-ælfadl* ('watery-, or moisture-elf-disease'). None of these words occur in the other medical collections from Anglo-Saxon England. In some cases the terminology remains uncertain. Hall for instance translates *ælf-sogoþa* as 'internal pain caused by elves'. Simek, however, suggests that *sogoþa* 'might simply refer to "illness", corresponding to the most common MHG term for illness, *suhtin*'.[32] *Wæter-ælfadl* also presents some challenges. The Bosworth and Toller dictionary renders *wæter* as a modifier of *ælfe*, suggesting the interpretation that this designation refers to an illness caused by a particular category of elf. This reading is certainly possible. However, as there is no other evidence for 'water elves' and there are examples of *wæter* being used as a modifier for illnesses in Old English it seems more likely that this term instead is meant to represent a particular subtype of *ælf-adl*, as Hall and Bonser have argued.[33] In both cases, these terms only appear once in the corpus.

Although it is easy to see that *Leechbook III* contains more remedies, and reflects a more variegated terminology related to elf-ailments, identifying these ailments is a difficult task. In some cases it is problematic to know whether a difference in terminology reflects a perceived difference in ailment. This difficulty is exacerbated by the lack of description of symptoms in most of the remedies found in the Old English medical corpus. The degree to which *ælf-siden*, *ælf-cynne*, and *ælf-adl* represented different afflictions is unclear from texts. As Hall has noted, *Leechbook III*'s remedy *wiþ ælfcynnne ond nihtgengan ond þam mannum þe deofol mid hæmð* ('against elf-kind, *nihtgengan*, and those persons who have sex with the devil') has a high degree of textual similarity to the earlier remedy found in Chapter 41 against *feondes costunga ond ælfsidenne ond lencten adle* ('temptations of the Enemy, and *ælf-siden*, and spring sickness').[34] This at least suggests that *ælf-siden* and *ælf-cynne* were similar enough afflictions to be remedied

---

[32] R. Simek, 'Elves and Exorcism: Runic and Other Lead Amulets in Medieval Popular Religion', in *Myths, Legends, and Heroes: Essays on Old Norse and Old English Literature*, ed. D. Anlezark (Toronto, 2011), pp. 25–52, at 40. All these terms are discussed in more detail by Hall (*Elves*, pp. 105–07, 126–27).

[33] *An Anglo-Saxon Dictionary*, s.v. 'wæterælf-adl'; Hall, *Elves*, pp. 106–07; Bonser, *The Medical Background of Anglo-Saxon England*, pp. 162–63.

[34] Hall, *Elves*, p. 127.

with the same type of treatment (and perhaps furthermore a relationship between these ailments and malaria or fever, signified by *lencten adl*). However, *Leechbook III* is unique in positing a degree of distinction in at least some cases of elf-related diseases.

The remedies for *ælf-sogoþa* and *wæter-ælfadl* are the only entries for elf-related ailments in the corpus to come with a description of symptoms. The entry for *wæter-ælfadl* begins: *Gif mon biþ on wæter ælfadle, þonne beoþ him þa hand næglas wonne and þa eagan tearige, and wile locian niþer* ('If one has water/moisture elf-disease, then the fingernails will be dark and the eyes tearful, and he/she will look down').[35] The symptoms described here remain somewhat mysterious. It has been suggested that the disease described could be a skin disease, possibly chickenpox or measles.[36] This might make sense, as there is some precedent for linking *ælfe* and cutaneous disorders more generally.[37] An equally mysterious, albeit more elaborate, description precedes the treatment for *ælf-sogoþa*:

> Gif him biþ ælfsogoþa him beoþ þa eagan geolwe þær hi reade beon sceoldon. Gif þu þone mon lacnian wille þænc his gebæra ond wite hwilces hades he sie. gif hit biþ wæpned man ond locað up þonne þu hine ærest sceawast ond se andwlita biþ geolwe blac. þone mon þu meaht gelacnian æltæwlice gif he ne biþ þær on to lange. gif hit biþ wif ond locað niþer þonne þu hit ærest sceawast. ond hire andwlita biþ reade wan þæt þu miht eac gelacnian. gif hit bið dægþerne leng on þonne .xii. monaþ ond sio onsyn biþ þyslicu þonne meaht þu hine betan to hwile. ond ne meaht hwæþere æltæwlice gelacnian.[38]

> [If someone has *ælf-sogoþa* their eyes will be yellow where they ought to be red. If you want to treat the person, consider their behaviour and know which sex they belong to. If it is a male person, and [he] looks up when you first examine him, and the face is yellow [or] colourless, you may be able to cure him completely, if he hasn't had it too long. If it is a woman, and looks down when you first examine it, and her face is red [or] dark, you can also treat it. If it has been going on a day longer than twelve months, and the appearance is like this, then you may be able to improve it for a while, but you will not be able to cure it completely.]

It is not my aim to attempt to provide a specific clinical diagnosis for these afflictions. What is instead significant for this discussion is the more basic fact that, while the vast majority of disorders occurring in the Old English medical corpus contain no description of symptoms, these two

---

[35] LBIII, 62.
[36] Hall, *Elves*, p. 107; Cameron, *Anglo-Saxon Medicine*, pp. 154–55.
[37] See Hall, *Elves*, p. 107; Simek,'Elves and Exorcism', p. 40. See also p. 71 n. 45.
[38] LBIII, 62.

remedies both list their symptoms, which in the case of *ælf-sogoþa* are quite elaborate.[39] This is suggestive on several accounts.

First, the level of description in these remedies at least implies that the compiler of the collection thought that these two ailments might not be recognisable to some potential users of his text. We can see this purpose evidenced in the table of contents entries for these remedies:

> LXII. Wiþ ælf adle læcedom ond eft hu mon sceal on þa wyrte singan ær hi mon nime ond eft hu mon sceal þa wyrta don under weofod ond ofer singan. ond eft tacnu be þam hwæþer hit sie ælf sogoþa ond tacn hu þu ongitan meaht hwæþer hine mon mæg gelacnian ond drencas ond gebedu wiþ ælcre feondes costunge.

> LXIII. Tacnu hu þu meaht ongitan hwæþer mon sie on wæter ælf adle. ond læcedom wiþ þam ond gealdor on to singanne ond þæt ilce mon mæg singan on wunda.[40]

> [LXII. A remedy against *ælf-adl* and also how one must sing on the herbs before he/she picks them and afterwards how one shall place the herbs under the altar and sing over [them] and also the signs by which [you can know] whether it is *ælf-sogoþa* and the signs how you can know if it is possible to cure him and drinks and prayers against each temptation of the Enemy.

> LXIII. Signs how you might understand whether one has *wæter-ælfadl* and a remedy against that and a *galdor* to sing over it and the same [*galdor*] one may sing over wounds.]

In both cases, *tacnu* ('signs') are necessary for the text's user to be able to correctly identify the disease in question. This seems to suggest that although there were widely known elf-related condition(s) designated by names such as *ælf-siden*, *ælf-cynne*, and *ælf-adl*, the diseases signified by *ælf-sogoþa* and *wæter-ælfadl* would only be known by some select group. This could either mean that these terms were old terms in the process of becoming obsolete at the time in which these remedies were written down, or that they represent a facet of elf-related mythology particular to a certain milieu or sub-culture in Anglo-Saxon England.

Secondly, by the simple fact of describing different symptoms, these remedies suggest that elves could be associated with a variety of conditions (rather than simply internal pains). The two remedies clearly distinguish themselves from one another, and both also, it seems, differentiate themselves from the more general *ælf-adl*, which is not accompanied by a

---

[39] An exception to this is the 'longer remedies' in *Bald's Leechbook*, discussed in Chapter 1, which sometimes contain descriptive passages borrowed from their Latin source.

[40] *LBIII*, 62, 63 (table of contents).

description of symptoms and thus presumably would have been generally recognisable. *Ælf-sogoþa* appears as part of the entry beginning with *wið ælfadl* and Hall has suggested that it might represent a sub-category of that condition.[41] The support for this suggestion comes from the table of contents, where the phrase *tacnu be þam hwæþer hit sie ælfsogoþa* ('the signs by which [you can know] whether it is *ælf-sogoþa*') occurs within the larger entry for *ælfadl*. It does not appear too much of a stretch to suggest that *wæter-ælfadl* might similarly represent a type of sub-category of the more general *ælf-adl*, as is reflected in its name. This stratification found in *Leechbook III* with a general ailment manifested in widely known forms, with two related but less widely known ancillary conditions, is certainly a more nuanced portrayal of the possibilities of elf-disease than found in the other medical collections extant from Anglo-Saxon England.

Continuity and Discontinuity in the Description of Ælfe

The questions 'what are *ælfe*?' and 'which diseases were they associated with?' have attracted the focus of several scholars, including two book-length studies, one produced by Karen Jolly and another more recently by Alaric Hall.[42] Jolly takes a historico-theological approach to the role of elves. She addresses early twentieth-century criticism, which tended to associate the elf-related remedies with the categories of paganism and magic. Instead, Jolly emphasises the Christian content found in the 'elf charms' and argues that they should be considered in the theological context of the period. Hall, by contrast, takes a more philological approach, exploring the changing conception of elves during the Anglo-Saxon period and beyond through linguistic analysis and comparative study from Scandinavian sources. Both of these studies contribute important perspectives to the question of how Anglo-Saxons might have conceived of *ælfe*. Yet in both cases, each author's principal concern is with the mythology of elves and their role in society and practice, rather than the medical texts *per se*. In keeping with this, neither Hall nor Jolly fully attempts to distinguish the presentation of *ælfe* in one medical context from another. Instead, they place more emphasis on creating a cohesive image of elves and their attributes. Nevertheless, there are some points of difference in the appearance of elf-remedies in the various medical

---

[41] Hall, *Elves*, pp. 105–06.
[42] Hall, *Elves*; Jolly, *Popular Religion*. For article length studies, see Simek, 'Elves and Exorcism'; R. Simek, 'Demons and Alfar', in *Conversions: Looking for Ideological Change in the Early Middle Ages*, ed. L. P. Slupecki and R. Simek (Vienna, 2013), pp. 321–42; L. Motz, 'Of Elves and Dwarfs', *Arv: Journal of Scandinavian Folklore* 29–30 (1973–74), 93–127; T. A. Shippey, 'Light-Elves, Dark-Elves, and Others: Tolkien's Elvish Problem', *Tolkien Studies* 1 (2004), 1–15.

collections; in particular there are differences between those remedies epitomised in *Leechbook III* but also found in *Bald's Leechbook*, and those of the *Lacnunga*.

In order to help illuminate these differences, I have compiled some information from these remedies into tables. Table 1 summarises the most common herbs used in the remedies for elf-diseases found in the medical collections. In the case of *Leechbook III* and *Bald's Leechbook* only the most frequently occurring herbs are listed; in the case of the *Lacnunga* all the herbs are listed. The relatively small numbers of remedies for these conditions limits the usefulness of this type of data analysis, as in the case of *Bald's Leechbook* or the *Lacnunga* the addition of a single remedy could change totals dramatically. However, this table is helpful in illustrating the fact that the majority of remedies against elf-diseases rely on a fairly stable selection of herbs in *Bald's Leechbook* and *Leechbook III*, but a quite different selection in the *Lacnunga* (a point that will be soon returned to). As Jolly has also indicated, the most frequently recurring herbs in the treatment of these types of diseases are *elehtre* and *bisceop-wyrt*.[43] Additionally, we could add *cropleac* and *wermod* to this list, although there are other herbs that also recur.

	Table 1: Herbs used against Elves	
	Herb Name	*Number of Occurrences*
Bald's Leechbook	elehtre	2
	bisceop-wyrt	2
	cropleac	2
	reademagþan	2
	armelu	2
	hegerifan corn	2
Leechbook III	elehtre	5
	bisceop-wyrt	4
	wermod	4
	cropleac	3
	elenan	3
	finol	3

[43] Jolly, *Popular Religion*, p. 135.

	Herb Name	Number of Occurrences
Lacnunga	cassoc	1
	cristallan	1
	disman	1
	feferfuige	1
	finol	1
	reade netele	1
	sidewaran	1
	wegbrædan	1

Table 2: Herbs used against Devils		
	Herb Name	*Number of Occurrences*
Bald's Leechbook & Leechbook III	elehtre	9
	bisceop-wyrt	6
	finol	6
	cassoc	5
	betonica	4
	gyþrife	4
	garleac	4
	wermod	4

Table 3: Herbs used in only Elf-Related Remedies		
	Herb Name	*Number of Occurrences*
Bald's Leechbook & Leechbook III	elehtre	6
	bisceop-wyrt	4
	finol	5
	cassoc	5
	betonica	4
	gyþrife	3
	garleac	3

The stability of identifying a particular group of herbs for treating elf-disease is enhanced when we consider the herbs used in treating ailments related to the demonic (Table 2). This analysis reveals a very similar breakdown of herbs in the remedies used for ailments against the *deofol* ('devil'), *deofles costunga* ('temptations of the devil'), *deofle-seocnysse* ('devil-sickness'), and *feond-seocnysse* ('Enemy-sickness'). Again, only the most commonly occurring herbs are listed in the table. The correlations between the herbs listed here and those used against elves is exaggerated by the fact that three remedies from *Leechbook III* and *Bald's Leechbook* list both devilish and elvish causes (of course, this is in itself telling). However, when we subtract these remedies from the totals (Table 3), the parallels in treatment between these two types of diseases are still clear. In these remedies, we see a general stability across the herbs used to deal with these afflictions. *Elehtre* and *bisceop-wyrt* remain the most consistently used. *Finol* also reappears. Further connections are found when we consider that *betonica* may be another name for *bisceop-wyrt* and that *garleac* and *cropleac* both appear to be words for types of garlic.[44] Outside of remedies for ailments directly associated with *ælfe* or demons, these herbs most frequently occur in remedies for mental ailments or headache and for skin conditions.[45] This is in keeping with the link sometimes made between *ælfe* and mental and cutaneous disorders.

This basic similarity of treatments for these types of ailments is suggestive from various angles about the relationship between the Christian category of the demonic and the figure of *ælfe*. This will be the focus of later discussion. However, for the moment we can observe that *Bald's Leechbook* and *Leechbook III* demonstrate an established set of herbs used in the treatment of elf-related or demonic ailments, and that the remedies of the *Lacnunga* do not adhere to this pattern. In the case of *ælfe*, we see an entirely different group of herbs being used in the *Lacnunga*, with the

---

[44] See DOE, s.v. 'crop-lēac', 'betonice', 'bisceop-wyrt'. See also *Dictionary of Old English Plant Names*, ed. P. Bierbaumer and H. Sauer with H. Klug, and U. Krischke (2007–09), consulted at <http://oldenglish-plantnames.org> (accessed 15 March 2016), 'bisceop-wyrt', for a discussion on the difficulties associated with identifying this plant-name.

[45] I have counted 20 remedies within the larger corpus that contain two or more of these herbs (for this purpose I considered only the most recurrent herbs: *elehtre*, *bisceop-wyrt*, *cropleac/garleac*, *wermod*, and *finol*). For remedies against mental ailments or head pain involving these herbs, see BLB I 53, BLB I 62.2, BLB I 63 [two recipes], BLB I 66 [two recipes], BLB II 65.5, LBIII 68, and LAC 49. For treatments for skin conditions or *þeor*, see BLB I 31.7, BLB I 39.3, BLB I 47.3, and LAC 49. Other remedies involving these two or more of these herbs include: a remedy for *lencten adle* (BLB I 62.2), three recipes for *leoht drencas* ('light drinks') or *unspiwol drencas* ('non-emetic drinks') (BLB II 53 [three remedies]), three remedies for sudden sickness or death in animals or people (BLB II 55.2, LAC 134, LAC 136), a remedy for side pain (LAC 50), a recipe for a green salve (LAC 15), a recipe for a holy salve (LAC 63).

only overlap being *finol*. I have not given a formal tabulation of herbs used against demonic agents in the *Lacnunga*, because there is only one remedy purporting to treat such an affliction, which is also one of the two remedies for treating elf-diseases in the collection. So, again we would see *cristallan*, *disman*, *sidewaran*, *cassuc*, and *finol*, a group clearly divergent from the established herbal practices seen in the other collections. It might also be worth mentioning that the herbs whose powers are extolled in the 'Nine Herbs Charm' do not align with the herbs typical of these afflictions in the other collections, again with the exception of *finol* and less significantly *mægðe*, which is likely a related herb to *reademagþan* listed in Table 1.

Certainly it is difficult to talk about routine practice or convention in treating these conditions when we only have such a tiny selection of remedies as in the *Lacnunga*. However, the paucity of remedies for these ailments is itself suggestive. In a text that has been described by Singer as 'our best source of the primitive medicine of this country', by Bonser the most 'pagan' of the medical texts, and 'reflect[ing] more of the actual practice' by Jolly, it is noteworthy that we find the fewest remedies related to *ælfe*, and none at all for the seemingly related conditions of *maran* and *nihtgengan*.[46] This is not to suggest that there is no 'popular' or 'Germanic' element in the *Lacnunga*, only that its extent might perhaps have been exaggerated in some cases. As discussed in Chapter 3, the fact that many of the remedies in the *Lacnunga* diverge from the standard presentation of Old English prose might not be the result of them being more 'native', but instead shows a heavier influence from foreign or literary traditions, including early Insular texts. Overall, this serves to emphasise again the distinctiveness of each of the extant collections of medical material from Anglo-Saxon England.

In the cases where typically 'Germanic' ailments are presented, the *Lacnunga* appears to bear witness to a medical tradition separate from the other collections. As mentioned above, there is one occurrence of the term *ælf-siden* in the *Lacnunga*, but the ailment is treated with decidedly different herbs from those typically used in the other collections. It is perhaps significant that the other reference to elves in the collection (occurring in *Wið færstice*) uses the term *ylfa* (gen. pl. of **ylf*), identified by Hall as the West Saxon form.[47] The spelling *ælf*, by contrast, which appears in every instance in *Leechbook III* and generally in *Bald's Leechbook*, is the Anglian form. The only other instance of the West Saxon *ylfa* within the medical texts occurs in *Gif hors gescoten si*, of *Bald's Leechbook*. In both cases, then, the (late) West Saxon *ylf** appears to be used in the context of shooting

---

[46] C. Singer, 'Early English Medicine and Magic', *PBA* 9 (1919–20), 341–74, at 342; Bonser, *The Medical Background of Anglo-Saxon England*, p. 25; Jolly, *Popular Religion*, p. 107.

[47] Hall, *Elves*, pp. 4–5.

pains – although that is not to say other elf-diseases might not also relate to internal pain, as Hall has argued.[48] Also in both cases the disease in question appears to be only potentially rather than necessarily linked with elves and is treated primarily through incantation (*Wið færstice*) or inscription (*Gif hors ofscoten sie*) rather than through application of any of the herbs normally associated with elf-afflictions. Moreover, in *Wið færstice* elves do not occur with the *maran* or *nihtgengan* of *Bald's Leechbook* and *Leechbook III* but instead *hægtessan* and *esa*, figures not mentioned in any other collection. This provides an interesting parallel instead to Old Norse, where *álfar* and the *Æsir* are routinely evoked together.[49] Taken together these points could perhaps provide some evidence to the influence of different traditions on the *Lacnunga*.

Additionally, the *Lacnunga* is the only medical collection in Old English to testify to a different and perhaps also traditionally northern affliction: *dweorh* ('dwarf'). This term occurs three times in the *Lacnunga*, in two separate remedies.[50] Cameron argues that we should understand the word *dweorg* as an Old English word for 'fever'. This is because there is a series of Latin remedies against fever with close textual relationships to the first part of the remedy in *Wið dweorh*; additionally, in the *Medicina de Quadrupedibus*, *ad fugandam febrem* ('to banish fever') is translated as *dweorg onweg to donne* ('to get rid of *dweorg*').[51] As a result of this reasoning, Pettit translates *dweorh* (in its various forms) as 'fever' throughout his edition; this is in distinction to his treatment of *ælf-siden* which he translates as '(?)elvish magic'. Although Cameron's argument about the association between *dweorg* and fever is persuasive, there is no reason for doubting at least the original association of this ailment with a creature known as dwarf.[52] In Norse lore, dwarves and elves are related entities. Although it is difficult to know its meaning to the compiler of the *Lacnunga*, these remedies are among the only extant evidence of an ailment known as *dweorh*.

Although it does not occur frequently enough to be considered one of the most-used herbs listed above, a herb called *ælf-þone* occurs only in *Leechbook III* and *Bald's Leechbook*.[53] The first element in this name is clearly

---

[48] Hall, *Elves*, pp. 105–08.
[49] The collocation *æsir ok álfar* (and its variants) occurs 14 times in Old Norse. This is discussed by Hall in *Elves*, pp. 35–39. See also Shippey, 'Light-Elves, Dark-Elves, and Others', p. 3.
[50] Two of these references occur in *LAC*, vol. I, LXXXI. For discussion over whether they should be treated as a single entry or two distinct pieces, see *LAC*, vol. II, LXXXI. The other remedy contains a metrical charm and is widely known as *Wið dweorh* ('against dwarf'), *LAC*, LXXXVI. The term *dueorge* also appears once in the twelfth-century *Peri didaxeon*, but this later text is beyond the scope of my study.
[51] *MDQ*, 10.17 (MS V), see also the note, p. 337, cf. Cameron, *Anglo-Saxon Medicine*, p. 152.
[52] For a more detailed study of this relationship, see C. Doyle, '*Dweorg* in Old English: Aspects of Disease Terminology', *Questio Insularis* 9 (2008), 99–117.
[53] See DOE, s. v. 'ælf-þone'.

ælf; the second appears to mean 'vine or creeper', being cognate with the Old High German *thona*.⁵⁴ This term appears in *Bald's Leechbook* in a remedy against *lyft-adl* (probably 'paralysis') and in a recipe for a *leoht drenc* ('light drink').⁵⁵ It appears in *Leechbook III* in a remedy for *micel lic* ('large body', possibly elephantiasis) and in another remedy for a *leoht drenc wiþ wedenheorte* ('*leoht drenc* against mad-heart'), and finally in a remedy for *ælf-adl*. Hall has argued that this herb is likely woody nightshade and was used to heal ailments associated with elves, particularly fever and altered mental states, and, in extreme doses, possibly was also seen to cause these types of symptoms.⁵⁶ If *ælf-þone* is a traditional and archaic herb name, as Hall argues, then again it is interesting to note its complete absence from the *Lacnunga*.

I would like to suggest that the *Lacnunga* should be viewed as participating in a different tradition of folk belief than that exhibited by *Leechbook III*. *Leechbook III* testifies to the existence of a complex network of ailments associated with elves. These diseases in turn were treated by a generally stable assortment of particular herbs. The influence of these same traditions is also exhibited, although to a lesser extent, within *Bald's Leechbook*. However, the *Lacnunga* diverges from this standard. In the *Lacnunga*, diseases involving *ælfe* are decidedly less prominent, the herbal reflex *ælf-þone* is entirely absent, and there is at least residual attestation to another creature known as *dweorh*. This is possibly reflective of regional differences within England and might suggest that depictions of *ælfe* and their relationship to disease may not have been as stable across Anglo-Saxon England as has been assumed in previous studies.

Elves and Demons in the Medical Collections

Across the Anglo-Saxon medical corpus, elves are clearly presented as agents of disease and bodily harm. Traditionally, this has been viewed as the result of a process whereby an element of native belief became 'demonised' through its encounter with Christianity. Bonser, for example, expresses this view clearly: 'when Christianity came, the elves of heathendom were equated with demons, and therefore elf-shot and flying venom were thought to be the same as demonical possession (*deōfol-seōcnes*).'⁵⁷ This

---

⁵⁴ A. Hall, 'Madness, Medication—and Self-Induced Hallucination? *Elleborus* (and Woody Nightshade) in Anglo-Saxon England, 700–900', *Leeds Studies in English* New Series XLIV (2013), 43–69, at 55.

⁵⁵ For discussion of the first term, see L. Bezzo, 'Parallel Remedies: Old English "Paralisin þæt is lyftadl"', in *Form and Content of Instruction in Anglo-Saxon England in the Light of Contemporary Manuscript Evidence*, pp. 435–45. For the second term, see p. 25 n. 11.

⁵⁶ Hall, '*Elleborus*', pp. 58–59, 61–62.

⁵⁷ W. Bonser, 'Magical Practices against Elves', *Folklore* 37.4 (1926), 350–63, at

general perspective has characterised discussion of *ælfe* in Anglo-Saxon England. Recent scholarship, however, has led to a more nuanced reading of this relationship. Alaric Hall and Rudolf Simek have both emphasised that the association between elves and disease probably reflects an older tradition and pre-dates the coming of Christianity to England.[58] However, the fact that there exists a clear connection between *ælfe* and demons within the Old English medical corpus is nonetheless widely acknowledged.

As has already been seen, several remedies against elf-related afflictions state that they also benefit demonic afflictions. A clear example of this is the entry in the *Lacnunga* which records the recipe for a holy salve, useful *wið ælfsidene ond wið eallum feondes costungum* ('against *ælf-siden* and against all temptations(?) of the Enemy').[59] The meaning of *feondes* (or sometimes *deofoles*) *cost[n]unge* has been the occasion of some discussion as 'costung' generally has the meaning of a mental test or temptation rather than a physical condition clearly associated with a particular disease.[60] This is the word, for instance, that Ælfric uses to describe the temptation of Christ by the Devil in the desert.[61] However, although the symptoms suggested by this condition are uncertain, it appears to involve demonic agency. The relation between those illnesses which are *ælf*-related or demon-related is also seen in several remedies from *Leechbook III*. For instance, a remedy discussed above details a salve useful against *ælfcynne nihtgengan þam mannum þe deofol mid hæmð* ('elf-kind, *nihtgengan*, and those persons who have sex with the devil'). In this remedy these various afflictions are placed in parallel, seemingly functioning as independent afflictions but ones apparently closely enough linked to benefit from the same treatment.[62] The remedy beginning *gif him biþ ælfsogoþa* ('if a person has *ælf-sogoþa*') concludes with the statement *þes cræft mæg*

---

359. See also: Jolly, *Popular Religion*, pp. 136, 160, 164; S. Zavoti, 'Blame it on the Elves: Perceptions of Illness in Anglo-Saxon England', in *Medieval and Early Modern Literature, Medicine and Science*, ed. R. Falconer and D. Renevey (Tübingen, 2013), pp. 67–78, at 74–75.

[58] Hall, *Elves*, pp. 97–98; Simek, 'Demons and Alfar', pp. 336–37.

[59] *LAC*, vol. I, XXIX.

[60] DOE, s.v. 'costung, costnung', 1, 2.b.ii. Meaney has suggested that perhaps we should think of this as some type of hallucination caused by the devil: A. Meaney, 'The Devil Can Seriously Damage Your Health: Reflections on Anglo-Saxon Demonology', in *The Devil in Society in Premodern Europe*, ed. R. Raiswell and P. Dendle (Toronto, 2012), pp. 69–108, at 96. For further discussion, see also A. Meaney, 'The Anglo-Saxon View of the Causes of Illness', in *Health, Disease and Healing in Medieval Culture*, ed. S. Campbell, B. Hall, and D. Klausner (Basingstoke, 1992), pp. 12–33, at 17–18; A. Hall, 'The Meaning of Elf and Elves in Medieval England', unpublished PhD dissertation (University of Glasgow, 2004), p. 113.

[61] Ælfric, *Ælfric's Catholic Homilies: The First Series. Text*, ed. P. Clemoes, EETS s.s. 17 (Oxford, 1997), p. 270. This edition will be used throughout for citations from the first series of homilies. This will be referred to as Clemoes in the footnotes.

[62] See also *LBIII*, 41.

wiþ ælcre feondes costunge ('this craft is strong against every temptation of the Enemy').[63] This statement might suggest that *ælf-sogoþa* is here being included under the (presumably broader) category of *feondes costunge*. It is unclear whether *cræft* in this remedy refers to the entire remedy or only to some part – or whether it could alternatively carry a more general meaning such as 'strength' or 'power'. In any case, the two conditions are clearly related within the remedy.

The relationship between ailments involving *ælfe* and those involving demonic agencies is demonstrated at an even more fundamental level in the ingredients employed in these remedies. Treatments for elf-ailments in *Leechbook III* and *Bald's Leechbook* rely on a relatively stable group of herbs, and these same herbs occur routinely and pervasively in remedies said to address demon-related sicknesses. The only herb from Table 2, 'Herbs used against Devils', not to occur in Table 1, 'Herbs used against Elves', is *garleac*. The herbs *elehtre* and *bisceop-wyrt* are the most frequently occurring in both types of remedies. However, if some sort of relationship between elves and demons in these texts is clear, the features of this relationship are still obscure. As Hall has suggested, a variety of beliefs concerning *ælfe* appear to have survived throughout the Anglo-Saxon period and although elves and demons appear to occupy a similar category in the medical collections, it does not necessarily follow that they were synonymous.[64] Ultimately, while we cannot know precisely what an Anglo-Saxon would have thought about *ælfe* and the devil, it is clear that at least within the existing medical tradition the same treatments were seen as effective against both.

The real but obscure relationship between demons and elves within the medical texts has no doubt contributed to the common identification of elf-remedies with demonic possession and the practice of exorcism in critical scholarship.[65] Frequently this association appears to rest on the following syllogism: one of the main attributes of demons is their ability to possess human victims; demons are equivalent to elves in the medical texts; therefore elves also should be considered as possessing their victims. Yet, as plausible as this conclusion appears, there are reasons for questioning the correlation of the remedies in the medical collections and the practice

---

[63] *LBIII*, 62.

[64] Hall, *Elves*, p. 173.

[65] For examples of the use of these terms in relationship to elf remedies, see Singer's preface to the 1961 reprinting of Cockayne's editions, *Leechdoms, Wortcunning, and Starcraft* (London, 1961), vol. I, p. xxxvi; Bonser, 'Magical Practices Against the Elves', p. 358; Meaney, 'The Devil Can Seriously Damage Your Health', p. 95; N. Thun, 'The Malignant Elves', *Studia Neophilologica* 41 (1969), 378–96, at 381; Jolly, *Popular Religion*, p. 136; Zavoti, 'Blame it on the Elves', p. 74; Hall, 'Calling the Shots', p. 201; R. North, *Heathen Gods in Old English Literature* (Cambridge, 1997), p. 52; Arthur, *'Charms', Liturgies, and Secret Rites*, pp. 110–14.

of exorcism. Although this may appear a minor issue, I would suggest that a clear understanding of this topic is important for a nuanced discussion of the relationship of these texts to liturgical practice during the period.

Certainly it must be acknowledged that terms such as exorcism and possession are difficult to define. Some scholars use these terms loosely; for instance, 'exorcism' is sometimes used to mean the removal or expulsion of something damaging from the body, without it necessarily following that an indwelling spirit was involved. In this sense, anything involving some type of purge could be viewed as 'exorcistic'. There is no difficulty with using the word in this sense. However, instead of debating the applicability of a particular word, my intention is to consider the remedies of the medical texts against a particular concept present in medieval thought. In keeping with this, I am using the terms exorcism and possession in a rigorous and specific way, as defined by Augustine:

> spiritus immundus [...] qui extrinsecus invadit animam sensusque conturbat, et quemdam hominibus infert furorem; cui excludendo qui praesunt, manum imponere vel exorcizare dicuntur, hoc est, per divina eum adiurando expellere.[66]
>
> [An unclean spirit ... invades the soul from the outside, perturbs the senses, and brings on men a certain madness; the ones who preside over removing it are said to impose hands or to exorcise, that is, they expel it, adjuring it by divine things.]

In this paradigm, possession involves the indwelling of a demon within a person, generally resulting in a recognisable set of symptoms. In his recent monograph, *Demon Possession in Anglo-Saxon England*, Peter Dendle defines the traditional symptoms of demonic possession as 'falling to the ground, thrashing about, lashing out violently, shouting abusively, raving'.[67] Exorcism, then, is the expulsion of this spirit normally through a formula of adjuration, generally involving the command *adjuro te* ('I command you') or *exorciso te* ('I exorcise you'). This same meaning is echoed in Ælfric's description of the role of an exorcist in his *Pastoral Letter to Wulfsige*: *exorcista is on englisc: se þe mid aðe halsað þa awyrgedan gastas, þe wyllað menn dreccan þurh þæs hælendes naman, þæt hy þa men forlæton* ('exorcist is in English: he who with oaths adjures cursed spirits – those who wish to torment men – through the name of the Saviour that they

---

[66] Augustine, *De beata vita* (Turnhout, 2010), 3.17.
[67] P. Dendle, *Demon Possession in Anglo-Saxon England* (Kalamazoo, 2014), p. 1. See also F. Chave-Mahir, 'Medieval Exorcism: Liturgical and Hagiographical Sources', in *Understanding Medieval Liturgy: Essays in Interpretation*, ed. H. Gittos and S. Hamilton (Farnham, 2015), pp. 159–75, at 159: she describes the symptoms of possession as 'consisting of fits, shouting incomprehensible words in an unknown language, or committing acts of extreme violence'.

depart from the men').⁶⁸ Of course, even in the Middle Ages there was no single systematic categorisation of demons and their influence in human lives.⁶⁹ What I term 'demonic possession', then, is only one of several ways demons were seen to afflict human persons and societies. However, it does reflect a real and influential facet of the medieval understanding of demons and one present in Anglo-Saxon England.

Exorcism in Anglo-Saxon England

There are numerous examples of exorcism within the New Testament, performed both by Jesus and by the Apostle Paul. In the early Church, the ability to discern and cast out demons was not limited to the ordained but instead was seen as a spiritual gift that could be practised by all Christians. However, between the third and fifth centuries, the practice of exorcism increasingly became the domain of the clergy, with 'exorcist' becoming an established ecclesiastical office in its own right.⁷⁰ The fifth-century Gaulish *Statuta Ecclesiae Antiqua* contains the first example of the ordination rite for an exorcist:

> Exorcista cum ordinatur, accipiat de manu episcopi libellum in quo scripti sunt exorcismi, dicente sibi episcopo: accipe et commenda, et habeto potestatem imponendi manus super energumenum sive baptizatum sive catechumenum.⁷¹

> [When the exorcist is ordained, let him accept from the hands of the bishop a little book (libellum) in which are written exorcisms, [while] the bishop says to him: 'Accept, and cherish, and have the power to lay hands on the possessed, whether baptised or catechumens.']

This office was considered one of the minor orders of a church, alongside reader (lector), doorkeeper, and acolyte, for instance.⁷² The fact that the exorcist in the quotation above is presented with a *libellum* ('little book' or 'booklet') of exorcisms suggests that by this time exorcism was meant

---

⁶⁸ *Die Hirtenbriefre Ælfrics in Altenglischer und Lateinischer Fassung*, ed. B. Fehr (Darmstadt, 1966), Brief I.32. This is reading in MS O (CCCC 190). MS X (Bodley Junius 121) reads: *exorcista is on englisc: se-þe mid aðe halsað þa awyrgedan gastas, þe wyllað men dreccan Him be-beodeð þurh þæs ælmihtigan naman* ('he who with oaths adjures cursed spirits, those which wish to torment me, [he] commands them through the name of the Almighty').

⁶⁹ For a general description of demons in the Middle Ages, see A. Franz, *Die kirchlichen Benediktionen im Mittelalter*, 2 vols. (Frieburg i. B., 1909), vol. II, pp. 19–37.

⁷⁰ E. A. Leeper, 'Exorcism in Early Christianity', unpublished PhD dissertation (Duke, 1991), pp. 318–25. Leeper links the clericalisation of exorcism with the increasing role of exorcism as part of the baptismal ceremony in this period.

⁷¹ Leeper, 'Exorcism in Early Christianity', p. 324.

⁷² This is a general list of potential offices (cf. Ælfric's list below). Of course,

to be confined to established written rituals rather than charismatic inspiration.[73] Although there are some early examples of exorcism formulas from the East, the oldest datable ecclesiastical formulas from the Western Church date to the turn of the eighth century.[74]

It is difficult to know how widely established was the office of exorcist in this period. There is only one exorcist known by name from Anglo-Saxon England, a certain Pinewald, who is recorded as a witness on a seventh-century charter.[75] Dendle suggests that this paucity relates in part to the insignificant status of the office, as 'exorcists were usually too low a rank to appear as signatories in official documents'.[76] Ælfric mentions an exorcist in his description of the seven orders of the Church, which he lists in apparently ascending order of importance as: *hostiarius* ('door keeper'), *lector* ('reader'), *exorcista* ('exorcist'), *acolitus* ('acolyte'), *sub-diaconus* ('sub-deacon'), *diaconus* ('deacon'), and *presbiter* ('priest').[77] This, alongside the fact that some Anglo-Saxon liturgical books contain rubrics for the ceremony of ordination, suggests that at least in some regions Anglo-Saxon churches would have followed the practice of ordaining exorcists.[78]

Presumably these exorcists would have made use of the exorcism rituals recorded in liturgical books. There are many examples of these types of rituals found in existing service books from Anglo-Saxon England. The most prevalent of these types of formulas are 'exorcisms' of sacramentals used in the Church and as part of the mass. Throughout the Middle Ages, formal rituals of exorcism could be addressed towards inanimate objects such as water and salt (during the creation of holy water) or even bread and cheese (to be used in the judicial trial of ordeal).[79] In this case, 'exorcism' appears to mean something more like purification than expulsion of

---

    different offices and their responsibilities varied from place to place in the early Church.

[73] See Dendle, *Demon Possession*, p. 134, n. 174, for a discussion on what these *libelli* might have contained.

[74] Franz, *Die kirchlichen Benediktionen*, vol. II, p. 577.

[75] W. Birch, *Cartularium Saxonicum: A Collection of Charters Relating to Anglo-Saxon History*, 3 vols. (London, 1885–93), item 77, vol. I, p. 113 (Sawyer 75).

[76] Dendle, *Demon Possession*, p. 104.

[77] *Die Hirtenbriefre Ælfrics*, Brief I.29. This is also mentioned in Meaney, 'The Devil Can Seriously Damage Your Health', p. 88.

[78] For examples of rubrics in liturgical books, see *The Leofric Missal*, ed. N. Orchard (London, 2002), vol. II 2309–11, p. 394, and *Pontificale lanaletense*, ed. G. H. Doble (London, 1937), p. 51.

[79] For general background on the types of exorcisms performed in Anglo-Saxon England and where those rituals are recorded, see S. L. Keefer, 'Manuals', in *The Liturgical Books of Anglo-Saxon England*, ed. R. W. Pfaff (Kalamazoo, 1995), pp. 99–110. For the use of exorcism within the trial of ordeal, see S. L. Keefer, 'Ut in omnibus honorificetur Deus: the *corsnæd* ordeal in Anglo-Saxon England', in *The Community, the Family and the Saint: Patterns of Power in Early Medieval Europe*, ed. J. Hill and M. Swan (Turnhout, 1998), pp. 237–64.

an indwelling spirit.[80] The second most common type of exorcism ritual is that involved in the baptismal ceremony; in this instance, once again, exorcism appears to achieve something more general than the expulsion of an indwelling spirit. Finally, there are those rituals to be said over an *energumen* (demoniac). These various rituals were clearly related, and in practice the formulas associated with the various types of exorcism were often adapted or reused for different purposes. Indeed, Franz suggests that baptismal exorcisms of the Latin Church were originally derived from exorcisms for the possessed.[81]

However, if the rituals employed were similar, conceptually these types of exorcism probably differed. Dendle makes a distinction between 'procedural exorcism' (including those used during baptism and in the preparation of sacramentals), which occur as a normal part of life in the Church, and 'solemn exorcism' (practised on a demoniac), which occurs only as need arises. A further point of contrast between these ceremonies is that 'procedural exorcisms' can be seen as types of speech acts, as Dendle puts it: 'it is inconceivable that a correctly performed prebaptismal exorcism will not work.'[82] Solemn exorcisms on the other hand were known to occasionally fail or need to be repeated several times. These fundamental differences justify treating the exorcism of a demoniac as a separate action from other types of exorcisms.

In general, it is difficult to know how solemn exorcisms would have actually been performed in this period. In most cases, exorcism formulas occurring in early medieval liturgical books do not come with corresponding *ordines*. This means that we can know the words recited during the ceremony, but it is more difficult to know the rituals that would have accompanied these words. There is one, reasonably late, example of an *ordo* for an exorcism in the *Lanalet Pontifical*.[83] In this pontifical, the bishop (who performs the exorcism) is to fast and pray for three days. The possessed person is then meant to eat food containing specially prepared holy water and salt, following which the priest recites a number of exorcism formulas over the patient. It is hard to determine the degree to which this would have represented normal practice in this period. However, there is evidence elsewhere for the importance of fasting and prayer prior to the exorcism ritual.[84] I would suggest that the use of formulas of command by an ordained member of clergy (or possibly an official exorcist), preceded

---

[80] *Handbook for Liturgical Studies*, IV Sacraments and Sacramentals, ed. A. J. Chupungco (Collegeville, MN, 1997–98), pp. 400–01; Keefer, 'Manuals', p. 108.

[81] Franz, *Die kirchlichen Benediktionen*, vol. II, p. 577.

[82] Dendle, *Demon Possession*, p. 107, 109. See also Keefer, 'Manuals', p. 108.

[83] *Pontificale lanaletense*, pp. 111–16. The *Lanalet Pontifical* (Bibliothèque de la ville de Rouen MS A. 27) is an English pontifical of the late-tenth or early-eleventh century.

[84] Chave-Mahir, 'Medieval Exorcism', p. 166; Leeper, 'Exorcism in Early Christianity', pp. 223–26.

by fasting, and perhaps accompanied by other rituals, probably defined the practice of exorcism within the Church in the Anglo-Saxon period. This rough outline will form the foundation for discussion of the relationship between exorcism and the elf remedies of the Old English medical corpus.

Exorcism and the Medical Texts

Many of the remedies described in this chapter are occasionally referred to by scholars as being 'liturgical' or containing liturgical elements, with one scholar going so far as to suggest that certain types of ailments associated with the demonic, including dementedness and fever, 'required Christian liturgy'.[85] Given this frequent usage, it is useful to consider what 'liturgy' or 'liturgical' means in the context of the medical collections. Liturgy itself is a modern term used to encompass a wide variety of activities related to Christian worship. In the Middle Ages, however, there was no such blanket term, and it was instead usual to refer to particular types of texts, such as prayers or *ordines*, or types of collections, such as sacramentaries, rituals, and pontificals.[86] When medical remedies from this period are sometimes described as 'liturgical', I believe this term should be understood in the very general sense of containing rituals associated with the Church (most notably the use of sacramentals such as holy water or the sign of the cross), and should not generally be taken to imply that these remedies mirror any specific liturgical ceremony performed within the Church. Rather than comment on the generally Christian nature of the remedies considered within this chapter, which I do not dispute, I will consider these cures against the very specific liturgical practice of exorcism, at least in so far as it can be understood in the Anglo-Saxon period.[87] This discussion is relevant to the wider use of learned ecclesiastical material within the medical corpus.

As has been suggested, one possible point of connection between the demonic and elf-related remedies of the medical texts and the practice of exorcism is the widespread use of sacramentals related to the mass. Aside from a core group of herbs that are characteristic of the remedies from the medical corpus involving elves, slightly more than half of these remedies

---

[85] Jolly, *Popular Religion*, p. 145, see also 165, 167–68. See also K. Jolly, 'Cross-Referencing Anglo-Saxon Liturgy and Remedies: The Sign of the Cross as Ritual Protection', in *The Liturgy of the Late Anglo-Saxon Church*, ed. H. Gittos and M. B. Bedingfield (Woodbridge, 2005), pp. 213–43; K. Jolly, 'Tapping the Power of the Cross: Who and for Whom?', in *The Place of the Cross in Anglo-Saxon England*, ed. C. Karkov, S. Keefer, and K. Jolly (Woodbridge, 2006), pp. 58–79, at 59.

[86] H. Gittos and S. Hamilton, 'Introduction', in *Understanding Medieval Liturgy*, pp. 1–10, at 4.

[87] For a general overview of the Christian elements found within the elf-related remedies, see Jolly, *Popular Religion*, Chapter 5.

make use of either holy water or holy salt. The remedy against *ælf-sogoþa* also calls for *oleum infirmorum* (the oil of unction) and a remedy from the *Lacnunga* involves holy wine. The situation is very similar in demon-related remedies, where half use either of these substances. In most cases, these sanctified substances are used in the preparation of drinks or salves to be given to the patient. This practice bears some likeness to the ritual described in the *Lanalet Pontifical* where the possessed person is made to eat food prepared with holy water and salt. However, it is difficult to know how widespread this practice would have been or whether it was unique to exorcism. If we take the presence of either a priest or an official exorcist, a preparatory period of fasting and prayer, and the use of a command formula as the defining features of exorcism in our period, the dissimilarity between this ceremony and those detailed in the medical texts becomes striking.

The adjuration (or formula of command) is arguably the most defining feature of exorcism. This is the prayer in which the indwelling spirit is commanded to leave its host, normally through the invocation of the power of Christ over the Devil. The statement of command is a common feature in some form or another of nearly every prayer of exorcism found in liturgical texts, even those for the inanimate objects of salt or water. However, in all the remedies lexically linked to elves or demons in *Leechbook III* and *Bald's Leechbook* only one contains a formula of command.[88] This occurs in the remedy against *ælf-sogoþa*. The appearance of this type of formula in this remedy is certainly interesting and will be a topic of later discussion. However, this is a unique occurrence and is not echoed in any of the other remedies for elf- (or even demon-) related illness in these texts.

Interestingly, some episodes from early Anglo-Saxon saints' lives depict the curing of a possessed person without the use of a command formula. In Felix's *Life of Guthlac*, the saint heals a demoniac by blowing on his face, an action associated with exorcism, but without verbally adjuring the spirit (or at least this is not mentioned).[89] Even more strangely, in the anonymous *Life of St Cuthbert*, a woman *a demonio vexatam* ('vexed by a demon') is cured by touching the bridle of Cuthbert's horse.[90] These episodes and others like them present a much more charismatic vision of exorcism than

---

[88] There are more adjurations in the *Lacnunga* than in the other collections. These occur in entries 25, 63, and 158. None of these, however, occur in remedies explicitly stated to be for a demonically- (or elvishly-) induced ailment, although entry 63 is for the creation of a holy salve, which could imply some of these influences.

[89] *Felix's Life of Saint Guthlac*, ed. and trans. B. Colgrave (Cambridge, 1985), p. 131. For background on insufflation (or blowing air) as part of exorcism, see: Leeper, 'Exorcism in Early Christianity', pp. 150–52; S. Foot, '"By Water in the Spirit": The Administration of Baptism in Early Anglo-Saxon England', in *Pastoral Care Before the Parish*, ed. J. Blair and R. Sharp (Leicester, 1992), pp. 171–92, at 177.

[90] *Two Lives of Saint Cuthbert: A Life by an Anonymous Monk of Lindisfarne and Bede's*

that defined within liturgical manuscripts. They shift the focus away from particular rituals to the power and charisma of the holy man.

Yet the hagiographical record too presents a point of noticeable contrast with the remedies of the medical texts. Although the office of exorcist was probably somewhat accepted during the ninth and tenth centuries (when *Leechbook III* and *Bald's Leechbook* were probably compiled) there is no evidence that any of these cures for elf- or demon-related afflictions would have involved someone of this order. Indeed, there is little hard evidence to prove that these remedies would have necessarily been carried out by a priest. The involvement of masses in several remedies (normally to be said over certain ingredients) and the use of sacramentals associated with the Church imply some level of involvement by ordained clergy.[91] However, the only remedy of this type that explicitly addresses the question of performer appears to directly contradict that a priest is necessary for its function. This occurs at the end of the remedy for *ælf-sogoþa*, where the remedy directs:

> wæt þæt gewrit on þam drence ond writ crucem mid him on ælcum lime ond cweð signum cruces christi conseruate In uitam eternam. amen. Gif þe ne lyste hat hine selfne oþþe swa gesubne swa he gesibbost hæbbe ond senige swa he selost cunne. þes cræft mæg wiþ ælcre feondes costunge.[92]

> [Wet that writing in the drink and write a cross for him on each limb, and say: *signum cruces Christi conseruate in vitam eternam, amen*. If you do not wish [to do this], have him [do it] himself or such relative as he is most closely related to, bless [him] as best he can. This remedy is powerful against every temptation of the Enemy.]

It is unclear why exactly the reader of this remedy would not want to perform these rituals on the patient. Storms suggested that a priest might have had qualms about carrying out the remedy because it was not sufficiently orthodox.[93] Yet Jolly argues that there is no reason for reading the instruction this way as all elements in the remedy are clearly Christian. Instead she suggests that perhaps there was some hesitation or repugnance around touching the sick man.[94] Nevertheless, irrespective of the reason for this instruction, it is clear that this remedy could be performed by a variety of possible figures, without any indication that

---

Prose Life, ed. B. Colgrave (Cambridge, 1985), p. 93.

[91] Jolly discusses the employment of specifically ecclesiastical rituals and equipment in a number of remedies lacking overt mentions of clergy: *Popular Religion*, pp. 119–20, 142–43, 148, 153–54.
[92] *LBIII*, 62.
[93] Storms, *Anglo-Saxon Magic*, p. 233.
[94] Jolly, *Popular Religion*, p. 164.

they need have prior ecclesiastical training. Indeed, none of the other remedies explicitly invoke the figures of exorcist, or bishop, whom we would normally associate with exorcism. There is also no evidence that a preparatory period of fasting and prayer was required (or even recommended) before the performing of these remedies. When we consider this lack of fasting, coupled with the absence of command formulas, and the only questionable involvement of ordained clergy, I would suggest that the elf- and demon-related remedies of the medical texts bear no clear relationship to the formal practice of exorcism as it was known in the Anglo-Saxon period.

It is furthermore unclear that the afflictions signified by terms such as *ælf-adl* or *deofol-seocnysse* would have been seen as similar in their symptoms to demonic possession. There is some agreement that in some cases elves appear linked to causing mental problems in their victims, and the remedies for elf-related or demon-related illnesses sometimes also explicitly relate that they can cure mental disorders.[95] Madness is a traditional and perhaps the most widespread sign of demonic possession. It is possible this might have encouraged some semantic overlap between some of these illnesses and the concept of demonic possession. However, it is also worth noticing that the other symptoms traditionally associated with possession (such as frenzy, lashing out violently, thrashing about, or shouting abusively) do not occur in these remedies, although they do occur in hagiographical sources from the Anglo-Saxon period. Such an observation is complicated by the fact that in general the remedies of the Old English medical collections do not describe their symptoms, and that many of the words for mental conditions in Old English are difficult to define with confidence.[96] Yet internal evidence within these remedies suggests that frenzy and loss of control were not among their assumed symptoms. Fourteen of the elf- or demon-related remedies in *Bald's Leechbook* and *Leechbook III* call for the patient to be given something to eat, or more commonly, to drink. On several occasions, it is instructed that the patient only receive the drink at night after fasting. This type of treatment presupposes cooperation of the patient. There is no hint in any of these remedies that the patient would have to be bound, or in any other way restrained, as would be expected at least in some cases involving frenzy or loss of control. This type of argument is somewhat speculative given the general lack of description offered within the medical collections. However, it is worth remarking that in the two instances where

---

[95] Hall, *'Elleborus'*, pp. 60–62. See also Hall, *Elves*, pp. 119–56; Jolly, *Popular Religion*, pp. 132–33.
[96] This is due in part to the difficulty of assigning distinct definitions to different Anglo-Saxon terms related to the mind. For a discussion of this difficulty, see A. Low, 'Approaches to the Old English Vocabulary for "Mind"', *Studia Neophiliologica* 73 (2001), 11–22.

symptoms of an elf-disease are described in detail – in the remedies for *ælf-sogoþa* and *wæter-ælfadl* – these look nothing like demonic possession. Even if it is difficult to know what conditions these remedies actually describe, change of skin colour or nail colour and watery eyes are hardly the quintessential traits of possession. Ultimately, I would suggest that, although firm conclusions are impossible, there are reasons for doubting the clear correlation of the ailments described in the medical remedies with the symptoms of demonic possession, at least when this is understood in a formal and rigorous sense.

If the elf-remedies of the medical collections do not appear to include the defining elements found in the formal practice of exorcism and the symptoms treated do not clearly parallel those of demonic possession, it is perhaps best not to refer to these remedies as 'exorcisms' and the victims as 'possessed', unless these terms are being used in a very loose sense. Rather, if we would like to look for a closer parallel to these types of remedies among the liturgical ceremonies practised at this time, it might be more useful to consider the rituals for the infirm.

Some of the manuscripts brought together under the title of the *Romano-Germanic Pontifical* contain elaborate rituals for the sick.[97] For instance, the *ordo ad visitandum et unguendum infirmum* ('order for visiting and anointing the sick') includes sprinkling the infirm with holy water, the recitation of prayers and psalms, the use of incense, and the blessing of the sick person by the priest. Another rite, *ordo ad unguendum infirmum* ('order for anointing the sick') involves anointing the sick person with oil.[98] Similarly, the *Leofric Missal* also contains an *ordo ad visitandum et unguendum infirmum* which includes the singing of various prayers including the Pater Noster and the sprinkling of the sick with holy water.[99] All of these actions occur with varying degrees of repetition in the remedies directed towards *ælfe* in the medical corpus.

The medical procedures of *Leechbook III* and ecclesiastical rituals such as the *ordo ad visitandum et unguendum infirmum* should not be seen as equivalent. One of the chief characteristics of the remedies against elves (or demons) in the medical texts is their use of a stable group of particular herbs, and these herbs are never used in liturgical rituals for treating the sick. The parallels between these two types of rites do suggest, however, that the 'liturgical' elements occurring in certain medical remedies need

---

[97] For a current assessment of the difficulties in talking of the *Romano-Germanic Pontifical* as testimony to a single tenth-century exemplar, see H. Parkes, 'Questioning the Authority of Vogel and Elze's *Pontifical romano-germanique*', in *Understanding Medieval Liturgy*, pp. 75–101.

[98] *Le pontifical romano-germanique du dixieme siècle*, ed. C. Vogel and R. Elze, 3 vols, ST 226, 227, 229 (Vatican City, 1963), vol. I, pp. 246–56, see also vol. II, pp. 258–70.

[99] *Leofric Missal*, 'Incipit ordo ad visitandum et unguendum infirmum', 2507–22, vol. II, pp. 444–47.

not be linked to a specific ritual (such as exorcism), as has been widely surmised, but can also be thought of as common elements of the treatment of the sick within an ecclesiastical community.

Ælf-sogoþa *and the* Leofric Missal

Leechbook III boasts a particularly fascinating example of the careful incorporation of learned material into a remedy for an apparently traditional ailment, *ælf-sogoþa*. This remedy is also the only example where a command formula or adjuration is used in the elf- or demon-related remedies found in the medical corpus. The fact that this remedy employs a command formula does not mean that the term *ælf-sogoþa* should be taken as synonymous with demonic possession, as there are other uses of command formulas within the medical corpus which occur in remedies clearly unassociated with the normal symptoms of possession.[100] Additionally, the symptoms described at the beginning of this remedy bear no resemblance to the traditional symptoms associated with an indwelling spirit. If this disease is not seen as a case of 'possession', we could interpret the words of exorcism as possibly generally enhancing the efficacy of the cure, perhaps in the more general sense of purification or blessing, although it is difficult to know how this would have been understood. Nevertheless, this formal ecclesiastical formula is clearly coming from a written source, likely a liturgical handbook of some type, and was then carefully and purposefully rewritten for its place in this remedy. This remedy thus provides a window into the interaction possible between established liturgical rites and a medical procedure that is unparalleled in the other remedies.

The instructions for preparing the treatment against *ælf-sogoþa* are quite complex. After the instructions for identifying the ailment, quoted above, the remedy prescribes:

Writ þis gewrit:
Scriptum eSt rex regum et dominus dominantium. byrnice. beronice. lurlure. iehe. aius. aius. aius. Sanctus. Sanctus. Sanctus. dominus deus Sabaoth. amen. alleluiah.

 Sing þis ofer þam drence ond þam gewrite:
'Deus omnipotens pater domini nostri iesu cristi. per Inpositionem huius scriptura expelle a famulo tuo N. Omnem Impetum castalidum. de capite. de capillis. de cerebro. de fronte. de lingua. de sublingua. de guttore. de faucibus.

---

[100] These include remedies for the 'black blains' (or blisters) (*LAC*, vol. I, XXV), tooth pain (*LAC*, vol. I, CLVIII), and fever (*BLB*, I 62). For a general discussion of the use of formulas of command in medieval charms, see Olsan, 'Latin Charms of Medieval England', p. 133.

de dentibus. de oculis. de naribus. de auribus. de manibus. de collo. de brachiis. de corde. de anima. de genibus. de coxis. de pedibus. de compaginibus. omnium membrorum intus et foris. amen.'

Wyrc þonne drenc font wæter. rudan. Saluian. cassuc. draconzan. þa smeþan wegbrædan niþewearde feferfugian. diles crop. garleaces .iii. clufe. finul. wermod. lufestice. elehtre. ealra emfela. writ .iii. crucem mid oleum infirmorum ond cweð 'Pax tibi.' Nim þonne þæt gewrit writ crucem mid ofer þam drince ond sing þis þær ofer.

'Deus omnipotens pater domini. nostri. iesu cristi per Inpositionem huius scripturæ et per gustum huiuS expelle diabolum a famulo tuo .N.'

ond credo. ond pater. noster. wæt þæt gewrit on þam drence and writ crucem mid him on ælcum lime and cweþ *'signum cruciS christi conseruate In uitam eternam. amen.'* Gif þe ne lyste hat hine selfne oþþe swa gesubne swa he gesibbost hæbbe and senige swa he selost cunne. þes cræft mæg wiþ ælcre feondes costunge.[101]

['Write this writing:

'It is written, King of kings and Lord of lords. Veronica, Veronica, lurlure(?) Yahweh (?) holy holy holy [in Greek], holy holy holy [in Latin], Lord, God of Hosts. Alleluia.'

Sing this over the drink and the writing:

'All-powerful God, father of our Lord Jesus Christ, through the imposition of this writing expel from your servant N. every attack of *castalidae*, from the head, from the hair, from the brain, from the forehead, from the tongue, from below the tongue, from the throat, from the neck, from the teeth, from the eyes, from the nostrils, from the ears, from the hands, from the neck, from the arms, from the heart, from the mind, from the knees, from the thighs, from the feet, from the joints of all the limbs internal or external. Amen.'

Work then a drink [with] font water, *rudan, saluian, cassuc, draconzan*, the lower part of the smooth *wegbrædan, feferfugian, diles'* top, three cloves of *garleac, finul, wermod, lufestice, elehtre*, of all the same amount. Write three crosses with oil of unction and say 'peace to you'. Take then this writing, write a cross over [it] with the drink. Then sing this over:

'All-powerful God, father of our Lord Jesus Christ, through the imposition of this writing and through the taste of this, expel the devil from your servant N.'

And [then] the Creed, and the Pater Noster. Wet that writing in the drink and write a cross on each limb and say 'May the cross of Christ keep you in life eternal, amen.' If you do not wish [to do this], have him [do

---

[101] *LBIII*, 62. I have accepted Cockayne's emendations in his edition of this section (although not those made in his 'translation' of the Latin), additionally quotation marks have been added by me for clarity; my translation of the garbled *gewrit* is dependent upon Jolly's translation in *Popular Religion*, p. 164. For a discussion of the meaning of *castalidae*, see below.

it] himself or whichever relation that is closest to him, sign [him] as best he can. This remedy is powerful against every temptation of the Enemy.]

As can be readily observed, this remedy contains two (I would suggest related) exorcisms. These exorcisms are variants of an exorcism also found in the *Leofric Missal* and other sources.[102] Patrick Sims-Williams has argued that this exorcism is probably Irish in origin, as two of the earliest copies are found in the *Stowe Missal* and the *Antiphonary of Bangor*, and there appears to be a fragment of the same exorcism in an eighth-century Irish liturgical fragment.[103] The closest versions to the *Leechbook III* formula are those in the *Leofric Missal* and the French *Sacramentary of Ratoldus*. The editor of the *Sacramentary of Ratoldus* suggests that that text relied in part on an English pontifical, and that this prayer was most likely borrowed from an English source.[104] In the *Leofric Missal* the exorcism is titled *alia* ('another') under the larger heading *item super energumino baptizato* ('in the same way [to be said] over a baptised demoniac'):

Domine sancte pater omnipotens aeterne deus, per impositionem scripture huius et gustum aquae, expelle diabolum ab homine isto. De capite, de capillis, de uertice, de cerebro, de fronte, de oculis,/ de auribus, de naribus, de ore, de lingua, de sublingua, de gutture, de collo, de corpore toto, de omnibus membris, de compaginibus membrorum suorum, intus et foris, de ossibus, de uenis, de neruis, de sanguine, de sensu, de cogitationibus, de omni conuersatione, et operetur in te uirtus christi, in eo qui pro te passus est, ut uitam aeternam merearis. Per.[105]

[Lord, holy father, all-powerful eternal God, through the imposition of this writing [or scripture] and taste of water, expel the devil from this man, from the head, from the hair, from the top, from the brain, from the forehead, from the eyes, from the ears, from the nostrils, from the mouth, from the tongue, from under the tongue, from the throat, from the neck, from the whole body, from all the limbs, from the joints of all his limbs, internal or external, from the bones, from the veins, from the

---

[102] This is also noted by Jolly, *Popular Religion*, p. 163.
[103] P. Sims-Williams, 'Thought, Word, Deed: An Irish Triad', *Ériu* 29 (1978), 78–111, at 88–91. Sims-Williams notes that versions of this exorcism also occur in *The Collectar-Pontifical of Baturich*, edited in *Das Kollektar-Ponifikale des Bischofs Baturich von Regensburg*, ed. F. Unterkircher (Freiburg, Switzerland, 1962), p. 128; Munich, MS Bayerische Staatsbibliothek, Clm. 17027, edited in Franz, *Die kirchlichen Benediktionen*, vol. II, pp. 601–02; *The Ritual of St Florian*, edited *in Das Rituale von St Florian aus dem zwölften Jahrhundert*, ed. Á. Franz (Freiburg, 1904), p. 18. However, he does not note the version in *Leechbook III* or that found in the *The Sacramentary of Ratoldus*, ed. N. Orchard (London, 2005), 2231, p. 419.
[104] *The Sacramentary of Ratoldus*, pp. cxci, clxxxii.
[105] *Leofric Missal*, vol. II, 2479, pp. 437–38. This exorcism occurs as part of *Leofric A*, the oldest part of the compilation, dating from the late-ninth or early-tenth century: *Leofric Missal*, vol. I, p. 23.

tendons, from the blood, from the senses, from the thoughts, from every habit, and let Christ's virtue work in you, who died for you, that you may merit life eternal. Through.]

Although the exorcisms are clearly related, there are several significant points of contrast between the remedy in *Leechbook III* and the other versions of the formula. Though presented separately, the second command formula in the remedy for *ælf-sogoþa* seems to be drawn originally from this same exorcism, as can be seen from its close similarity to the first line of the *Leofric* formula. In the first version of this exorcism, *expelle diabolum* (present in all other known versions of this exorcism) has been replaced with *expelle* [...] *omnem impetum castalidum* ('expel [...] every attack of elves'). *Castalidae* here appears to be a reference to the Castalian spring on Parnassus; the term is ultimately derived from Aldhelm, who uses it to refer to the Muses.[106] In glossaries, however, *castalidae* is sometimes glossed by *dun-ælfa* ('mountain-ælfe'), where the mountain presumably refers to Parnassus. The term *dun-ælfa* is probably a nonce-form and occurs nearly exclusively in glossaries.[107] The only exception to this occurs in a passage from Byrhtferth of Ramsey's *Enchiridion*. Yet he also uses the term effectively as an intertextual gloss for *castalidae*: *Ic hate gewitan fram me þa meremen, þe synt sirene geciged, ond eac þa Castalidas nymphas (þæt synt dunylfa)* ('I order to leave from me those sea-people (who are called sirens), and also the Castalian nymphs (who are called dunylfa)').[108] Nevertheless, the glossary entries do suggest that *castalidas* was a known translation for the term *ælf*, and, given the exorcism's context within the remedy for *ælf-sogoþa*, it seems very likely that this is the intended meaning here.

The existence of this formula could be interpreted as evidence of belief in elvish possession, and of the general synonymy of demons and elves in this period.[109] However, it is perhaps worth stressing again that this is the only elf-related remedy in any of the medical collections to contain such a formula. The inclusion of this ritual in the remedy for *ælf-sogoþa* confirms the unusual nature of this remedy (and that for *wæter-ælfadl*), not only for being directed towards otherwise unattested conditions, but also for their elaborate descriptions of symptoms and the careful and complex treatments offered. Moreover, as noted by Hall, the fact that the remedy presents two separate formulas, one for a demon and one for elves, could

---

[106] E. Thornbury, 'Aldhelm's Rejection of the Muses and the Mechanics of Poetic Inspiration in Early Anglo-Saxon England', *Anglo-Saxon England* 36 (2007), 71–92, at 89–91.

[107] Hall, *Elves*, pp. 78–83; see also Shippey, 'Light-Elves, Dark-Elves, and Others', pp. 2 3.

[108] *Byrhtferth's Enchiridion*, ed. P. S. Baker and M. Lapidge, EETS s.s. 15 (Oxford 1995), pp. 134–36; cf. Thornbury, 'Aldhelm's Rejection of the Muses', p. 91.

[109] See, for instance, Zavoti, 'Blame it on the Elves', pp. 74–75.

be taken to suggest that these two causes needed to be treated separately.[110] Additionally, while in one case we have the demon itself being expelled, in the other only the *attacks* of elves are being expelled, which may reveal a fundamental difference between these afflictions. As the reference to *castalidae* does not occur in any other version of this exorcism, this appears to be evidence for how this type of liturgical formula could be adapted to a new context.

There are other examples of how this general exorcism formula was adapted within the remedy. The formula in the *Leofric Missal*, and the (nearly identical) formula found in the *Sacramentary of Ratoldus*, state that the demon is to be expelled *per impositionem scripture huius et gustum aquae* ('by the placing of this writing and the taste of water'). Aside from the remedy for *ælf-sogoþa*, none of the other versions of this exorcism include similar instructions. The phrase appears to some degree unusual in itself and does not regularly appear in exorcisms.[111] It appears to suggest that some type of writing, likely holy scripture, is placed on the sufferer prior to (or possibly during) the exorcism and that he or she is given to drink a sip of holy water as part of the ceremony.

However, in its place in the medical remedy, the phrase appears to take on a wholly different meaning. The instruction within the exorcism that it is to be done *per inpositionem huius scriptura* occurs in close proximity to instructions for creating a *gewrit* ('piece of writing') containing a string of somewhat scrambled Latin and Greek words. When the exorcism formula indicates that *this* writing is to be placed on the patient, it is hard to avoid the conclusion that this should refer to the piece of writing just prepared. The fact that this may be a purposeful adaption is supported by the second exorcism formula in the remedy where *per impositionem scripture huius et gustum aquae* has been replaced with *per inpositionem huius scriptura et per gustum huius* ('through the placing of this writing and the tasting of this'). This formula is immediately preceded by a recipe for creating a herbal drink, and reference to this drink also immediately follows the formula. It seems very likely that this drink is the referent meant by *huius* ('this') in the formula. I would suggest that what we have here is an example of an exorcism formula being adapted to a specifically medical scenario. This would suggest the possibility for intersection between formal liturgical rituals and a medical procedure.

The other major difference between the exorcism within the remedy for *ælf-sogoþa* and how this remedy occurs in other sources is that the final part of the remedy has been reduced. Although the other extant versions

---

[110] Hall, *Elves*, p. 106.
[111] I have not been able to find another example of its use in an exorcism formula. Its unusual nature is also remarked on by Nicholas Orchard in his edition of the *Leofric Missal*, vol. I, p. 112.

of this formula vary to some degree from one to another, all other versions continue beyond the listing of physical body parts to include non-corporeal aspects. This can be seen in the *Leofric Missal*'s instruction that the demon also be expelled *de sensu, de cogitationibus, de omni conuersatione* ('from the senses, from the thoughts, from all habits'). Some other versions also include *de verbis* ('from words') and *de operibus* ('from deeds') in this list.[112] Sims-Williams has argued that these non-corporeal elements formed a part of the exorcism in its original form.[113] With the single exception of *anima* ('spirit/mind'), which is listed alongside parts of the body, the *Leechbook III* exorcism excludes these elements to focus entirely on the physical. It is possible this was not a deliberate choice and could reflect changes in an exemplar of the exorcism prior to its inclusion in this remedy. Yet it is also possible that this could be yet another adaptation of this formula to a specific medical scenario. As seen above, the symptoms of *ælf-sogoþa* appear to have been physical rather than mental, in which case the author of the remedy might have viewed the more psychological elements of the exorcism unimportant.

References to elves normally occur only within poetic or medical texts from Anglo-Saxon England and are not treated in ecclesiastical texts. However, in this remedy we see a traditional exorcism adapted specifically to a medical condition related to *ælfe*. The only other example similar to this from Anglo-Saxon England occurs in the *Royal Prayerbook*, which contains an adjuration that begins: *adiuro te satanae diabulus aelfae* ('I conjure you, Satan, devil, elves'). The *Royal Prayerbook* is also known to be the most medically concerned of the early Insular prayerbooks, which might suggest a similar type of adaption of an existing formula.[114] As has been seen, however, the revision of the exorcism in *Leechbook III* is deeper than simply changing the addressee, and involves altering the nucleus of the ritual to include a herbal drink and written incantation, both of which would normally have no place in an ecclesiastical ritual. Rather than simply including liturgical elements, such as holy water or incense, this remedy effectively creates a medical *ordo* for treatment of the disease that includes both prayers and actions.

The remedy for *ælf-sogoþa* provides an example of how contemporary ecclesiastical ritual could be specifically adapted for a medical scenario. The changes made to this formula indicate that the remedy must have

---

[112] These are the versions found in the *Stowe Missal*, and the *Antiphonary of Bangor*.

[113] Sims-Williams, 'Thought, Word, Deed', p. 90. He lists this as among some of the earliest evidence for the use of the 'thought, word, deed' triad in liturgical sources.

[114] *The Prayer Book of Aedeluald the Bishop, Commonly Called the Book of Cerne*, ed. A. B. Kuypers (Cambridge, 1902), p. 221. The translation is with reference to Simek's in 'Elves and Exorcism', p. 43. Simek argues that *aelfae* should be read as a vocative, rather than Hall's suggestion that it is a genitive singular modelled after *satanae*, cf. Hall, *Elves*, p. 72.

passed through the hands of (or possibly originated with) someone literate in Latin. This person was almost certainly not a person 'not resident in monastery' who spent their days collecting 'charms, incantations, and rituals' from the people, a description Grattan and Singer imagine for one of the compilers of the *Lacnunga*, for instance. Whoever redacted this text was confident and skilled in composing Latin text, adapting the remedy in several ways and also supplying the learned word *castalidae* to provide a Latin translation of the Old English term *ælfe*. The extremely complex nature of this remedy calls into question the clear connection between the 'native' or 'Germanic' ailments found in the medical texts and popular practices and folk traditions. Although elements of this entry may have their origin in popular traditions – including perhaps the herbs used here and elsewhere for treating elf-related ailments – the remedy as it exists is clearly a learned piece, part of the wider literary and ecclesiastical tradition of the period.

The Testimony of Leechbook III

Although the shortest of the Old English medical collections, *Leechbook III* provides an invaluable testament to particular facets of medical practice in Anglo-Saxon England. While containing the short, Latinate remedies common to all the medical collections, *Leechbook III* also contains our greatest testament to a category of diseases understood to be caused by *maran*, *nihtgengan*, and *ælfe*. Although these types of ailments occur in the other medical collections, they do so only rarely and sporadically. Without the testimony of *Leechbook III* it would be impossible to make general inferences about these ailments and how they might have been treated.

From the evidence of *Leechbook III* we are able to conclude that there was a consistent approach to these ailments, one that is also attested in *Bald's Leechbook*. In these remedies we can see that a certain core group of herbs was used in the treatment of these conditions. An analysis of the 12 remedies related to elves in *Bald's Leechbook* and *Leechbook III* also highlights the exceptional nature of the *Lacnunga's* remedy *Wið færstice*. Although this is indisputably the most famous 'elf-remedy' from the medical corpus, and comprises the first entry discussed in Hall and Jolly's books on elves, we should not take this remedy as typical of medical responses to elves in the Anglo-Saxon period. Although the attraction of the vibrant narrative in this remedy is obvious, it stands in distinction to the majority of remedies involving *ælfe* that contain herbal cures accompanied by simple rituals including the sign of the cross or the use of holy water. Indeed, the singularity of the testimony of the *Lacnunga* with regard to these types of diseases is only made clear when the Old English medical collections are treated individually, rather than as one homogeneous body of evidence.

The witness of *Leechbook III* also provides evidence of the interrelation of traditional figures such as *ælfe* and the Christian demonic within the practical sphere of medicine. The remedies of *Leechbook III* point towards a significant overlap between these types of afflictions, as they frequently receive the same type of treatment and occasionally are even featured within the same remedy. The fact that these afflictions are treated with the same group of herbs, but without the presence of exorcism, furthermore suggests that the traditional paradigm of elves undergoing 'demonisation' after the coming of Christianity, and the assertion that 'elf-shot' was 'the same as demonical possession', at best represent only a partial truth. There is in fact very little evidence that elf-related diseases were understood as instances of possession by an indwelling spirit in need of exorcising. The medical texts appear to testify instead to demons being treated with remedies for elves. If elves were indeed undergoing the process of being demonised, it appears demons were also being 'elfified'. This type of paradigm might also explain the general lack of exorcism accounts in hagiography and preaching material dating from after the eighth century.[115] The permeability of the terms for *ælfe* ('elves') and demons in the Old English medical texts is yet another testimony to the syncretic nature of Anglo-Saxon culture and society.

The example of exorcism also highlights the complex nature of the relationship of the remedies found in the medical corpus to ecclesiastical practice. Too often this has been assumed to be a one-to-one relationship where medical remedies can be closely identified with specific liturgical rituals. This is not always the case, and such an approach can disguise the complexity of understanding sicknesses in the period and the multifarious ways they were treated.

Furthermore, *Leechbook III* demonstrates that even the entries targeted at what appear to be the most clearly 'native' or 'Germanic' types of diseases reveal the influence of a learned environment. One elf-related remedy, for instance, directed at the disease *ælf-sogoþa*, contains, alongside instructions for the preparation of what may be a traditional herbal drink and common church rituals such as the sign of the cross, a variety of textual passages that are clearly neither Germanic nor 'popular' in their content. The first is an inscription of holy words and names of God deriving from languages including Latin, Greek, and Hebrew. The second is an exorcism formula, probably of Irish origin, which appears to have been specifically adapted for its use in this remedy. The redactor of this piece not only made certain changes within the body of this Latin text but was likely also responsible for inserting the learned word *castalidae*, a term ultimately derived from Aldhelm, into the formula as a translation of the Old English term *ælfe*. This person instead must have had a quite high-

---

[115] For a discussion of this trend, see Dendle, *Demon Possession*, pp. 149–74.

level command of Latin and a variety of texts on hand. While elements in the remedies directed towards *ælfe* and related concerns may have their origin in traditional or popular practices, the literary elements in these texts testify to the influence of a learned (and very likely monastic) setting.

Finally, these remedies show the incorporation of liturgical elements and ritual into the process of medical treatment. This incorporation could involve the use of individual rituals or elements associated with the Church, such as holy water, holy salt, and certain prayers, but could also extend to the inclusion and adaptation of complex rites to the specific needs of a medical environment. Overall this demonstrates the close connection between medical expertise and ecclesiastical practice in this period.

3

The *Lacnunga* and Insular *Grammatica*

The British Library manuscript Harley 585 is significant for containing two distinct collections of medical material. It begins with a copy of the *Old English Pharmacopeia*; this collection is then followed immediately by a second, independent collection of cures in Old English. The second text is the only extant copy of the medical collection known to scholars today as the *Lacnunga*. 'Lacnunga' is the Old English word for 'remedies', a title given to the collection by Cockayne, who first edited the text in the 1860s. The manuscript contains no formal illustrations, even in the *Old English Pharmacopeia* which in other manuscripts is sometimes illustrated. Ker dates the majority of the manuscript to the end of the tenth or beginning of the eleventh century, with the table of contents to the *Herbarium* and the final part of the *Lacnunga* as perhaps slightly later; this agrees with the chiefly late Old English linguistic features of the text (even if these features are somewhat mixed).[1]

A date in the late tenth or early eleventh century would position the compilation of the *Lacnunga* as later than *Bald's Leechbook*, and perhaps not too distant in time from the translation of the *Herbarium Complex*. However, the *Lacnunga* has frequently been treated as somewhat different in character from these other collections. It lacks the sophisticated system of organisation observed in *Bald's Leechbook* and is the only extant collection to not have a table of contents. It is also the smallest manuscript, measuring only 192 x 115 mm, which may indicate that it was meant to be a portable aid.[2] However, the collection has mostly attracted attention for its 'magical' or 'superstitious' content, which is generally considered to be popular in its origin.

In his influential book on Anglo-Saxon medicine, Cameron describes the *Lacnunga* as 'folk medicine at its lowest level'. He contrasts this collection with *Bald's Leechbook* and *Leechbook III*, arguing that together these repre-

---

[1] Ker no. 231; *LAC*, vol. I, pp. 135 and 201. Citations from Pettit's edition are generally given by entry number in Roman numerals. Translations given from the *Lacnunga* are also Pettit's unless otherwise stated (although herb names have been retained in Old English to reflect the practice elsewhere in this book); translations from other sources are my own unless otherwise stated.

[2] This measurement is taken from the British Library's catalogue of digitised manuscripts <www.bl.uk/manuscripts> (Accessed 30 June 2016).

sent 'examples of the two sides of the Anglo-Saxon medical world, the learned against the popular'.[3] Although not all scholars would defend such a binary division, the general idea that the *Lacnunga* is more representative of popular or folk practice is widespread. The two most recent editions of the text have emphasised this aspect. The full title of Grattan and Singer's edition is *Anglo-Saxon Magic and Medicine: Illustrated Specifically from the Semi-Pagan Text* Lacnunga. Within, the authors describe the text as being 'on as low a cultural level as any in the Anglo-Saxon language' and suggest that at least one compiler of the text was a doctor, not resident in any monastery, who 'collected charms, incantations and rituals that were used by his brother leeches and by the people themselves'.[4] Pettit, the most recent editor of the collection, also introduces the text as 'a repository of much presumably "popular" lore'.[5] Although some have found the 'superstitious' nature of the collection as worthy of praise rather than censure, this general portrayal has characterised much scholarship of the collection.

The majority of remedies found in the *Lacnunga* are the simple, herbal remedies common in some measure to each of the Old English medical collections. That many remedies found in the *Lacnunga* have variant versions in the other collections (38 or 39 are shared with *Bald's Leechbook* and nine with *Leechbook III*) indicates that the compiler (or compilers) was drawing, in part at least, on the same body of pre-translated cures used by the compilers of these other texts.[6] These short, simple (mostly herbal) remedies are primarily translated from Latin sources such as *Physica Plinii* (or other derivative Plinian sources) and Marcellus's *De medicamentis*.[7] Such cures are similar to many dealt with in the previous chapters, even if in the *Lacnunga* they often appear less well organised. Remedies of this type are always presented in Old English prose. Indeed, vernacular prose is the form taken by the majority of remedies in the Old English medical corpus.

However, the *Lacnunga* also contains a variety of material that differs from this typical format. It contains for instance much more text in Latin than the other collections. It also contains a number of remedies that include words in other languages such as Greek, Hebrew, and Old Irish. Finally, it includes a number of cures written entirely or partially in Old English metre. Entries matching these descriptions are also found in other Old English medical collections. However, they appear in significantly greater numbers within the *Lacnunga*. These varieties of cures in particular

---

[3] Cameron, *Anglo-Saxon Medicine*, p. 34.
[4] Grattan and Singer, *Anglo-Saxon Magic and Medicine*, pp. 7, 19–21.
[5] Pettit, vol. I, p. xxvii.
[6] *LAC*, vol. I, pp. 163–65; Meaney, 'Variant Versions', pp. 238–39. Meaney's table records 39 remedies from the *Lacnunga* found in the *Leechbook*, and Pettit's similar table records 38 variants with two additional possible variants. The count for *Leechbook III* is taken from Pettit's table.
[7] Pettit's edition provides a helpful summary of the Latin sources occurring in the *Lacnunga*'s remedies: *Lac*, vol. I, pp. 160–62.

have attracted attention for being illustrative of popular practice, or in the case of the metrical pieces, representative of historic Germanic tradition. However, while it is possible that some of these remedies may resemble practices popular among wider Anglo-Saxon society, overall the impression given is of a compiler with an ultimately learned interest in foreign languages, letters, and the alphabet, or, at the very least, a milieu where such material was available.

Latin in the Remedies of the Lacnunga

At first glance, the increased presence of Latin text in the *Lacnunga* is conspicuous. Although *Bald's Leechbook* and the *Old English Herbarium* draw significantly upon Latinate sources, the preponderance of these texts is written in Old English. While Old English is still the primary language of the *Lacnunga*, more than 40 of the *Lacnunga*'s 190 remedies are in Latin or call for the recitation of Latin words. This is in comparison to eight such treatments in *Bald's Leechbook* and two in the *Old English Herbarium*.[8] Latin, of course, was not the native language of the Anglo-Saxons. It was, however, the language of the universal Church and of literary education more generally. Because of its relationship to the Church, Latin was considered to be one of the *tres linguae sacrae* ('three sacred languages'), alongside Greek and Hebrew. These languages were considered 'not only as the languages of scholarship, but in a deeper, mystical way as *tres linguae sacrae*, sacred indeed, because they were employed in the suprascription of the cross of Christ'.[9] This trinity of languages held significance since the Patristic period, but were particularly revered in the early Insular Church.[10] The employment of all three sacred languages is found in the *Lacnunga*, but Latin is by far the most common and extensively used. Because of its status as the language of the Church and of intellectual thought in the West, it would also have been certainly the most familiar to any literate user or reader.

Much of the Latin employed in the remedies of the *Lacnunga* is closely related to the liturgy and common prayers of the early medieval Church. The *Pater Noster* and the *Credo* are the most frequently called for Latin prayers, but calls for ten separate Latin psalms also occur throughout

---

[8] These numbers are my own estimate and do not include treatments where the names of herbs, ingredients, or illnesses are given in Latin.

[9] R. E. McNally, 'The *Tres Linguae Sacrae* in Early Irish Biblical Exegesis', *Theological Studies* 19 (1958), 395–403, at 395.

[10] For more information, see D. R. Howlett, '"Tres Linguae Sacrae" and Threefold Play in Insular Latin', *Peritia* 16 (2002), 94–115; McNally, 'The *Tres Linguae Sacrae*', pp. 395–96.

the text.[11] Aside from specific prayers, some remedies also call for readings from the gospels or Old Testament, from the divine office, from the prayers and hymns used during the celebration of mass, or the recitation of litanies. These passages are hardly ever given in full, and instead are generally referred to by name or by their first words.

Entry XXIX provides a good example of how prayers and passages are referenced in some of the remedies:

> Þis is se halga drænc wið ælfsidene ond wið eallum feondes costungum: Writ on husldisce: 'In principio erat uerbum' usque 'non conprehenderunt', et plura 'Et circumibat Ihesus totam Galileam docens' usque 'et secuti sunt eum / turbe multe'; 'Deus in nomine tuo' usque in finem; 'Deus misereatur nobis' usque in finem; 'Domine Deus in adiutorium' usque in finem.
>
> Nim cristallan ond disman ond sidewaran ond cassuc ond finol, ond nim sester fulne gehalgodes wines; ond hat unmælne mon gefeccean swigende ongean streame healfne sester yrnendes wæteres; nim þonne ond lege ða wyrta ealle in þæt wæter ond þweah þæt gewrit of ðan husldisce þærin swiðe clæne; geot þonne þæt gehalgade win ufon on ðæt oþer.
>
> Ber þon to ciricean; læt singan mæssan ofer, ane / 'Omnibus', oðre 'Contra tribulatione', þriddan 'Sancta Marian'.
>
> Sing ðas gebedsealmas: 'Miserere mei Deus', 'Deus in nomine tuo', 'Deus misereatur nobis', 'Domine Deus', 'Inclina Domine', ond 'Credo', ond 'Gloria in excelsis Deo', ond letanias, 'Pater noster'; ond bletsa georne in ælmihtiges Drihtnes naman ond cweð, 'In nomine Patris et Filii et Spiritus Sancti sit benedictum'; bruc syþþan.[12]

> [This is the holy drink for (?)elfish magic and for all the temptations of the Devil: Write on a paten: 'In the beginning was the word' as far as 'comprehended it not', and furthermore 'And Jesus went about all Galilee teaching' as far as 'and great crowds followed him'; 'God in your name' until the end; 'May God have mercy on us' until the end; 'Lord God to my aid' until the end.
>
> Take *cristalle* and *disme* and *sideware* and *cassuc* and *finol*, and take a full sextarius of consecrated wine; and have a virgin fetch in silence against the current half a sextarius of running water; then take and place all the plants in the water and wash the writing off the inside of the paten very cleanly; then pour the consecrated wine from above onto the other [liquid].
>
> Then carry it to the church; have masses sung over it, first 'By all [the saints]', second 'Against trouble', third 'Holy Mary'.

---

[11] This estimation relies on Pettit's identification of psalms in the commentary to his edition. It is possible that other psalms also occur in the collection but references to them are corrupted or unclear.

[12] *LAC*, vol. I, XXIX.

Sing these precatory psalms: 'God have mercy on me', 'God in your name', 'May God have mercy on us', 'Lord God', 'Turn, Lord', and the Creed, and 'Glory to God in the highest', and litanies, the Our Father; and zealously bless [it] in the name of the almighty God and say, 'In the name of the Father and of the Son and of the Holy Spirit let it be blessed'; then use it.]

In this example, the recitations required are referred to in a kind of shorthand, rather than given in full (these types of shortened forms are also found in liturgical books and preaching materials). In the first paragraph, a number of texts are meant to be written on a paten, the dish upon which the consecrated host sits. The first two texts are sections from the gospels. The first is the beginning of the Gospel of John, a text frequently granted special power in the Middle Ages. The second is from the Gospel of Matthew and describes Jesus in Galilee, 'healing all manner of sickness and every infirmity, among the people'.[13] The next three texts to be written are all psalms calling on the help of the Lord.[14] Later in the entry a number of additional psalms are referenced along with other prayers including a litany, the Creed, and the Pater Noster.

The prayers referenced here are used differently than the Latin passages found in the remedy for *ælf-sogoþa* (discussed in Chapter 2), where a particular liturgical formula has been specifically adapted for a medical scenario. These prayers have not been specifically adapted for their use in this remedy, although most of them do generally relate to seeking healing or help from God. Certainly, this remedy would have still required a reasonable degree of knowledge on the part of a practitioner, who is expected to recognise the psalms and other prayers by their first words. It is also possible that the biblical references would have assumed that a text of the gospels was available to the user. Together these references suggest a monastic or ecclesial environment for the use of these remedies.

In conclusion, the use of Latin throughout the *Lacnunga* has a clear association with the power of God to bring about healing through the instruments of the Church. However, there also appears to be a recognition of Latin as a sacred language, its words becoming powerful in their own right. This is particularly evident in some cures where Latin words or saints' names are used totemically: for instance, the use of the names of the four evangelists (or a Latin phrase which includes their names) which appear in several entries, in one case with the instruction that they be written on a stick used in a remedy.[15] The same notion seems to be present when short Latin phrases and allusions are appended to otherwise vernacular

---

[13] Matthew 4:23, Douay-Rheims 1899 American Edition.
[14] These are vulgate psalms 53, 66, 70.
[15] *LAC*, vol. I, LXIII. Other uses of the names of the four evangelists include: CXXVI, XXXI.

remedies. For instance, *in nomine Patris et Filii et Spiritus Sancti* is sometimes appended to incantations otherwise in Old English or Old Irish, and the Hebrew word 'amen' is used similarly.[16] In other instances longer passages of Latin prose or poetry are found quoted in their entirety. The longest, and most famous, of these texts is the Hiberno-Latin prayer known as the *Lorica of Laidcenn*. This exceptionally difficult Latin metrical composition is chiefly concerned with bodily and spiritual health and in particular protection from demonic assailants. The poem was probably written in Ireland in the seventh century.[17] The inclusion of this piece within a medical text is unusual, and no comparable entries are found in the other collections. This prayer was probably drawn from a devotional collection or florilegium. Together these various types of pieces testify to the availability of quite a variety of material to a compiler(s) of the collection and suggest the overall assumption of Latin learning and a familiarity with liturgical material.

Other Languages used in Remedies

The other two 'holy languages', Greek and Hebrew, also occur, albeit infrequently, in remedies in the *Lacnunga*. This infrequency is no doubt partially due to the fact that knowledge of Greek and Hebrew was extremely limited in the later Anglo-Saxon period and tended to be confined to the knowledge of specific words without an understanding of syntax.[18] The remedies utilising words in these languages are normally garbled and difficult to understand, which probably reflects a low-level knowledge of these languages in whoever wrote or copied these entries. It appears that someone involved in producing some of the material found in the Old English medical collections knew Greek, as Latinised Greek words are often translated correctly in medical material (seen, for instance, in the long passages of *Bald's Leechbook*). However, the garbled nature of these remedies in the *Lacnunga* makes it doubtful that the meaning of their words would have been understood, even by an exceptionally learned reader. Instead, the inclusion of these remedies demonstrates an interest in powerful words and perhaps foreign tongues more generally on the part of the compiler.

Greek occurs alongside Latin in remedy LXXXVIII, *wið omum ond blegnu[m]* ('for erysipelas and boils') which reads: *Cristus natus aaius sanctus*

---

[16] For examples, see *LAC*, vol. I, XXII, XXV, XXXI, LXIV, LXXXVI, CXLIX, CXXVI.
[17] This prayer has sometimes been attributed to Gildas and known under the name *Lorica Gildae*, but this attribution is very likely incorrect: see M. Herren, 'The Authorship, Date of Composition and Provenance of the so-called *Lorica Gildae*', *Eriu* 24 (1973), 35–51.
[18] M. C. Bodden, 'Evidence for Knowledge of Greek in Anglo-Saxon England', *ASE* 17 (1988), 217–46; D. Fleming, '"The Most Exalted Language": Anglo-Saxon Perceptions of Hebrew', unpublished PhD dissertation (Toronto, 2006).

a Cristus passus aaius a Cristus resurrexit a mortuis aaius sanctus aa superare potens, where 'Aaius' appears to be a misspelling of the Greek Ἅγιος.[19] The Greek letter omega is also evident in remedy LXXXI: *writ ðis ondlang ða earmas wiþ dweorh: +T+ Aω. ond gnid cyleðenigean on ealað; Sanctus Macutus, Sancte Uictorici* ('write this along arms for fever: +T+ ωA. And (?)crush *celeþonie* in ale; Saint Machutus, Saint Victoricus').[20] Other exotic tongues are discernible in other entries. For instance, Greek, Hebrew, and possibly Aramaic all appear to occur in remedy CLX. This remedy purports to record the content of a letter sent from heaven that will cure diarrhoea.[21] The letter reads:

> Ranmigan adonai. Eltheos. mur. O ineffabile. O miginan. midanmian. misane. / dimas. mode. mida. memagartem. Orta min. sigmone. beronice. irritas. uenas quasi dulaþ. feruor. fruxantis. sanguinis. siccatur. fla. fracta. frigula. mir gui. etsihdon. segulta. frautantur. in arno. midomnis. abar uetho. sydone. multo. saccula pp pppp. sother. sother. miserere mei Deus Deus mini. Deus mei. AMEN. Alleluia, Alleluia.[22]

According to Pettit, *ranmigan adonai* can be translated as 'shout, my shield is the Lord God' in Hebrew, and the Greek *theos* is probably intended in *Eltheo*. He also suggests that *etsihdon. segulta* might translate as Latin *et* (and) and Aramaic *sader ian segulta* ('send us a remedy') and *mur* might correspond to the Aramaic *mar* ('Lord'), although these connections are not certain. I have discussed these terms with an expert in Aramaic who has expressed doubts that *etsihdon. segulta* derives from Aramaic, unless possibly *segulta* is a corruption of Syriac *asyuta* ('remedy'). *Mar* ('Lord'), however, which occurs in First Corinthians 16:22 (*maran atha*, 'Come, Lord!'), may well be the intended meaning of *mur* as it occurs in the entry in what is apparently a list of terms for God.[23] Several Latin words are also easily discernible in this same remedy.

However, more commonly than Greek or Hebrew, Old Irish is likely to appear in these unintelligible types of cures. By my own measure, I have counted 11 cures in the *Lacnunga* that either involve the recitation of words that are either completely incomprehensible or are in languages

---

[19] *LAC*, vol. I, LXXXVIII.
[20] *LAC*, vol. I and II, LXXXIII. An expanded version of this follows later in the remedy: T + þ + T + N + ω + T + UI + M + ωA.
[21] For a background on heavenly letters as a wider genre, see R. Hebing, 'The Textual Tradition of Heavenly Letters Charms in Anglo-Saxon Manuscripts', in *Secular Learning in Anglo-Saxon England: Exploring the Vernacular*, ed. L. S. Chardonnens and B. Carella (Amsterdam, 2012), pp. 203–22.
[22] *LAC*, vol. I, CLX.
[23] I am very thankful to Dr Salam Rassi for his help on these points in personal correspondence.

foreign to England.[24] Out of these 11, six have been discerned by earlier scholars to likely contain Old Irish words.[25] This is a markedly higher percentage than in the other medical collections, which only contain two such cures combined. One of the clearest examples of this is found in *Lacnunga* entry XXVI:

> Wið ðon þe mon oððe nyten wyrm gedrince, gyf hyt sy wæpnedcynnes sing ðis leoð in þæt swiðre eare þe heræfter awriten is; gif hit sy wifcynnes sing in þæt wynstre eare: 'Gonomil orgomil marbumil marbsai ramum tofeð tengo docuillo biran cuiðær cæfmiil scuiht cuillo scuiht cuib duill marbsiramum.' Sing nygon/ siðan in þæt eare þis galdor ond 'Pater noster' æne.[26]

> [In the event that man or beast drinks an insect, if it is male sing this song which is written hereafter into the right ear; if it is female sing it into the left ear. *Gonomil orgomil marbumil marbsai ramum tofeð tengo docuillo biran cuiðær cæfmiil scuiht cuillo scuiht cuib duill marbsiramum.* Sing this incantation nine times into the ear and the Our Father once.]

The majority of the words of the song in the centre of this remedy have been reconstructed, with some emendation, from Old Irish. Pettit, drawing on the work of scholars of Old Irish, offers a very provisional translation:

> I wound the animal, I hit the animal, I kill the animal. Kill the (?)persistent creature! Its tongue will fall out. I destroy the little spear with verse. Against the (?)dear-beast (?)An ending. I destroy. (?)An ending. (?to the) (?)dear-animal. Kill the (?)persistent creature![27]

However, as in several of the remedies seen above, the Old Irish appearing in these charms is most often corrupted to the point of near or total unintelligibility, leaving Pettit's translations highly tentative. It seems unlikely that even an Anglo-Saxon medical practitioner with some knowledge of Irish would have been able to understand the literal meaning of these cures. What is more likely is that, when articulated, these cures would have carried a generally exotic 'Irish sound' to their reciters. Pettit suggests that the reasons for the inclusion of these cures in the *Lacnunga* could possibly stem from a belief in the healthfulness of Ireland; he cites

---

[24] These are entries XXII, XXV, XXVI, LXIII, LXXXIII, CXXXVII, CLIV, CLX, CLXIV, CLXVIII, and CLXXXII. However, entries LXXXVIII and CLXV might be considered borderline cases that come much closer to being comprehensible with only a few illegible or foreign words.

[25] H. Meroney, 'Irish in the Old English Charms', *Speculum* 20 (1945), 172–82; H. Zimmer, 'Keltische Studien, 13. Ein altirischer Zauberspruch aus der Vikingerzeit', *KZ* 33 (1895), 141–53.

[26] *LAC*, vol. I, XXVI.

[27] *LAC*, vol. II, XXVI.

Bede's description of Ireland as a land whose very air drives away snakes, and whose products are useful against poison.[28] However, one would not have to look far for reasons why 'Irish-ish' might have been an appealing sound to an Anglo-Saxon listener, as in the early centuries particularly of the Anglo-Saxon period the Irish were distinguished for their great learning and erudition. It appears that the compiler may have been particularly interested in Irish and Hiberno-Latin material, an interest that will be explored at greater length below.

There is a final category of remedies found within the *Lacnunga* that differs from the standard format of Old English prose. These remedies are not distinguished by language, but by form. These are remedies found written in Old English alliterative verse. There are by my count seven entries in the *Lacnunga* containing discernible Old English verse.[29] This is an exceptionally high number in comparison to the other Old English medical collections. The metrical remedies found in the *Lacnunga* differ from one another substantially in both purpose and form, apparently treating a wide variety of ailments or conditions. These seven entries are easily the most studied texts in the *Lacnunga*. Though clearly different from the remedies discussed above, the fact that these remedies (or, in some cases, parts of the remedies) are written in verse again seems to indicate a level of importance being attached to the form and words in these remedies above and beyond their semantic content. Several examples of this type of remedy will be discussed later in this chapter.

This has only been a very brief survey of the varied and complex contents of this collection. However, even such a brief survey is suggestive that a general preoccupation with words, language, and esoteric knowledge is characteristic of the *Lacnunga* to an extent not found in the other Old English medical collections.

---

[28] Bede, *Bede's Ecclesiastical History of the English People*, ed. B. Colgrave (Oxford, 1969), bk. 1.1, cited in *LAC*, vol. I, XXXI. The use of Irish-influenced material in the *Lacnunga* (as well as to a lesser extent in *Bald's Leechbook* and *Leechbook III*) is noted by Jolly, who traces the veneration of the cross from Irish monastic practices into Anglo-Saxon medical texts and wider practice: Jolly, 'Tapping the Power of the Cross'.

[29] *LAC*, vol. I, entries: LXXVI, LXXXVI, CXXVII, CXLIX, CLXI, CLXII, CLXIII. There is some debate over which remedies in the collection contain verse or simply patterned prose. Additionally, the final three entries listed above have sometimes been classified by editors as a single remedy. Pettit argues for the original independence of the three cures, yet the similarity of theme (childbirth and child rearing) and form has led most commentators to treat them together.

Manuscript Context, Sources, and Analogues

As a compilation of pieces taken from other texts and collections, the *Lacnunga* forms the centre of an intricate web of connections to other texts from Anglo-Saxon England. Pettit, in his edition, offers a list of 27 Anglo-Saxon manuscripts containing sources, variant versions, or analogues to remedies found in Harley 585.[30] This list is more varied than those of the other collections, which contain a higher proportion of clearly medical material. Pettit writes that the predominant dialect of the *Lacnunga* is Late West Saxon, although 'such clusters of linguistic features untypical of LWS – combined with the haphazard ordering and presentation of the text in MS – lend support to the common opinion that the compiler(s)/scribe(s) of the *Lacn.* were working from more than one (and probably many) exemplars, which may well have had distinguishing linguistic features.'[31] This proliferation of relationships can make drawing closer connections, assessing provenance, and dating the compilation more difficult. In such a varied mix of sources, it is easy to over-value the significance of particular analogues. Bearing this in mind, I will nonetheless explore the relationship of the *Lacnunga* to certain texts with the goal of envisioning the type of milieu in which the development of such a collection could take place.

The *Lacnunga* shares a variety of content with contemporary liturgical and ecclesiastical collections, to an extent not seen in the other Old English medical collections. Passages from the *Lacnunga* find analogues in the *Leofric Missal*, the *Gelasian Sacramentary*, and most significantly the tenth-century *Durham Ritual* (in which six remedies of the *Lacnunga* have either analogues or variant versions).[32] Together these works contain a diverse variety of liturgical material, including not only prayers and directives for the mass but also for other rites such as the consecration of a church or exorcism, as well as collects for the divine office.

Some of the most interesting parallels are found in much earlier material, including a set of codices known as the early Insular prayerbooks. Three of these collections have content shared with the *Lacnunga*. These are the *Book of Cerne* (Cambridge, University Library MS L1.1.10), the *Royal Prayerbook* (London, BL, MS Royal 2 A. xx), and the *Book of Nunnaminster* (London, BL, MS Harley 2965).[33] A fourth, fragmentary, collection, the

---

[30] See *LAC*, vol. I, pp. 151–57.
[31] *LAC*, vol. I, p. 201.
[32] For parallels with the *Leofric Missal* or the *Galesian Sacramentary*, see *LAC*, vol. II, LXIII, CLI. For parallels or analogues in the *Durham Ritual*, see *LAC*, vol. II, LXIII, LXIV, CL, CLXXXV, CLXXXVI, CLXXXVIII.
[33] See *LAC*, vol. II: entries LXIV, LXV have direct parallels in the prayerbooks; entries XXIX, LXXXVI, CLIX, CLX have analogous examples or passages. The *Book of Cerne* (Ker no. 28; G&L no. 27) was edited by Kuypers, *The Prayer Book of Aedeluald the Bishop*. The *Royal Prayerbook* (Ker no. 207; G&L no. 450) is also found

Harleian Prayerbook (London, BL, MS Harley 7653), is also generally included in this group of interrelated texts.[34] These codices bring together texts apparently chosen for private devotion, rather than for a public liturgical use. All four date from the late eighth or early ninth century and were likely copied in Western England. Irish influence on these collections is evident, even though there are no extant collections for private prayer dating from early Ireland.

Some of these collections contain remedies or prayers of a medical nature; the *Royal Prayerbook* in particular contains several entries related to blood staunching, a fact that has led some to speculate that it may have been a physician's book.[35] Patrick Sims-Williams suggests that the *Royal* and *Harleian Prayerbooks* are especially preoccupied with 'the theme of protection against illness, death, and supernatural adversity'.[36] There are clear links between these early collections and the *Lacnunga*, first through actual overlaps in content, and secondly through general preoccupations with physical and spiritual health. These similarities can also be seen in the fact that the two biblical passages to be written on the paten in the recipe for a holy drink given above are both found in the gospel extracts found at the beginning of the *Royal Prayerbook*, extracts that overall appear to highlight Christ's role as a miracle worker and healer. The emphasis in the *Lacnunga* is generally on physical healing, but in some cases this shares a permeable border with spiritual afflictions, as can be apparently seen in remedies *wið eallum feondes constungum* ('for all temptations of the Enemy'), for instance.[37] Similarly, although spiritual salvation and health are what is emphasised in the prayerbooks, their compilers apparently did not find occasional remedies for ailments such as eye problems or formulas for staunching bleeding out of place.

---

in Kuypers' edition. The *Book of Nunnaminster* (Ker no. 237; G&L no. 432) was edited by W. Birch, *An Ancient Manuscript of the Eighth or Ninth Century; Formerly belonging to St. Mary's Abbey, or Nunnaminster, Winchester* (London, 1889).

[34] The *Harleian Prayerbook* (Ker no. 245; G&L no. 443) was edited by F. E. Warren, *The Antiphonary of Bangor: An Early Irish Manuscript in the Ambrosian Library at Milan* (London 1893–95), appendix. For more information on this group of texts, see P. Sims-Williams, *Religion and Literature in Western England, 600–800* (Cambridge, 1990), pp. 275–76, 279–82.

[35] M. Brown, *The Book of Cerne: Prayer, Patronage and Power in Ninth-Century England* (London, 1996), p. 152; M. Brown, 'Female Book-Ownership and Production in Anglo-Saxon England: the Evidence of the Ninth-century Prayerbooks', in *Lexis and Texts in Early English: Papers in Honour of Jane Roberts* (Amsterdam, 2001), pp. 45–68, at 57. Brown suggests that the collection may have belonged to a female physician.

[36] Sims-Williams, *Religion and Literature*, p. 285. See also J. Morrish, 'Dated and Datable Manuscripts Copied in England During the Ninth Century: A Preliminary List', *Medieval Studies* 50 (1988), 512–38, at 519–21.

[37] *LAC*, vol. I, XXIX.

A different manuscript containing a variety of shared content with the *Lacnunga* is MS Cambridge Corpus Christi College 41. This manuscript is most famous for containing a copy of the Old English version of Bede's *Ecclesiastical History*. However, it has also long been of interest to scholars for a collection of entries in its wide, ruled margins. Almost all of these entries appear to have been written by a single scribe, but one distinct from the two scribes responsible for copying the Old English *Bede*. It has been proposed that the margins in the manuscript functioned as a sort of archive for storing and organising texts.[38] The contents of this marginal archive are varied but not unrelated, with entries being written both in Old English and in Latin. Grant describes the Old English contents as being: six charms, selections from a martyrology, a portion of the *Solomon and Saturn*, six homilies, rubrics for Latin masses and for Latin charms, the *Metrical Epilogue* to the *Ecclesiastical History*, and the record in Old English of the gift to Exeter. In Latin there is also a version of the record of the gift to Exeter as well as five charms, church offices, and rubrics for two of the Old English homilies.[39] In his *Catalogue*, Ker dates these marginal additions to the first half or middle of the eleventh century.[40] This dating is similar to the proposed dating of the *Lacnunga*, although potentially slightly later, and the content of these marginal additions bears a similarity to some portions of the *Lacnunga*, particularly the classes of remedies mentioned above. The relationship between these two texts has never been thoroughly explored, yet there are multiple points of comparison between CCCC 41 and Harley 585 with regard to both the general characteristics shared between the two manuscripts and in individual entries and sources.

The marginal additions of CCCC 41 and Harley 585 both represent eclectic collections of various types of texts. Of course, the *Lacnunga* is, first and foremost, a medical collection. Nearly all of its 200 entries relate in some way to either spiritual or physical health. However, as we have seen, the form taken by its entries ranges widely, from simple herbal remedies to long metrical incantations in Old English, to Latin prayers, to extracts from liturgical rites, to passages in Old Irish. The compiler of CCCC 41 also apparently had no qualms about collecting seemingly incongruous pieces: storing prayers, incantations, homilies, and liturgical rubrics all in one place; placing Latin texts side by side with vernacular.[41]

---

[38] See S. Keefer, 'Margin as Archive: The Liturgical Marginalia of a Manuscript of the Old English Bede', *Traditio* 51 (1996), 147–77, at 148–49.

[39] R. Grant, *Cambridge, Corpus Christi College 41: The Loricas and the Missal* (Amsterdam, 1979), p. 2.

[40] Ker no. 32.

[41] K. Jolly, 'On the Margins of Orthodoxy: Devotional Formulas and Protective Prayers in Cambridge, Corpus Christi College 41', in *Signs on the Edge: Space,*

Indeed, the aims of the two collections may not be as distant as they appear at first glance. Grant proposed that the liturgical material found in the margins of CCCC 41 was perhaps copied from an otherwise no-longer extant Anglo-Saxon missal. This theory, however, has been rejected by Keefer and Jolly, both of whom consider the liturgical material to be derived from a variety of texts.[42] Jolly argues that the wide variety of apparently disparate types of texts in the collection is instead motivated by the broader theme of protection and protective texts:

> Viewing the Latin and Old English formulas together regardless of their liturgical pedigree reveals that the protection theme is central not only in placement but in the way it connects the earlier liturgical and later homiletic strands. Inter-related elements of protection from spiritual forces visible in CCCC 41's marginalia include the Pater Noster, the cross, the Resurrection and Last Judgment, and angelic beings.[43]

A similar perspective is shared by Richard Johnson, who examines the protective presence of angels in several of the marginal texts.[44] This focus on spiritual and physical protection in these entries is markedly similar to the early Insular prayerbooks and, most importantly for this study, to the *Lacnunga*. I would suggest that the early Insular prayerbooks, and very likely no-longer extant collections of a similar nature, represent an earlier generation of texts that provided a share of the source material used in the compilation of the *Lacnunga* and in the marginalia found in CCCC 41, and that the latter collection thus provides a useful point of comparison for the medical text.

The Lacnunga *and CCCC 41:* Variant Versions

Grant describes CCCC 41 as having 11 charms, six in Old English (three of which have some Latin passages) and five in Latin.[45] The Old English entries relate to varying topics including eye ache, protection against theft of one's possessions, theft of bees, and protection on a journey. The Latin formulas deal with a variety of medical conditions including eye and ear pain, stomach sickness, and one that is against the cruelty of all enemies (*wið ealra feonda grimnessum*); finally there is an incantation for giving birth

---

Text and Margins in Medieval Manuscripts, ed. S. L. Keefer and R. H. Bremmer (Leuven, 2007), pp. 135–83, at 145–46.

[42] Grant, *The Loricas and the Missal*, p. 28; Keefer, 'Margin as Archive', p. 148; Jolly, 'On the Margins of Orthodoxy', pp. 142–43.

[43] Jolly, 'On the Margins of Orthodoxy', p. 145.

[44] R. Johnson, 'Archangel in the Margins: St. Michael in the Homilies of Cambridge, Corpus Christi College 41', *Traditio* 53 (1998), 63–91, at 67–69.

[45] Grant, *The Loricas and the Missal*, p. 2.

that includes the 'sator' formula.[46] Many of these remedies are comparable to types of passages found in the *Lacnunga* or in the Old English medical corpus more broadly. However, three in particular are of interest to this study because they have variant versions in the *Lacnunga*. In my discussion below I will be referring only to the most pertinent parts of these passages, but their full text is listed alongside the relevant entries from the *Lacnunga* as an appendix (1-B).

Lacnunga entry CXLIX addresses a situation in which one's cattle have been stolen. The remedy contains both a metrical and prose component in Old English.

> Þonne þe mon ærest secge þæt þin ceap sy losod, þonne cweð þu ærest ær þu elles hwæt cweþe:
>
> 'Bæðleem hatte seo buruh þe Crist on acænned wæs.
> Seo is gemærsad geond ealne middangeard;
> Swa þyos dæd for monnum mære gewurþe,
>   Þurh þa haligan Cristes rode. Amen.'
>
> Gibide þe þonne þriwa east ond cweþ þonne þriwa: 'Crux Cristi ab oriente reducað'; gebide þe þonne þriwa west ond cweð þonne þriwa: 'Crux Cristi ab occidente reducat'; gebide þe þonne þriwa suð ond cweþ þriwa: 'Crux Cristi ab austro reducat'; gebide þonne þriwa norð ond cweð / þriwa: 'Crux Cristi ab aquilone reducað; Crux Cristi abscondita est et inuenta est; Iudeas Crist ahengon, dydon dæda þa wyrrestan, hælon þæt hy forhelan ne mihtan; swa þeos dæd nænige þinga f[o]rholen ne wurþe, þurh þa haligan Cristes rode. Amen.'

> [As soon as someone tells you that your cattle are lost, then before you say anything else say: 'The city is called Bethlehem in which Christ was born. It is glorified throughout the whole world; so may this deed become notorious in the sight of men, through the holy Cross of Christ. Amen'.
>
> Pray then thrice eastwards and then say thrice: 'May the Cross of Christ bring (them) back from the east'; pray then thrice westwards and then say thrice: 'May the Cross of Christ bring (them) back from the west'; pray then thrice southwards and say thrice: 'May the Cross of Christ bring (them) back from the south'; pray then thrice northwards and say thrice: 'May the Cross of Christ bring (them) back from the north; the Cross of Christ was lost and is found; the Jews hung Christ, did the worst of deeds, hid that which they could not fully conceal; so may this deed not be concealed by any means, through the holy Cross of Christ. Amen.']

---

[46] The 'sator' formula is an ancient palindromic square reading 'sator arepo tenet opera rotas'. The origins of the formula are unknown, but it dates back at least to Pompeii as several versions are found inscribed there on walls (see also p. 123).

This was apparently a popular remedy in Anglo-Saxon England, appearing in various forms in several manuscripts.[47] However, the closest parallel to the version found in Harley 585 is one occurring in the margins of CCCC 41. I have listed both entries side by side in an appendix (1-B), along with the other variant versions discussed in this section.

In his analysis of the different versions of the cattle theft charm, Grant proposes a rough stemma; the closest connection he finds is between the version found in the *Lacnunga* and that found in CCCC 41, which he suggests were copied from 'a common exemplar or a close copy of it'.[48] However, it seems unlikely that the variations between the metrical components of the two charms reflect differences arising in written transmission. This can be seen in a comparison of the metrical sections of the charms:

Harley 585:
Bæðleem hatte seo buruh þe Crist on acænned wæs.
Seo is gemærsad geond ealne middangeard;
Swa þyos dæd for monnum mære gewurþe,
Þurh þa haligan Cristes rode. Amen.[49]

[The city is called Bethlehem in which Christ was born.
It is glorified throughout the whole world;
So may this deed become notorious in the sight of men,
Through the holy Cross of Christ. Amen.]

CCCC 41:
Bathlem hattæ seo burh ðe Crist on geboren wes.
Seo is gemærsod ofer ealne middangeard;
Swa ðeos dæd wyrþe for mannum mære,
per crucem Cristi.

[The city is called Bethlehem where Christ was born.
She is celebrated throughout the whole earth;
As this deed may become notorious among men,
Through the cross of Christ.]

As Dendle also notes, some of the differences between these two poems can be considered 'substantive variants' and cannot be explained by scribal corruption.[50] The most notable example is in the first line, where

---

[47] Aside from MSS Harley 585 and CCCC 41, versions occur in CCCC 190, CCCC 383, BL MS Cotton Tiberius A. iii, and Textus Roffensis. See Grant, *The Loricas and the Missal*, p. 7.
[48] Grant, *The Loricas and the Missal*, pp. 8–9.
[49] For citations and the entire text, see the appendix. Translations from CCCC 41 are my own; translations from the *Lacnunga* are Pettit's.
[50] P. Dendle, 'Textual Transmission of the Old English "Loss of Cattle" Charm', *JEGP* 105 (2006), pp. 514–39, at 519–21. For a discussion of the term 'substantive

the Corpus example uses the word *geboren* ('born') to form an AABA alliterative pattern, and the Harley version employs the word *acænned* ('born'), resulting in an AABB alliterative pattern. These two lines relate the same semantic content, but to very different metrical effect. Similar deviations can be seen in the third lines, which also convey the same meaning but with different alliterative patterns. These differences suggest that the two charms reflect the same living tradition, rather than necessarily a shared exemplar as Grant proposed. This is suggestive about the relationship between the two collections and perhaps indicates that they were copied in geographic proximity to one another.

However, discussion of the two charms is confused further by another remedy immediately following in the Corpus manuscript. This second remedy, also apparently against the theft of cattle, has an introduction in Old English followed by a longer passage in Latin. The last few lines of the Latin formula provide a striking parallel to the final lines of the Old English theft charms, which read in the Corpus version (and very similarly in the *Lacnunga*): *Iudeas Crist ahengon, gedidon him dæda þa wyrstan, hælon þæt hi forhelan ne mihton; swa næfre ðeos dæd forholen ne wyrðe; per crucem Cristi* ('the Jews hanged Christ, they did to him the worst of deeds, they concealed what they could not conceal, so may this deed never be concealed at all, through the cross of Christ'). The Latin text following in the Corpus manuscript reads by comparison: *Iudei Christum crucifixerunt pessimum sibimet ipsum perpetrauerunt. Opus celauerunt quod non potuerunt celare; sic nec hoc furtum celatum nec celare possit. Per dominum nostrum* ('the Jews crucified Christ, they performed for themselves the worst thing itself, they concealed the deed which they could not conceal; so may this theft not be concealed, nor may he be able to conceal it. Through our Lord.').[51] The correspondences between these passages appear too close for mere coincidence, and Grant has suggested these lines likely represent the original Latin source for part of the Old English formula found earlier in CCCC 41 and also that in the *Lacnunga*. While these passages do not appear to be directly copied from one another and show evidence of oral variation, the existence of this Latin source passage suggests some type of written connection between these pieces as well.

The Latin passage containing these lines begins after the instruction in Old English *sing ærest uprihte hit* ('first, sing standing erect'): *ond Petur, Pol, Patric, Pilip, Marie, Brigit, Felic, in nomine dei, ond Chiric. Qui queri inuenit* ('and Peter, Paul, Patrick, Philip, Mary, Brigit, Felix, in the name of God and the Church. Who seeks finds'). After this follow the final three stanzas of the *Hymnus S. Secundini in Laudem S. Patricii*, an Irish hymn in praise of

---

variants', see K. O'Brien O'Keeffe, *Visible Songs: Transitional Literacy in Old English Verse* (Cambridge, 1990), p. 66.

[51] 'Grant, *The Loricas and the Missal*, p. 6.

St Patrick. This poem is found recorded in full only in the eleventh-century Irish *Liber Hymnorum*.[52] As Stephanie Hollis has suggested, it is strange that a statement meant to be read aloud begins with the word 'and' as though completing a list. She has argued that the occurrence of the hymn lines within the charm resulted from an error in the recording process in which pages of the exemplar being copied were erroneously flipped.[53] She suggests that part of the passage *ond Petur, Pol, Patric, Pilip, Marie, Brigit, Felic, in nomine dei, ond Chiric. Qui queri inuenit* is actually meant to be the end of the formula, but was miscopied because the exemplar which the scribe was using had a reversed page. The final verses to the hymn of St Patrick were then listed following the end of the formula, with the middle section of the formula on the following page. This sequence of events or something similar seems likely. It is probable that the hymn was never intended to be part of this theft charm; it seems, however, very likely that all three entries were copied from the same exemplar text. As Jolly notes, the theft formulas and the hymn are set apart by blank pages from other marginal contents, presumably indicating that they were copied from a single exemplar.[54] These pieces may well have come from a selection of broadly devotional material, similar to some of the items found in the Insular prayerbooks. The invocation of the Irish saints Patrick and Bridget in the second cattle theft charm also indicates Irish origin or influence, a common theme in both the Corpus manuscript and the *Lacnunga*.

Immediately following the formula against theft found in the *Lacnunga* is another remedy paralleled in CCCC 41. Both remedies are for eye problems and recount the apocryphal story of Tobit, who was miraculously cured of his blindness by fish gall. As in the case of theft formulas, the relationship between these two prayers appears to be very close. The main difference between the passages seems to be the result of an eye-skip on the part of CCCC 41's scribe, who jumped from *cecorum* to *caecorum*, omitting Harley 585 *Domine tu es oculos* ('Lord you are the eyes').[55]

The final remedy from the *Lacnunga* that is paralleled in CCCC 41 is a Latin prayer forming part of entry LXIII, a recipe for making a *haligre sealfe* ('holy salve'). The instructions for making this salve are complex, calling for a long list of ingredients and many passages to be recited. Following the instructions for physically crafting the salve are several extended passages and prayers in Latin including the passage paralleled in CCCC 41, which begins with *cedita a capite*. The beginning of this text

---

[52] Grant, *The Loricas and the Missal*, pp. 9–10.
[53] S. Hollis, 'Old English "Cattle-Theft Charms": Manuscript Contexts and Social Uses', *Anglia* 115 (1997), 137–64, at 147–49.
[54] Jolly, 'On the Margins of Orthodoxy', p. 154.
[55] It is possible that the scribe skipped even more text if, as Pettit believes, additional text is missing from the Harley 585 version following *quos*, see *LAC*, vol. II, CL.

is closely connected with the exorcism discussed in Chapter 2, occurring in both the remedy for *ælf-sogoþa* and the *Leofric Missal*.[56] As mentioned in my discussion in that chapter, it is likely that the original formula behind these variants was of Irish origin (something indicated by its manuscript tradition). This sort of extended enumeration of body parts has also been more generally associated with Irish tradition.[57] The two versions of this formula are not as close as in the previous examples examined in this chapter, with many more variants existing between the two manuscript copies, suggesting several degrees of removal between the exemplars for the two entries. The remedy reinforces, however, the probability that both compilers had a variety of Hiberno-Latin (or otherwise Irish-influenced) material on hand.

A final point of comparison between these two collections is that both are unusual for containing long metrical formulas in Old English. As mentioned above, seven entries in the *Lacnunga* contain discernible Old English verse. Some of these entries only contain a few lines of verse; for instance, the first theft formula seen above is partially in verse. However, some entries provide examples of the longer metrical compositions possible in Old English medicine, with the longest and also most studied being the 'Nine Herbs Charm' and *Wið færstice*.

The 'Nine Herbs Charm' is a metrical piece to be sung in the preparation of a herbal salve. It devotes most of its length to extolling the virtues of different herbs and is followed by a prose remedy that details how these herbs can be used to make a salve.[58] The text appears to aspire to a stanziac form, with the purpose of the remedy to be found in a line quoted (with slight variation) at the end of the first three stanzas: *þu miht wiþ attre ond wið onflyge,/ þu miht wiþ þa[m] laþan ðe geond lond færð* ('you have power against poison and against flying disease,/ You have power against the loathsome one that travels throughout the land').[59] This sentiment is also repeated later in the poem: *Nu magon þas VIIII wyrta wið nygon wuldorgeflogenum/ wið VIIII attrum ond wið nygon onflognum* ('now these nine plants have power against nine (?)fugitives from glory,/ against nine poisons

---

[56] See Chapter 2, pp. 86–92.
[57] C. Wright, *The Irish Tradition in Old English Literature* (Cambridge, 1993), p. 263; A. Frantzen, *The Literature of Penance in Anglo-Saxon England* (New Brunswick, 1983), pp. 86–88; *Hisperica Famina II: Related Poems*, ed. and trans. M. W. Herren (Toronto, 1987), p. 25.
[58] *LAC*, vol. I, LXXVI. The poem itself declares that there should be nine herbs, but scholars differ over exactly what those nine herbs are. The situation is slightly complicated by the fact that several of the herbs have a second name in the poem. Additionally, there is a crab-apple which may or may not have been intended to count as one of the herbs. For a detailed discussion of this question, see Pettit's commentary in *LAC*, vol. II, LXXVI.
[59] *LAC*, LXXVI, ll. 4–5, 12–13, 18–19.

and against nine flying diseases').[60] *Onflyge* probably indicates some type of flying contagion, but the 'nine fugitives from glory' and the 'loathsome one' who roams across the land are harder to identify. Some light might be cast on this second peril by a formula found in the margins of CCCC 41.

Significantly, the 'Journey Charm' provides the only close analogue for the 'loathsome one' of the 'Nine Herbs Charm'. This long composition, also in Old English metre, is found in the margins of pages 350–53 of CCCC 41. The formula was apparently intended to grant protection on a journey or undertaking. The first lines of this formula bear some resemblance to the 'Nine Herbs Charm', in particular lines 2–5:

wið þane sara stice, wið þane sara slege,
wið þane grymma gryre,
wið ðane micela egsa þe bið eghwam lað,
and wið eal þæt lað þe in to land fare.[61]

[Against the painful stitch, against the painful blow,
 against the cruel horror,
Against the great dread that is loathsome to all.
And against all that loathsomeness which may enter the land.]

The final line quoted provides an almost direct parallel to the 'Nine Herbs Charm': *miht wiþ þa[m] laþan ðe geond lond færð*. Additionally, the clustering of various dangers, each preceded by *wið*, is evocative of the *Lacnunga's* text. In both cases, the threats addressed are obscure or very general. In the 'Journey Charm' it is difficult to know if the 'gruesome horror' and the 'frightful terror' are supposed to be identified with the 'loathsomeness' or if they represent different perils.

A separate metrical remedy, also from the *Lacnunga*, possibly provides another parallel for these loathsome travellers. Although the word *laþan* ('loathsome' or 'impure') is not used, the formula beginning *Wið færstice* and sometimes called 'For Sudden Stabbing Pain' also describes enemies travelling across the land. The remedy begins: *hlude wæran hy, la hlude, ða hy ofer þone hlæw ridan,/ wæran anmode ða hy ofer land ridan* ('loud were they, lo, loud, when they rode over the mound,/ they were fierce when they rode over the land').[62] It is tempting to imagine these riders as embodying a similar Anglo-Saxon belief to the 'loathsome one' in the 'Nine Herbs Charm' and the 'Journey Charm' but it is difficult to be sure. There may be a point of contrast between the shadowy horrors present in the 'Journey Charm' and the loud named figures of the elves, *ese*, and *hægtessan* of *Wið færstice*. The latter remedy appears to be directed towards either real or

---

[60] *LAC*, vol. I, LXXVI, ll. 45–46.
[61] 'A Journey Charm', *ASPR*, vol. VI, p. 126.
[62] *LAC*, CXXVII [b].

symbolic projectiles being hurled by this variety of hostile forces, although it is unclear which (if any) of these figures ought to be identified with the loathsome traveller(s).[63]

Together the 'Nine Herbs Charm', the 'Journey Charm', and *Wið færstice* represent three of the longest metrical charms from Anglo-Saxon England. Only four extant metrical charms exceed 25 lines – the fourth is the *æcerbot* formula, or 'Field Remedy', which is found in BL MS Cotton Caligula A. vii. The three described above are each distinctive pieces. In particular, the use of Christian imagery, including the names of the evangelists and Old Testament figures, is much more pronounced in the 'Journey Charm', although these elements can be seen elsewhere in remedies from the *Lacnunga*. Nevertheless, it is interesting to see the presence of this same unidentified menace ('the loathsome one') in Harley 585 as well as CCCC 41. It is possible that they arose out of a similar cultural milieu which was particularly troubled by these concerns. If not, the presence of these three unusually long metrical formulas in the two manuscripts suggests at the very least that this type of vernacular composition was available to compilers of each collection.

I would argue that the compilers of the *Lacnunga* and the marginalia of Cambridge Corpus Christi College 41 had strikingly similar source material on hand. Parallels in the Old English compositions, between the 'Journey Charm' and the 'Nine Herbs Charm' as well as in the two theft charms, may even suggest the two works were compiled at some geographic proximity to each other. More generally, I would suggest that these two compilations reflect similar underlying interests. Although the texts differ significantly, primarily in the *Lacnunga*'s clearly medical intention and in CCCC 41's much greater proportion of liturgical and homiletic material, they both appear to reflect a broader preoccupation with divine protection for spirit and body. Both collections continuously mix Latin and the vernacular, liturgical material and charm-like formulas, and, on an even more fundamental level, I will suggest the selection of material in both collections reflects shared intellectual and literary interests.

Literary Context and Grammatica

In her work on the early Insular prayerbooks, Jennifer Reid has examined their testimony to the idea of the power of words to effect bodily change. This principle is grounded in biblical and Patristic understandings of the

---

[63] Finding modern definitions of these words is difficult. Pettit offers 'gods [or spirits]' for *esa*, a word seemingly etymologically related to the Norse Æsir, and 'witch [or witches]' for *hægtessan*. For a discussion of this second term, see Meaney, 'Women, Witchcraft and Magic in Anglo-Saxon England', pp. 15–18.

efficacy of words and prayer, with a particular emphasis on the idea of Christ as the living word, the word made flesh – a concept coming from the beginning of John's gospel, evoked in the recipe for a holy drink mentioned above.[64] Yet although this theme is traditional, and even fundamental, it is articulated in these texts within the particular context of early Insular conceptions of *grammatica*. In the medieval period, *grammatica* (unlike the modern term 'grammar') was a broad category that extended beyond rules for the proper usage of language and could include methods of reading and approaching texts. Many early Insular authors make use of a hermeneutic of *grammatica*, which Reid defines as one characterised by 'enumeration, definition, and distinction' and the principle of analogy.[65] Vivian Law, in her work on Insular grammatical commentaries, suggests that several characteristics in these texts correspond with traits found in Irish biblical exegesis, including, among other things, an interest in the three holy languages and a tendency to compile word lists.[66] These descriptions, although representative only of general tendencies, can help us to conceptualise some distinctive characteristics of early Insular prose.

This hermeneutic of *grammatica* also extends to the use of individual letters as signifiers. Reid draws attention to the use of the alphabet as a tool used within the entries of the prayerbooks for 'transcending corporeality' by allowing the abstraction of the physical body. The alphabet 'suggest[s] to the poet a world of interconnection, often with spiritual and metaphysical implications'.[67] She gives an example from Byrhtferth's *Computus*, in which the first letters of the cardinal directions in Greek (*Anatole, Didis, Arcton* and *Mesembellos*) form the name ADAM, thereby 'interconnecting the letters of the alphabet with the constitution of man in the elements, and in relation to the unity of the microcosm and the macrocosm in Christ crucified'.[68] This conception of the alphabet might take some inspiration from the description of the role of letters in Isidore's *Etymologiae*:

> Litterae autem sunt indices rerum, signa uerborum, quibus tanta uis est, ut nobis dicta absentium sine uoce loquantur. (Verba enim per oculos non per aures introducunt.) Vsus litterarum repertus propter memoriam rerum. Nam ne obliuione fugiant, litteris alligantur.
>
> [Indeed, letters are tokens of things, the signs of words, and they have so much force that the utterances of those who are absent speak to us

---

[64] Cf. John 1:14; J. Reid, '"Caro Verbum Factum Est": Incarnations of Word in Early English and Celtic Texts', unpublished PhD dissertation (Toronto, 2007), pp. 25–39.
[65] Reid, 'Incarnations of Word', pp. 124, 126.
[66] V. Law, *The Insular Latin Grammarians* (Woodbridge, 1987), pp. 83–85; cf. Reid, 'Incarnations of Word', pp. 123–24.
[67] Reid, 'Incarnations of Word', p. 130; see also Frantzen, *The Literature of Penance*, pp. 85–87.
[68] Reid, 'Incarnation of Word', p. 131.

without a voice (for they present the words through the eyes, not through the ears). The use of letters was invented for the sake for remembering things, which are bound by letters lest they slip away into oblivion.][69]

The *Etymologiae* were known to the Irish at a very early date, and the idea of letters as the signs of words might help us to understand the popularity of acrostic and acronymic features in early Insular prose.[70]

The potential for conveying meaning through an alphabetic scheme appears in several entries from the Insular prayerbooks, but most impressively in the *Royal Prayerbook* where a number of individual prayers were combined to create a long abecedarian piece containing 23 sections.[71] This codex is also noteworthy for its use of Greek, which occurs both as transliterated Latin script and in Greek characters. Several prayers also make use of Hebrew and Aramaic words (particularly names for God). Interest in the alphabet can also be seen in similar poetic forms used in these collections, such as the acrostic, where letters beginning lines or stanzas are used to form words. An example of this can be seen in the dedicatory prayer found in the *Book of Cerne*, which spells the name AEDELVALD EPISCOPUS.[72] Although acrostics, abecedarials, and other grammar-focused poetic tools certainly exist outside Insular tradition, there seems to be a particular emphasis on *grammatica* amongst Hiberno-Latin and early Anglo-Latin authors.

The features found in the remedies examined above and typical of the *Lacnunga* have been previously thought to exhibit superstitious or 'magical' interests on the part of the compiler. However, it is also possible that these remedies demonstrate instead a common belief in the healing power of words alongside an interest in language, letters, and the alphabet consonant with early medieval ideas of *grammatica*, and that these same ideas may have (at least partially) guided the compilation of the marginalia in CCCC 41. Irish influence on the *Lacnunga* and the Corpus manuscript is explicit in many instances, including those remedies demonstrating knowledge of Old Irish or texts of Irish origin, such as the *Lorica of Laidcenn*, yet even some of the less obviously Irish-influenced

---

[69] Text and translation taken from *Etymologies of Isidore of Seville*, ed. and trans. S. Barney et al. (Cambridge, 2006), vol I.iii., p. 39; cf. Anlezark's discussion of this passage in *Old English Dialogues of Solomon and Saturn*, ed. D. Anlezark (Woodbridge, 2009), pp. 29–30. Isidore follows this with a description of the alphabets of the holy languages, beginning with Hebrew (which he believed to be the originator of the Greek and Latin alphabets).

[70] Some Irish texts from the mid- to late seventh century demonstrate knowledge of the *Etymologiae*, and the earliest manuscript fragments of the *Etymologiae* are written in an Irish scribal hand (*Etymologies of Isidore of Seville*, p. 24).

[71] *The Prayer Book of Aedeluald*, ff. 29a–38b; cited in Reid, 'Incarnations of Word', pp. 138–39.

[72] Brown, *The Book of Cerne*, pp. 131–36, 182–84; cf. Reid, 'Incarnations of Word', pp. 148–49. This is presumably the name of the owner of the collection and very possibly refers to bishop Aedeluald of Lichfield, although this remains uncertain.

remedies in these two collections may implicitly reflect an early Insular preoccupation with grammar, words, and letters.

The Insular focus on detail and proclivity to compile lists of words or synonyms can be easily associated with the *lorica* tradition of prayer shared between these collections. This type of prayer is generally considered to be originally an Irish tradition which later spread to England.[73] Godel offers the traditional definition of this genre of prayer:

> [a] litany form of prayer, usually fairly long, in a Latin or Celtic language, in which earnest expressions are used to invoke the protection of the three Divine Persons, the angels and the saints, in times of material or spiritual danger. The dangers are minutely detailed, mentioning various organs of the body for which protection is specifically asked. The petitioner asks God or the saints to shield him as a defensive wall against all hostile attack: hence the name *lorica* ('breastplate').[74]

The most famous example of this type of prayer is St Patrick's Breastplate, a portion of which reads:

Crist do'mm imdegali indíu
[...]
Crist lim, Crist rium,
Crist i'm degaid, Crist innium,
Crist íssum, Crist úasum,
Crist dessum, Crist tuathum[75]

[Be Christ this day my strong protector
[...]
Christ beside me, Christ before me,
Christ behind me, Christ within me,
Christ beneath me, Christ above;
Christ to the right of me, Christ to the left of me]

This same desire to, as it were, cover all of one's bases is also present in the *Lorica of Laidcenn*, a text common to the *Book of Cerne*, the *Book of Nunnaminster*, and the *Lacnunga*. This listing tendency can be seen even in this short except:

---

[73] *Hisperica Famina II*, p. 26. See also the discussion in Franzten, *Literature of Penance*, pp. 84–88.

[74] W. Godel, 'Irish Prayer in the Early Middle Ages', *Milltown Studies* 4 (1979), 60–99, at vol. 5, p. 85. See also T. Hill, 'Invocation of the Trinity and the Tradition of the *Lorica* in Old English Poetry', *Speculum* 56 (1981), 259–67.

[75] *Irish Liber Hymnorum*, ed. J. H. Bernard and R. Atkinson (London, 1898), vol. I, p. 135. Translation by N. D. O'Donoghue, 'St Patrick's Breastplate', in *An Introduction to Celtic Christianity*, ed. J. P. Mackey (Edinburgh, 1989), pp. 45–63, at 48.

Gigram ceph(a)le   cum iäris et conas,
Patham liz(a)nam   sennas atque michinas,
cladum carsum   madianum talias
bathma exugiam   atque binas idumas.

[(Deliver) my skull, head with hair, and eyes
mouth (?), tongue, teeth, and nostrils (?),
neck, breast, side, and limbs,
joints, fat, and two hands.][76]

The detailed enumeration of the parts of the body to be protected follows in the next 12 stanzas. Herren notes that this type of prolonged anatomical listing gives one 'the impression of reading a medical tract rather than a prayer'.[77] Although poetical and devotional, this prayer also has a practical and apotropaic element. Herren suggests that *loricae* may have originally arisen to counter heathen magic or curses. He compares them to enumerative lists found in some early curse tablets.[78] Yet the *Lorica of Laidcenn* acts as a repository not only for members of the body, but for unusual vocabulary more generally. It is considered to be 'Hisperic', that is, belonging to a group of texts related to the seventh-century *Hisperica Famina* and principally characterised by a playful use of obscure and arcane vocabulary. 'Hisperic' texts also display an interest in the sacred languages, and frequently employ words of Greek or Hebraic origin, often giving them Latin inflections. The *Lorica of Laidcenn*, as part of this tradition, exhibits a highly literate interest in words, their form, and their power as tools in a spiritual battle.

In the versions found in both the *Lacnunga* and the *Book of Cerne* the prayer has an Old English gloss, increasing its legibility to a wider audience. However, the glosses found in the *Lacnunga* do not appear to be derived directly from those in the *Book of Cerne*. Herren suggests that the versions of the *lorica* found in the *Book of Cerne* and *Book of Nunnaminster* were both copied from an earlier, probably eighth-century, Mercian exemplar and that the scribe of the *Lacnunga*'s *lorica* appears to have worked simultaneously from that original exemplar as well as the *Book of Nunnaminster*.[79] This provides further evidence for the link between these earlier collections and the material found in the *Lacnunga*.

CCCC 41's marginalia are also sometimes referred to as containing *loricae*. This term has been applied to both the hymn to St Patrick (which forms part of the theft charm) and the 'Journey Charm'.[80] However, in this

---

[76] *Hisperica Famina II*, 'The *Lorica* of Laidcenn', ll. 35–38 (trans. Herren).
[77] *Hisperica Famina II*, p. 25.
[78] *Hisperica Famina II*, pp. 26–31.
[79] *Hisperica Famina II*, p. 9.
[80] Grant, *The Loricas and the Missal*, p. 13; M. Amies, 'The *Journey Charm*: A Lorica for Life's Journey', *Neophilologus* 67 (1983), 448–62; Hill, 'Invocation of the

description the term is generally applied rather liberally to indicate the protective purpose of these texts. Not technically a *lorica*, the 'Hymnus S. Secundini in Laudem S. Patricii', also known as 'Audite omnes amantes', is a long abecedarial hymn in praise of the virtues of St Patrick. The version found in the Corpus manuscript contains the last three stanzas of this hymn (corresponding to X, Y, and Z) followed by the first stanza. Although the inclusion of these stanzas might have resulted from confusion in copying the exemplar, it is perhaps significant that the final stanzas of the hymn were credited with especial power against damnation and plague.[81] This suggests a similar concern with spiritual and bodily health seen in the *Lorica of Laidcenn* and elsewhere in the early prayerbooks.

The inclusion of the hymn within the theft charm indicates some relationship between these two pieces. Even if, as Hollis has argued, the hymn was miscopied out of sequence, then both pieces were travelling together in the same exemplar. This close positioning of charm-texts with Hiberno-Latin prayer is evocative of the position of the *Lorica of Laidcenn* within the *Book of Nunnaminster*. As Brown comments: 'Gospel extracts relating to the Passion were followed by a long cycle of meditative prayers which were apparently unrelated to the preceding or subsequent matter, which, from fol. 37r, consisted of an extraneous group of prayers of Irish origin: a charm against poison, the *Lorica of Laidcenn*; and a prayer to protect the eyes.'[82] It seems to me highly likely that this type of grouping – combining Hiberno-Latin hymns with prayer and charm material –was a source for portions of the *Lacnunga*, as well as for this section of CCCC 41's marginalia. These passages could have been drawn either from no-longer-extant prayerbook(s) related to the *Book of Cerne* group, or from florilegia which, in turn, reproduced their content. Another possibility would be that a collection more narrowly concerned with personal welfare (perhaps similar to the *Lacnunga*) could have been a source for portions of the prayerbooks. There are no examples of this type of collection from such an early date, but this is hardly surprising given the small number of surviving sources and does not rule out such a possibility.

The enumeration of the parts of the body seen in the *Lorica* could also be compared fruitfully to the enumerative exorcism discussed above and found in entry LXIII of the *Lacnunga* and page 272 in CCCC 41. This list of body parts begins when the demon is told to flee *a capillis, a capite, ab oculis, a naribus, a labis, a linguis* ('from the hair, from the head, from the

---

Trinity', pp. 262, 266; Jolly, 'On the Margins of Orthodoxy', p. 158.

[81] Grant, *The Loricas and the Missal*, pp. 12–13. Cf. also Orchard, 'Audite omnes amantes', p. 163; Jolly, 'On the Margins of Orthodoxy', p. 158.

[82] Brown, *The Book of Cerne*, p. 152. The first two of these entries have parallel versions in *LAC* LXIV, and LXV (although the *Book of Nunnaminster* was not the exemplar for either entry). See *LAC*, vol. II, LXIV, LXV, and vol. I, p. 157.

eyes, from the nose, from the lips, from the tongue [...]').[83] The textual enumeration of all of the parts of the body in this entry suggests a similar understanding of the interrelationship between word and body found within the *Lorica*. Both exorcisms share a basic similarity with an enumerative exorcism found in the *Stowe Missal* and the *Antiphonary of Bangor*, which reads:

> Domine sanctae pater omnipotens aeterne deus expelle diabulum et genitililitatem ab homine isto de capite de cappillis de uertice de cerebro de fronte de oculis de auribus de naribus de ore de lingua de sublingua de gutore de faucibus de collo de pectore de corde de corpore toto intus de foris de manibus de pedibus de omnibus membris de compaginibus membrorum eius et de cogitationibus de uerbis de operibus et omnibus conuersationibus hic et futuro per te iesu christus qui regnas.[84]

> [Lord, Holy Father, almighty, eternal God expel this devil and heathendom from this person from the head, from the hair, from the top, from the brain, from the forehead, from the eyes, from the ears, from the nostrils, from the mouth, from the tongue, from the under tongue, from the throat, from the windpipe, from the neck, from the chest, from the heart, from the whole body inside and outside, from the hands, from the feet, from all the members, from the joints of all his members, and from the thoughts, from the words, from the deeds, and from all habits now and in the future through you Jesus Christ who reigns.]

This passage is noteworthy as one of the earliest Insular instances of the thought-word-deed triad, which later became very popular in Irish and Anglo-Saxon sources. Sims-Williams argues that this exorcism is ultimately of Irish origin and draws attention to the fact that the purely physical listing of members of the body is followed by the immaterial concerns of thoughts and words.[85] This same structure is shared by the enumerative passages found in the Corpus manuscript and the *Lacnunga*, where physical parts of the body are followed by more immaterial actions such as speaking and laughing. However, it is in contrast to the treatment of the related exorcism in *Leechbook III*, in which immaterial actions are reduced. This would suggest that the two 'medical' exorcisms, while textually related, are performing differently in each collection. While the exorcism in *Leechbook III* appears to have been knowingly altered to focus on healing purely physical symptoms, the passages in the *Lacnunga* and CCCC 41 appear to link the spiritual and physical body, fundamentally emphasising the power of words and naming to heal afflictions of both types.

---

[83] The entirety of this prayer is given in the appendix to the chapter.
[84] *Antiphonary of Bangor*, fols. 30v–31r.
[85] Sims-Willams, 'Thought, Word, and Deed', pp. 88–89.

Although clearly different in meaning, it is also possible that the long, alliterative lists of herb types found in several remedies of the *Lacnunga* are also indicative of this general repository interest. Sims-Williams has suggested that the Irish drive towards enumeration has its origin in 'mnemonic techniques of the secular learned classes'.[86] If this were the case, herbs (an integral part of medical practice) would have been an excellent candidate for mnemonic attention. An example of one of these long lists is found in remedy XXXI, as part of the recipe *to godra bansealfe* ('for a good bone salve'). This section of the remedy calls for 36 separate herbs, which are listed in a broadly alliterative pattern beginning: *rude,/ rædic ond ampre, uane, feuerfuge, æscðrote, eoforðrote, cilðenige, bete ond betonican, ribbe ond reade hofe* [...] ('rude, radish and *ampre, uane, feuerfuge, æscðrote, eoforþrote,* beet and *betonica, ribbe* and *reade hofe*').[87] Although all this collection of herbs is ostensibly for use in creating a particular salve, one wonders if it may possibly have been drawn from an earlier, possibly oral, general mnemonic list of herbs. The 'Nine Herbs Charm' is another example of a piece with enumerative tendencies, detailing the powers of specific plants.[88]

It seems probable, given the significant evidence of Irish influence on these collections, that early Insular ideas about *grammatica* were also influential on other types of remedies found within the *Lacnunga* and the Corpus manuscript. For instance, the *Lacnunga* remedies which display garbled forms of different languages have been referred to as 'gibberish'[89] and more recently as 'spirit code';[90] yet might these remedies instead demonstrate a distillation of early Insular interest in language and etymology? Certainly, works such as the *Hisperica Famina* or *Lorica of Laidcenn* exhibit an exceptional degree of erudition, something lacking from the texts mentioned above. However, I would suggest that these pieces share an underlying interest in foreign tongues (in particular the *tres linguae sacrae*) and in the foundational belief that words have a spiritual power independent of knowledge of their semantic meaning.[91]

It is equally possible that the use of textual amulets might bear some relation to the popularity of Insular alphabetical traditions. In remedy LXXXI, mentioned above, the letters 'T + p + T + N + ω + T + UI + M +

---

[86] Sims-Williams, 'Thought, Word, and Deed', p. 78.
[87] *LAC*, vol. I, XXXI. For other examples, see *LAC*, vol. I, XIV, XXXI, LXIII; cf. also CLXX which lists 27 different types of seeds.
[88] See also the interesting discussion of this entry in J. Bolotina, 'Medicine and Society in Anglo-Saxon England: The Social and Practical Context of *Bald's Leechbook* and the *Lacnunga*', unpublished PhD dissertation (Cambridge, 2016), pp. 98–100.
[89] Grendon, 'The Anglo-Saxon Charms', pp. 105, 114; Cameron, *Anglo-Saxon Medicine*, p. 149.
[90] Arnovick, *Written Reliquaries*, p. 33.
[91] A similar perspective is advanced in Ciaran Arthur's recent book: *'Charms', Liturgies, and Secret Rites*, Chapter 5.

ωA' are meant to ward off fever. This charm features two of the sacred languages, with important theological concepts being rendered by their first letter, here 't' probably standing in for *trinitas* ('trinity'), and the Greek letters alpha and omega signifying God, the beginning and end of all things.[92] The meaning behind the writing is effectively encrypted, as is not unusual in charms, but could perhaps also be profitably compared to the tradition of concealing words and 'scrambling' strategies promoted by the Insular grammarian Virgilius Maro Grammaticus, who advised authors on how to conceal the meaning of their words from unworthy readers. He gives several reasons why this should be done:

> prima est ut sagacitatem discentium nostrorum in inquirendis atque inveniendis hiis quae obscura sunt approbemus; secunda est propter decorem aedificationemque eloquentiae; tertia ne mystica quaeque, et quae solis gnaris pandi debent, passim ab infimis ac stultis facile repperiantur.[93]

> [First, in order that the shrewdness of our students in inquiring and discovering those obscure things may be established; second, for the purpose of beauty and the cultivation of eloquence; third, lest secret things, which ought only be exposed to the skilful, are easily discovered everywhere by the foolish or lowest [of individuals].]

This same ideal can be seen in other Insular texts such as the commentary tradition of the Irish *Auraicept na néces* (of disputed date), which suggests letters in words should be re-ordered to reflect their alphabetical order, or the thirteenth-century Welsh treatise *Ymborth yr Enaid* which creates acronymic words out of the seven virtues and vices.[94] It possible that the remedy in question may be of Irish origin as the two saints indicated here by the first letters of their names are mentioned earlier in the remedy as Saints Macutus ('Machutus') and Uictorici ('Victoricus(?)'), one (or both?) of which appear to have connections with Ireland.[95]

Another interesting piece of possible relevance to this discussion is the SATOR formula of CCCC 41. This word square was very popular in

---

[92] *LAC*, vol. I & II, LXXXI.
[93] *Epitomi ed epistole: edizione critica*, ed. G. Polara (Gennaio, 1979), A X.1; cited in Reid, 'Incarnation of Word', pp. 139–40.
[94] For further discussion, see Reid, 'Incarnation of Word', pp. 140–41.
[95] St Machutus (also known as Malo) was a bishop in Brittany, probably of Welsh origin, who according to tradition travelled with St Brendan: S. Baring-Gould, *Lives of British Saints: The Saints of Wales and Cornwall and such Irish Saints as Have Dedications in Britain* (London, 1907), pp. 411–34. The identity of St Victoricus is less clear; Pettit suggests that the remedy might refer to a fourth-century French martyr of that name. However, this is also the name given to St Patrick's visionary visitor in the Confessions (*St. Patrick: His Writings and Muirchu's Life*, ed. and trans. A. B. E. Hood (London, 1978), ch. 23).

The Lacnunga *and Insular* Grammatica

the Late Antique and medieval world. It is unlikely that the charm was originally designed with a Christian meaning, yet in medieval practice it was clearly associated with the power of the cross. The letters of the charm can be arranged in several styles, including as a palindrome square and a cross, and rearranged to spell out 'PATER NOSTER A O' twice (with 'A' and 'O' understood to stand in for alpha and omega).[96] In the Corpus manuscript the letters of this charm are printed linearly as part of a longer charm for childbirth. However, it appears that the reader was intended to reconstruct the shape of a cross – a way the charm is popularly rendered – which is indicated by a cross on the left.[97] An example of this type of reconstruction might be:

```
                    P
                    A
      A             T             O
                    E
                    R
P   A   T   E   R   N   O   S   T   E   R
                    O
                    S
      A             T             O
                    E
                    R
```

Although not originally Insular, it is easy to see how this charm might appeal to an audience interested in encryptions, word games, and the protective power of the cross.

Taking into consideration the foreign provenance of the SATOR formula, it must also be remembered that many of the types of charm-texts found in the CCCC 41 and the *Lacnunga* are not unique to these collections

---

[96] The literature on the SATOR square is immense. For a brief discussion and summary, see R. Benefiel, 'Magic Squares, Alphabet Jumbles, Riddles and More: The Culture of Word-Games among the Graffiti of Pompeii' in *The Muse at Play: Riddles and Wordplay in Greek and Latin Poetry*, ed. J. Kwapisz, D. Petrain, M. Szymański (Berlin, 2013), pp. 65–79, at 67–70.

[97] Jolly, 'On the Margins of Orthodoxy', p. 169.

or even to Anglo-Saxon England. Indeed, some of the remedies found in the *Lacnunga* share partial analogues with continental manuscripts. Yet the fact that so many of these types of remedies are collected together in this particular compilation, exceeding that of any other medical collection extant from Anglo-Saxon England, indicates that they were both available and of interest to the compiler(s) of the text. I suggest the enthusiasm in this collection for these types of remedies might best be explained by the influence of early Insular ideas about language and grammar; a theory that is strengthened by the clear evidence of Irish influence upon the collection and its relationship to the early Insular prayerbooks.

The Solomon and Saturn Dialogues

Perhaps the best example from the Corpus manuscript of these intersecting interests in grammar, enumeration, and encryption is the *Solomon and Saturn Dialogues*. Alongside its other marginalia, CCCC 41 contains one of the two extant copies of the poem *Solomon and Saturn I*.[98] This is one of two poetic dialogues and one prose piece known collectively as the *Solomon and Saturn Dialogues*. All three pieces reflect similar themes and either share common authorship or are the work of a close circle.[99] These three texts exhibit highly literate wordplay and an interest in books and the power of words.

There is evidence for the influence of Irish texts and traditions on these dialogues both in individual detail and in choices of style and content.[100] Several passages from the *Solomon and Saturn Dialogues* are paralleled in the *Collectanea Pseudo-Bedeae*. It is uncertain where the *Collectanea* was compiled, but significant Irish influence on the collection is evident. The contents of the *Collectanea* are diverse and include trivia questions, riddles, and prayers. Several of the prayers included are in the abecedarial form, and some portions are shared with the *Book of Cerne*.[101] The *Solomon and Saturn Dialogues* also draw upon Christian apocryphal texts such as the *Visio S. Pauli*, which were probably transmitted to England via Ireland. The use of these Irish materials by the author(s) of the *Dialogues* is discussed by Anlezark in more detail in his edition.[102]

One of the most interesting aspects of the *Solomon and Saturn Dialogues*, however, is in their exploration of the power of books, words, and letters.

---

[98] *Solomon and Saturn*, p. vii. CCCC 41 does not contain the entire dialogue and drops off abruptly after 94 lines; a more-complete version is found in CCCC 422.
[99] See Anlezark's discussion in *Solomon and Saturn*, pp. 41–57.
[100] Some of these parallels are discussed in *Solomon and Saturn*, pp. 15–23, 26–28; Wright, *The Irish Tradition*, pp. 245–52.
[101] M. Lapidge, 'The Origin of the Collectanea', in *Collectanea Pseudo-Bedae*, ed. M. Bayless and M. Lapidge (Dublin, 1998), pp. 1–12, at 3–4, 10–11.
[102] *Solomon and Saturn*, pp. 12–41.

Solomon and Saturn I and the *Solomon and Saturn Pater Noster Prose* are both chiefly concerned with the power of the Pater Noster. The Pater Noster, the prayer given by Christ when his disciples asked him, 'Lord teach us to pray', has been one of the central prayers of Christianity since its beginnings.[103] The prayer was often seen as having a protective dimension and could function as a type of *lorica* that could protect its user from demonic attack. The power of the prayer against demonic attack became an especially prominent motif in Ireland.[104] It was not simply the prayer that was powerful, but its individual parts were sometimes given demon-fighting power, such as in the Old Irish *Geinemain Molling ocus a Bethae* ('Birth and life of St Moling'): *Pater noster ardom-thá. frisna huile eccrotá/ rop lemsa mo pater noster* [...] *Qui in celis, Dé bi. dom snadadh ar urbhaidhí, / ar demnaib co n-ilar. snaidsium sanctificetur* ('*Pater noster* is for me against all horrid(?) things! with me be my paternoster [...] *Qui es in caelis*, O living God, to protect me from bale: from demons with many sins(?) may *sanctificetur* protect me').[105] A similar synecdochical idea can be seen in Solomon's praise of the Pater Noster in *Solomon and Saturn I*:

> Gylden is se godes cwide   gymmum astæned,
> hafað seolofren <leaf>.   Sundor mæg æghwylc
> þurh gæstæs gife   godspellian.[106]

> [Golden is the word of God, decorated with gems, they have silver leaves. Separately each may tell the gospel, through the gift of the spirit.]

Solomon appears to suggest here that each individual utterance of God (in this case the Pater Noster) can convey the whole force of the gospel message. This concept is enhanced later in the poem when the individual letters of the Pater Noster become entities capable of warding off demonic attack. Solomon explains how the letters of the prayer become personified attackers of the *feohtende feond* ('hateful Enemy'):

> prologo prim   ðam is. P. nama;
> hafað guðmaga   gyrde lange,
> gyldene gade,   and þone grymmn feond
> swiðmod sweopeð.   And on swaðe filgið
> .A. ofermægene,   ond hine eac ofslehð
> .T. ***[107]

---

[103] Luke 11:1–4; cf. Mathew 6: 9–13.
[104] *Solomon and Saturn*, pp. 25–26; Wright, *The Irish Tradition*, pp. 240–41.
[105] *The Birth and Life of St. Moling*, ed. W. Stokes (London, 1907), p. 52, cited in *Solomon and Saturn*, p. 26 (trans. Stokes). See also Wright, *The Irish Tradition*, pp. 240–41.
[106] *Solomon and Saturn*, 'Solomon and Saturn I', CCCC 41, ll. 63–65.
[107] *Solomon and Saturn*, 'Solomon and Saturn I', CCCC 41, ll. 89–94.

[The first letter is that named 'P'; the warrior has a long staff with golden pointed head and, stout-hearted, he drives away the grim Enemy. And in the footsteps follows 'A' with overwhelming force, and also 'T' attacks him].

This is where the version found in CCCC 41 is cut off, but the full version continues through all the letters used in the words 'pater noster'. Given the known use of the Hiberno-Latin sources by the dialogue authors, it seems probable that this animated exploration of letters and their power for symbolism is rooted in Insular conceptions of the alphabet like those mentioned earlier in this chapter.

In the full version of this dialogue, found in CCCC 422, runic letters occur alongside the letters of the Pater Noster. The most recent editor of the text has agreed with previous scholarship that the runes were probably not part of the poem as it was originally written.[108] Even if this is the case (which seems likely), the presence of the runes in the poem suggests a milieu interested in the alphabet and alternative alphabet systems. Thomas Birkett has suggested that the designation *gepalmtwigude*, given to the Pater Noster, might refer to its being written in runes.[109] In the dialogue itself, the Latin letters appear to be implied in their descriptions; for instance 'P' is described as carrying a long staff with a golden goad (which he uses to attack the Devil), which appears to have taken inspiration from the letter's shape.[110] In this type of description we can see the author's fascination with the idea of letters not simply as sound or as pieces of a word but as objects in their own right.

Collectively, the inclusion of *Solomon and Saturn I*, the SATOR charm (which has its own relationship to the Pater Noster), the Irish abecedarial hymn to St Patrick, and the Old English 'Journey Charm', as well as other entries in Latin and Old English in the Corpus manuscript, suggest a preoccupation with the alphabet, enumeration, and the power of words for protection on the part of the compiler of the marginalia comparable to that found in the *Lacnunga*.

Situating the Texts

Little is known about the provenance of Harley 585, yet slightly more information is available relating to CCCC 41, which bears a donation notice from bishop Leofric to Exeter Cathedral. This indicates that it belonged to Exeter's library prior to Leofric's death in 1070, but that it was not originally com-

---

[108] *Solomon and Saturn*, pp. 28–29.
[109] T. Birkett, 'Rað Rett Runar: Reading the Runes in Old English and Old Norse Poetry', unpublished PhD dissertation (Oxford, 2011), pp. 141–42.
[110] Jonassen, 'The Pater Noster Letters', p. 1.

posed there. In his description, Ker attributes the main text of the *Bede* to a southern scriptorium in the early eleventh century. The marginal additions were probably added not long after (before mid-century) and thus predate its arrival in Exeter.[111] Two scholars have suggested that the manuscript may have its provenance in or around the monastery at Glastonbury.[112] The strongest case for this has been made by Robert Butler. He points to several reasons for attributing CCCC 41 to Glastonbury. These include the appearance of the Irish saints Patrick and Bridget in the second theft charm: by the tenth century Glastonbury was a cult centre for St Patrick and claimed to have not only his relics but also those of St Bridget (who was supposed to have lived for some time on an island near there).[113] Secondly, he points to a homily for the Feast of the Assumption, the second listed among CCCC 41's marginal homilies, and a feast day of special importance for Glastonbury.[114] Finally, he argues that the two Anglo-Saxon names found in CCCC 41, 'Ælfwine' and 'Ælfwerd', can easily be associated with Glastonbury, the first as either a bishop or monk based at Glastonbury, and the second as the name of two different abbots of the monastery.[115]

Although suggestive, none of these arguments are exceptionally compelling given the miscellaneous nature of the collection. However, it is worth noting that the most recent edition of the *Solomon and Saturn Dialogues* has suggested a Glastonbury origin for the composition of the dialogues.[116] If this is indeed the case, it would bolster the evidence for the Corpus manuscript also being compiled near there, where such texts were written and were presumably also in circulation. If Glastonbury is not after all the locus of the marginalia, it seems probable that it is not far removed. I would suggest that if the *Lacnunga* was compiled in a similar milieu as CCCC 41, then Glastonbury Abbey in the tenth century would provide an example of the type of intellectual climate that could have cultivated such a collection.

The pervasive influence of Irish and Irish-influenced material in both collections must reflect a centre containing a wide variety of such texts. The earliest life of St Dunstan (first a monk and later abbot of the monastery) records that Irish pilgrims would visit Glastonbury, bringing with them

---

[111] R. Butler, 'Glastonbury and the Early History of the Exeter Book', in *Old English Literature in its Manuscript Context*, ed. J. Lionarons (Morgantown, 2004), pp. 173–215, at 212. Butler quotes Grant's description: 'The greatest likelihood is that the additional matter was already in the margins when Leofric obtained the manuscript.'

[112] See C. Hohler, Review of Grant, *Cambridge, Corpus Christi College 41: The Loricas and the Missal*, *MÆ* 49 (1980), 275–78; Butler, 'Glastonbury and the Early History of the Exeter Book', p. 194.

[113] Butler, 'Glastonbury and the Early History of the Exeter Book', p. 213.

[114] Butler, 'Glastonbury and the Early History of the Exeter Book', p. 213.

[115] Butler, 'Glastonbury and the Early History of the Exeter Book', p. 214.

[116] *Solomon and Saturn*, pp. 49–57.

various books.[117] Intriguingly, the *vita* also hints that these books might not have been completely orthodox (or at least, that they might have seemed so to some), for reading them results in Dunstan being expelled from court. Dunstan's accusers charge him with learning *auitae gentilitatis uanissima* [...] *carmina* ('the vain spells of ancestral heathendom') and *histriarum friuoleas coluisse incantationes* ('cultivating the empty incantations of wizards(?)').[118] The author, anonymously known as 'B', vehemently asserts that there is no truth to this claim, yet the fact that this charge resulted in Dunstan's expulsion from court suggests that some at least took it seriously. Indeed, it seems unlikely that B would make up a story of such a damaging accusation being directed against the saint. I would not argue for this account as signifying that there was any truly heterodox material in Glastonbury, and, if there were, it is not at all certain what such a label would imply in this period.[119] Nevertheless, it may suggest that the library at the monastic foundation contained a particularly varied collection of types of texts.

Although a connection directly with Ireland would be an obvious channel for Irish incantations and Hiberno-Latin texts such as those included in the *Lacnunga*, it is also possible that the early Insular influences found in the *Lacnunga* and CCCC 41 could owe a debt to Welsh materials, as Wales was another main inlet by which Hiberno-Latin materials could reach English monasteries.[120] From the period of the conversion, the Church in Ireland and Wales maintained a close relationship. Indeed, distinctively 'Irish' traits are so common in Welsh manuscripts that it is frequently difficult to determine which culture influenced which; certainly intellectual traffic ran in both directions.[121] Once again, Glastonbury, with its location near to the border of South Wales, provides an example of this type of intellectual environment, although other English monastic houses (such as Canterbury) had similar connections.

Irish or Welsh material could have arrived at English monastic houses at any number of points in time across the period. However, given the presumably late dates of composition for both the *Lacnunga* and CCCC 41's marginalia, one might be reminded of the rise in popularity of the 'Hermeneutic style' in England during the tenth century.[122] This style of

---

[117] *The Early Lives of St Dunstan*, ed. M. Winterbottom and M. Lapidge (Oxford, 2012), pp. 18–20.
[118] *The Early Lives of St Dunstan*, p. 20 (text and translation by Winterbottom and Lapidge). An alternative translation of *histriarum* could be 'of jesters'.
[119] For greater discussion of this issue, see Chapter 5.
[120] M. Lapidge, 'Latin Learning in Dark Age Wales: Some Prolegomena', in *Proceedings of the Seventh International Congress of Celtic Studies*, ed. D. E. Ellis, J. Griffith, and M. Jope (Oxford, 1986), pp. 91–101, at 98–99; Wright, *The Irish Tradition*, p. 269.
[121] Lapidge, 'Latin Learning in Dark Age Wales', pp. 89, 102.
[122] Lapidge, 'The Hermeneutic Style in Tenth-Century Anglo-Latin Literature', pp. 73–76. See also Lapidge, 'Schools, Learning and Literature in Tenth-Century

Latin composition is heavily associated with that found in Irish Hisperic texts, although its success in England was mostly through the influence of Aldhelm, who was in turn at least partially influenced by Irish works.[123] Wright points to the popularity of this style during the reign of Athelstan and suggests that the extensive contact between England, Wales, and Brittany at this time would have allowed for the transmission of Hiberno-Latin texts.[124] Although beyond proof at this point, it may well be that the *Lacnunga* could reflect the intellectual climate of this era, and the marginalia of CCCC 41 (possibly dating slightly later) its aftermath. In any case, both collections demonstrate a literate interest in words, letters, and the alphabet that would be fitting in such an environment.

I suggest that it is in this context that we should view the *Lacnunga*. The collection has often been treated by scholars as outside of the 'mainstream', representing in particular the popular or superstitious side of Old English medicine. This can be seen, for instance, in the distinction drawn by Storms, who writes: 'the Leechbook may be characterised as the handbook of the Anglo-Saxon medical man, the Lacnunga may be characterised as the handbook of the Anglo-Saxon medicine man.'[125] However, the tendency to link the collection with popular, illiterate 'magical' practice is, I think, largely mistaken. The distinctive features of this collection, in particular the greater proportion of liturgical material, 'gibberish' foreign language charms, and Latin exorcisms and hymns need not reflect the presence of a superstitious and ill-educated compiler, but instead suggest a learned interest in the power of letters, words, and language consonant with early conceptions of *grammatica*.

England', in his *Anglo-Latin Literature, 900–1066* (London, 1993), pp. 1–48.

[123] D. R. Howlett, 'Aldhelm and Irish Learning', *Archivum Latinitatis Medii Aevi* 52 (1994), 37–75; B. A. E. Yorke 'Aldhelm's Irish and British Connections', in *Aldhelm and Sherborne: Essays to Celebrate the Founding of the Bishopric*, ed. K. Barker and N. Brooks (Oxford, 2010), pp. 164–80. It is worth noting that Aldhelm's style was not modelled on the *Hisperica Famina* although he was familiar with those texts.

[124] Wright, *The Irish Tradition*, p. 269. See also D. Dumville, *Wessex and England: From Alfred to Edgar* (Woodbridge, 1992), pp. 156–59.

[125] Storms, *Anglo-Saxon Magic*, p. 24; Talbot also expressed the view that the *Lacnunga* is 'nonsense' and is 'not typical of the culture of the period': Talbot, *Medicine in Medieval England*, pp. 22–23. For a fuller description of the history of scholarship of the *Lacnunga*, see Pettit, pp. xxxv–xliv.

4

The *Old English Herbarium* and the Monastic Reform

The *Old English Pharmacopeia*, known alternatively as the *Old English Herbarium Complex*, is distinctive among the Old English medical corpus for occurring in multiple manuscript copies. The manuscripts containing the *Pharmacopeia* date from the late tenth to the twelfth century. Most prominent among these is BL MS Cotton Vitellius C. iii, which, although damaged during the Cotton fire, is generally legible and contains beautiful illustrations. This manuscript has been used as the main text for the two published editions of the *Old English Herbarium* (first Cockayne's edition in the 1860s and, more recently, De Vriend's edition for the EETS series). Other copies of this text occur in Bodleian Library MS Hatton 76, whose version of the *Pharmacopeia* is closely related to the Cotton manuscript (although containing empty spaces intended for illustrations), BL MS Harley 585, which contains the oldest version of the text and also the only extant copy of the *Lacnunga*, and BL MS Harley 6258b, which dates from the twelfth century and is the latest extant copy of the text.[1] The fact that we have four separate complete editions of this text clearly testifies to the importance and popularity of this medical compilation in the late Anglo-Saxon period.

This work differs significantly from the other medical collections extant in Old English. The *Lacnunga*, *Bald's Leechbook*, and *Leechbook III* share basic structural similarities; each appears to aspire (to varying degrees) to follow a head-to-toe organisation. Additionally, each of these three collections contains cures drawn from a large variety of different medical texts, ranging from the works of Pliny or Dioscorides to Late Antique medical authors such as Marcellus. As we have seen, all three of these works also share entries apparently drawn from a pool of pre-existing remedies circulating in translated form, some of which are shared between two or more collections. These works can be aptly called 'compilations' as they bring together pertinent information more or less irrespective of source. In this sense, these texts are entirely different in character from the *Old English Pharmacopeia*.

The *Old English Pharmacopeia* is formed of two halves, the *Old English Herbarium* and the *Medicina de Quadrupedibus*, respectively. Transmitted

---

[1] For manuscript descriptions, see De Vriend, pp. xi–xxxviii. See also D'Aronco, 'L'erbario anglosassone', pp. 353–55.

together in all witnesses, these two texts made available in Old English a set of Late Antique medical treatises. These treatises were very popular medical pieces in the Early Middle Ages.[2] They often circulated together as a group in the Latin tradition, but the individual treatises maintained a separate identity. In the hands of Anglo-Saxon translators, however, these various treatises were combined to form two complementary units. In this process these translators effectively created a comprehensive, vernacular pharmacopeia for the late Anglo-Saxon period.

The method of translating entire texts, rather than individual remedies or passages from a work, sets this work in stark contrast to the other medical texts available in Old English. However, it also places the *Old English Herbarium* within a larger tradition of translated texts in Anglo-Saxon England, the majority of which are translations of individual texts. This chapter will highlight the careful and skilful nature of the translations found in this work and explore the most likely milieu for the creation of this text, the Benedictine reform movement of the tenth century. Understanding the *Old English Pharmacopeia* as a work created as part of this wider movement may also help explain the diffusion of this text and ultimately its survival even today in four copies.

The Sources of the Old English Pharmacopeia

The first half of the *Old English Pharmacopeia* is generally referred to as the *Old English Herbarium*, as it is essentially herbal in its focus. This text represents a coherent work formed from three separate Latin treatises. The majority of its content comes from the *Pseudo-Apuleius Herbal*; this herbal is probably of North African origin and was immensely popular in Late Antiquity and the Early Middle Ages. The herbal probably dates from the fourth century and was almost certainly not compiled by its namesake Apuleius, a second-century Roman orator.[3] Each chapter of the herbal is dedicated to a particular herb; following the title, remedies involving the herb are listed as well as general information about the appearance and character of the herb. Typically, there are 130 of these chapters in total. However, from an early point this herbal circulated in an enlarged form together with several additional treatises. This enlarged *Herbarium* enjoyed great popularity in the Early Middle Ages, with as many as 47

---

[2] D'Aronco, 'The Transmission of Medical Knowledge in Anglo-Saxon England', pp. 55–56; L. Voigts, 'The Significance of the Name "Apuleius" to the *Herbarium Apulei*', *Bulletin of the History of Medicine* 52 (1978), 214–27, at 214–15.

[3] Voigts, 'The Significance of the Name "Apuleius" to the *Herbarium Apulei*', p. 217; M. Collins, *Medieval Herbals: The Illustrative Tradition* (London, 2000), pp. 165–66; De Vriend, pp. l, lvii–lviii.

attested manuscript copies or fragments.[4] The Old English manuscripts of this text are translations of the enlarged *Herbarium* and the first to integrate these treatises together into a single work.[5]

The Old English translation of the *Herbarium* begins with a treatise on the herb betony, the *De herba vettonica liber*, which is appended to the beginning of the *Pseudo-Apuleius Herbal*. In its Latin versions this treatise is often attributed to the Roman physician Musa, but the Old English version lacks this attribution and presents the treatise as though it were the first chapter of the *Pseudo-Apuleius Herbal*. This results in the fact that the numbering of the chapters of the *Old English Herbarium* is off by one from most Latin recensions.[6] The actual author is unknown. Following the *Pseudo-Apuleius Herbal*, chapters 133–85 of the *Old English Herbarium* contain remedies taken primarily from Pseudo-Dioscorides's *Liber medicinae ex herbis femininis* and *Curae herbarum*. These texts represent an abridgment and revision of Dioscorides's immense work, *De materia medica*.[7] A few remedies in this section are also of uncertain origin. These chapters follow the same layout as the *Pseudo-Apuleius Herbal*, relating information about additional herbs. These pieces – the *De herba vettonica liber*, the *Pseudo-Apuleius Herbal*, and the remedies taken from *Liber medicinae ex herbis femininis* and *Curae herbarum* – are all presented as a continuous text within the Anglo-Saxon manuscripts. I will use the term *Old English Herbarium* to refer to this enlarged, composite collection, whereas the *Old English Pharmacopeia* will refer to the combination of this with its complement: the *Medicina de Quadrupedibus*.

Medicina de Quadrupedibus ('medicine from quadrupeds') is the appellation given by Cockayne to this second collection of medical material. The *Medicina de Quadrupedibus* consists of three originally distinct pieces: the *Liber de taxone* ('book of the badger'), an untitled treatise on the mulberry, and the *Liber medicinae ex animalibus* ('book of medicines from animals'). However, as is the case in the Old English version of the *Herbarium*, these distinct treatises are presented as one continuous text by their Anglo-Saxon translator. This group of texts began circulating together around the sixth century, with the texts individually dating to either the fourth

---

[4] De Vriend, p. l.
[5] D'Aronco, 'The Transmission of Medical Knowledge in Anglo-Saxon England', pp. 55–66.
[6] See for comparison *Antonii Musae de herba vettonica liber. Pseudoapulei herbarius. Anonymi de taxone liber. Sexti Placiti liber medicinae ex animalibus etc*, ed. E. Howald and H. E. Sigerist, Corpus Medicorum Latinorum, vol. iv (Leipzig, 1927). Henceforth referred to as Howald and Sigerist.
[7] Riddle, 'Pseudo-Dioscorides' *Ex herbis femininis*', p. 43; Bracciotti, 'Osservazioni sulla forma del latino lauer nell'edizione Wellmann di (pseudo-)Dioscoride', p. 46. For more information on Dioscorides and his influence, see the introduction, pp. 15–17.

or fifth century.⁸ The date of compilation for these treatises is later than the date normally ascribed to the Latin *Herbarium* complex; judging by its content, it may well have been compiled as a complementary group of texts. Aside from the anonymous tract on the uses of mulberry, these treatises supplement the herbal knowledge of the previous texts in the *Herbarium* by presenting the healing properties of animal-derived products (hence the title, 'medicine from quadrupeds'). The *Liber de taxone* is a short tract related to the healing properties of the badger, while the *Liber medicinae ex animalibus* mirrors the organisation of the *Herbarium*, with each chapter containing remedies derived from a specific animal listed together. This treatise is traditionally ascribed to Sextus Placitus, although attempts to identify this name with a historical author have been unconvincing. Evidently a translated aggregation of these treatises was seen to form a useful complement to the *Old English Herbarium*.

The texts of the *Old English Pharmacopeia* represent a different approach to their Latin source from the other extant Old English medical collections in that they render entire Latin treatises into Old English. However, although these two texts are similar to each other in this regard, and clearly complementary, they employ different translation techniques and should not be considered the work of a single compiling-translator. One of the chief differences between the two translation styles is that the *Herbarium* tends to take a more idiomatic approach to rendering Latin syntax (for instance rendering a Latin participial construction or ablative absolute with an imperative or subjunctive) whereas the *Medicina de Quadrupedibus* tends more frequently to imitate Latin syntax.⁹ To illustrate this we can consider an example of each text's style. The author of the *Old English Herbarium* translates *ad vulnera recentia. herba verminacia contrita cum butyro vulneri imponitur* ('for recent wounds, the herb *verminacia*, ground with butter, is placed on the wounds') as *wiþ niwe wundela genim þa ylcan wyrte ond cnuca mid buteran ond lege to þære wunde* ('for new wounds, take the same herb and cook with butter and lay [it] to the wound').¹⁰ This is typical of the style of that Anglo-Saxon translator, who often uses (*ge*) *niman* in his or her translations. In contrast, when translating *ad caliginem oculorum leporis fel cum melle mixtum et inunctum* ('for cloudiness of the eyes, the gall of a hare mixed with honey and anointed') the author of the *Medicina de Quadrupedibus* keeps the participle construction, translating as *wið eagena dymnysse haran geallan wið hunig gemencged ond mid gesmyre(d)* ('for dimness of the eyes, gall of a hare mixed with honey and anointed').¹¹ These differences are typical throughout the two collections and indicate

---

⁸ De Vriend, p. lxiv.
⁹ De Vriend, lxxiii–lxxiv; D'Aronco also includes several examples where this distinction is clear: 'L'erbario anglosassone', pp. 334–36.
¹⁰ *OEH*, 4.10 (MS Vo).
¹¹ *MDQ*, 5.7 (MS L).

that they are the work of two separate translators, although it is probable that they were created to be complementary pieces (as neither collection is ever attested to have travelled by itself).

Together these two composite works represent some of the most popular herbal and animal-based knowledge of the Early Middle Ages. The translation of these treatises constituted a major scholarly endeavour. Such a project would have required specialist knowledge and likely multiple exemplar texts. The work resulting from this scholarly and literary venture clearly became an important vernacular resource, as is testified to by its survival in multiple copies.

Dating the Old English Herbarium

As a translation, the *Old English Herbarium* differs significantly from *Bald's Leechbook* and the other medical collections in Old English, as these other works compile various pieces of material, at least some of which had been previously translated. Thus, these collections necessarily display inconsistency in their approach to translating Latin sources and are better thought of as independent compilations than as translations. These texts represent a different type of project from that involved in creating the *Old English Pharmacopeia*. Some portions of these other collections would have likely involved some new translation work, such as certain portions of *Bald's Leechbook*, which form an exception to the general inconsistency seen among the other collections. However, the style of these passages found in *Bald's Leechbook* should be contrasted with that employed in *Herbarium*, as these sections often deal quite freely with their source material, sometimes also combining material from more than one source. This translation style found within certain passages in *Bald's Leechbook* can perhaps be more profitably compared to some of the translations associated with the Alfredian programme, as I suggest in Chapter 1. However, the *Old English Herbarium* makes less sense in this context and likely dates to a later period.

The earliest manuscript containing the *Old English Pharmacopeia* is Harley 585, which is dated to either the late tenth or early eleventh century. The Cotton and Hatton manuscripts containing the collection both date to the eleventh century, and the most recent manuscript (Harley 6358) dates to the twelfth.[12] Scholars agree that the extant manuscripts ultimately relate back to the same exemplar, as they share several errors. Nevertheless, the relationship between the manuscripts is not entirely

---

[12] De Vriend, pp. xi–xxxvii. See also Van Arsdall, *Medieval Herbal Remedies*, pp. 101–05.

clear.[13] The Cotton manuscript (known as V) and the Hatton manuscript (B) have a close relationship: both follow exactly the same layout (although B only has empty spaces for illustrations). Additionally, as D'Aronco has shown, the oldest manuscript Harley 585 (H) is also related to the same illustrated original.[14] However, the question of when and where the text might have been originally translated has been the subject of some debate. De Vriend, in his edition of the *Herbarium*, argues that it was likely translated during the period of the Northumbrian ascendancy in the seventh and eighth centuries. This conclusion is largely due to the presence of what he sees as early Anglian characteristics in the text, especially in the *Medicina de Quadrupedibus*.[15] Such a dating would make sense, he argues, given that 'the study of herb medicine flourished throughout the post-classical and early medieval periods', and he imagines such a project fitting well in a monastic setting where herb gardens could have been cultivated.

More recently Maria D'Aronco has proposed a much later dating for the translation, one after the composition of *Bald's Leechbook*. She posits that the mainstay of De Vriend's argument – the Anglian features of the text – has been overstated. Drawing on Janet Bately's well-known arguments about the sometimes problematic nature of determining early Mercian works, D'Aronco suggests that the Anglian features of the text do not present conclusive evidence, as the features identified by De Vriend as Anglian are in fact very few in comparison to the vast majority of the text, which is written predominantly in a West Saxon dialect.[16] Further, she argues that the analysis of De Vriend (and later by Hofstetter) *non tenga conto della specificità dei testi di argomento medico e li consideri sullo stesso piano del resto della produzione anglosassone* ('does not take into account the specificity of texts on medical topics and considers them on the same level as the rest of the Anglo-Saxon corpus').[17] She suggests that it is not unusual if words considered to be part of the Winchester vocabulary (as defined by Hofstetter) are rare in the collection since these words mostly

---

[13] Two of these errors are identified by De Vriend, pp. xliii–xliv; for the third, see D'Aronco, 'The Transmission of Medical Knowledge in Anglo-Saxon England', p. 40. For more discussion of the relationship of the manuscripts, see Van Arsdall, *Medieval Herbal Remedies*, p. 103; De Vriend, p. x.

[14] H is not illustrated but contains some drawings of little snakes. Although these were previously taken to only be decorative embellishments, D'Aronco has shown that these snakes occur exactly where snake illustrations appear in the illustrated manuscripts: 'The Transmission of Medical Knowledge in Anglo-Saxon England', pp. 42–43.

[15] De Vriend, pp. lxii–lxxiii.

[16] For a detailed discussion of these features, see D'Aronco, 'L'erbario anglosassone', pp. 330–36; see also Bately, 'Old English Prose', p. 109.

[17] D'Aronco, 'L'erbario anglosassone', p. 332.

relate to abstract terms such as friendship or justice, few of which are likely to occur in a medical context.[18]

Moreover, the evidence from the glossaries instead suggests a later date, most likely in the tenth century. As D'Aronco's work on the botanical glosses found in the *Herbarium* demonstrates, the Anglo-Saxon compiler was not creating a vocabulary for his or her text, but using an accepted lexicon, and in instances where the compiler knew no equivalent, the Old English name was simply omitted.[19] In light of this, it is unusual that so few of the plant names found in the *Old English Herbarium* are recorded in the earliest Anglo-Saxon glossaries if the translation was known and used from the eighth century, as De Vriend suggests.[20] Instead, it is not until the eleventh century that we can find glosses of plant names which were left untranslated in the *Old English Herbarium*. This indicates that the lexicon used in the *Herbarium* was still being developed in the time before the tenth century and only began to be superseded in the eleventh. This conclusion is supported by the fact that, although *Bald's Leechbook* contains some remedies from the Herbarium Complex texts, it never relies on the translation given in the *Old English Herbarium* but instead contains independent translations of these remedies.[21] It seems unlikely that a compilation endeavour of the size required for the creation of *Bald's Leechbook* would have overlooked this text, whose popularity is demonstrated by its existence even today in several manuscript copies. These considerations together suggest that, as D'Aronco has argued, the *Old English Herbarium* was very likely translated in the tenth century subsequent to the compilation of *Bald's Leechbook*.

Dating the *Old English Herbarium* to the mid- or late tenth century would place this text in a different context from *Bald's Leechbook*, which is almost certainly an earlier work. I have suggested that *Bald's Leechbook* can be profitably compared to works connected to the translation project associated with King Alfred's court, which aimed to make essential texts available in the vernacular. The method of the compiler of *Bald's Leechbook* of supplementing the existing vernacular remedies with more theoretical material from Late Antique sources makes sense alongside translation projects with an encyclopaedic aim, such as the Old English *Orosius* or *Boethius* where the original Latin source has been heavily supplemented

---

[18] W. Hofstetter, *Winchester and der spätaltenglische Sprachgebrauch: Untersuchungen zur geographischen und zeitlichen Verbreitung Altenglischer Synonyme* (Munich, 1987), pp. 7–18, cited in D'Aronco, 'L'erbario anglosassone', pp. 332–33.

[19] M. A. D'Aronco, 'The Botanical Lexicon of the Old English *Herbarium*', *ASE* 17 (1988), 15–33, at 17–18.

[20] M. A. D'Aronco, 'The Old English Pharmacopoeia: A Proposed Dating for the Translation', *Avista Forum Journal* 13 (2003), 9–18, at 14–15. D'Aronco includes a table with all the herb names from the *Herbarium* and records their presence in each glossary in 'L'erbario anglosassone', pp. 357–66.

[21] D'Aronco, 'The Old English Pharmacopoeia', pp. 12–13.

with outside material. However, the *Old English Herbarium* is a different type of project; it is less a compilation of various pieces than a vernacular rendering of popular Latin medical treatises. The proposed dating of the translation places it in the second half of the tenth century, in what would have surely been a quite different political and scholarly environment from the creation of *Bald's Leechbook*. There is some evidence for suggesting that the special environment needed to foster the scholarly and complex project of translating the *Herbarium* and *Medicina de Quadrupedibus* would have been perhaps best offered by centres heading the Benedictine reform movement in England. D'Aronco has gone so far as to propose that a translation project of the scope and skill of the *Herbarium* would likely have taken place under the purview of Æthelwold, bishop of Winchester from 963–84, a suggestion that will be discussed in more depth at the end of this chapter.

Structuring the Text

The texts of *Old English Pharmacopeia* are formed from what were originally seven separate treatises. In most senses the *Herbarium* and the *Medicina de Quadrupedibus* appear to represent literal translations of their Latin source material, although in distinct styles. My focus in the following analysis is specifically on the first half of the *Pharmacopeia*, the *Old English Herbarium*. As there are four different manuscript copies of the *Old English Herbarium*, naturally there are slight differences from text to text, yet there are few major differences in content, except where one version may occasionally omit a remedy. The exception to this is MS Harley 6258b, the latest manuscript, which drastically reorganises the content to follow an alphabetical pattern. For my own analysis, I follow De Vriend's edition of the text, which is principally based on the Cotton manuscript. In this choice, De Vriend follows Cockayne's earlier edition, as this manuscript contains a complete version of the text in good condition.[22] Bodleian Library MS Hatton 76 also contains a good edition of the text but is missing four folios.

The particular Latin exemplar for the Old English edition of the *Herbarium* and the *Medicina de Quadrupedibus* has been lost and there is no extant Latin manuscript that parallels the English at all points. For this reason, De Vriend used seven different manuscripts to provide parallel texts in his edition. In this edition, however, De Vriend omits any sentences or remedies not paralleled in the Old English, so it is sometimes

---

[22] De Vriend, p. xliv.

necessary to also consult other printed editions of the Latin texts.[23] Even when consulting a variety of Latin manuscript versions, there is always the possibility of variations in the Latin exemplar texts used by our author giving rise to some of the differing versions in Old English. Nonetheless, it is still only by comparing the text of the *Old English Herbarium* with its known sources that the sensitive and careful nature of this translation is revealed.[24]

Because of the length of the *Old English Herbarium*, which contains in total 185 chapters and over 500 individual remedies, it is impossible within the scope of my analysis to highlight every passage of interest. However, I have chosen to discuss those aspects of the translation that seem to be most revealing of the translator's preferences. The chapter for *Clufwyrt*, the tenth herb listed in the *Herbarium*, acts as a useful illustration of a typical passage of this text and demonstrates the skill of its translator. I have included the Latin version for comparison before the Old English passage:

IX. Herba botracion statice.

1. Ad lunaticos. Herba botracion statice si lunatico in collo ligetur lino rubro luna decrescente cum erit signum tauri vel scorpionis parte prima, mox sanabitur.
2. Ad cicatrices nigras. Herba botracion tunsa cum sua radice, mixta cum aceto imponis [his] qui habent cicatrices nigras, eximit eas et similem corpori [reliquo] facit colorem.

Nascitur locis sablosis et campis arenosis. Radix eius verticulo est similis, radiculas paucas et tenuissimas habet.[25]

[IX *Botracion Statice*.

1. For lunatics, if the herb *botracion* is tied to a lunatic's neck with red thread, when the moon is waning, when it is the sign of Taurus or the first part of Scorpio, he will soon be healed.
2. For black scars, you lay the herb *botracion*, pounded with its root, mixed with vinegar, on those who have the black scars. It will take

---

[23] The printed edition of the *Pseudo-Apuleius Herbarium* is printed in the *Corpus Medicorum Latinorum* series and edited by E. Howald and H. E. Sigerist. H. F. Kästner has published the only printed edition of the *De herbis femininis*: 'Pseudo-Dioscorides *De herbis femininis*', *Hermes* 31 (1896), 578–635; 32 (1897), 160. In some circumstances I found the Latin text in either one edition or the other more appropriate to be cited; this choice is always made clear in my footnotes.

[24] An earlier version of the argument outlined below is found in E. Kesling, 'Translation Style and the *Old English Herbarium*', *Notes and Queries* 63 (2016), 9–14.

[25] *OEH*, 10.1–2 (MS Vo.) The Latin text is taken from De Vriend's edition, but has been reordered with reference to Howald and Sigerist to reflect the normal pattern in the Latin tradition.

The Old English Herbarium *and the Monastic Reform*

them away and make them the same colour as [the rest of] the body. It is found in sandy places and sandy fields. Its root is similar to a spindle, having few and thin root hairs.]

X. Clufwyrt

1. Ðeos wyrt þe man batracion ond oþrum naman clufwyrt nemneð bið cenned on sandigum landum ond on feldum, heo bið feawum leafum ond þynnum.
2. Wið monoðseoce genim þas wyrte ond gewrið mid anum readum þræde onbutan þæs monnes swyran on wanwegendum monan on þam monþe ðe man Aprelis nemneð ond on Octobre foreweardum, sona he bið gehæled.

Wiþ ða sweartan dolh genim þas ylcan / wyrte myd hyre wyrtwalan ond gecnuca hy, (m)engc eced þærto, lege to ðam dolchum, sona hyt fornimð hy ond gedeð þam oþrum lice gelice.[26]

[X Clufwort.

This herb which some call *batracion* and is also known as *clufwort* is found in sandy places and in fields. It has few leaves and thin ones.

1. For lunacy (lit. moon-sickness), take this herb and string it with a red thread around the person's neck during a waning moon in the month called April and in the beginning of October. He will be cured at once.
2. For black scars, take this same herb with its root and pound it. Mix this with vinegar and lay it to the scars. Immediately it takes them away and makes them like the rest of the body.]

One of the most easily noticeable changes between the Latin entry for *Batracion Statice* and the Old English entry is that in the Old English the physical description and the information regarding the herb's habitat have been moved from its place at the end of the chapter in the Latin version to the beginning. Linda Voigts comments upon this change elsewhere in the *Old English Herbarium*, emphasising how it could be counted as one of several organisational improvements of the Old English version of this text over its Latin counterparts.[27] Moving this information, found in Latin recensions at the end of the chapter, to the beginning of the Old English text makes this essential information easier to access and recognise. Voigts also mentions the table of contents, which forms a part of all four manuscripts of the Old English text. This table of contents is somewhat simplified from the *tituli morborum* found in some Latin recensions of the text.[28] The *tituli morborum* lists ailments in a head-to-foot order along with

---

[26] *OEH*, 10.1–2 (MS V). Translations from the Old English are my own but made with reference to Arsdall's translations in *Medieval Herbal Remedies*.
[27] Voigts, 'Anglo-Saxon Plant Remedies', p. 2.
[28] Collins, *Medieval Herbals: The Illustrative Traditions*, p. 166.

the numbers of the herbal chapters involving that condition. The table of contents in the Old English edition instead simply names the different herbal chapters with the remedies involving the plant listed following, often with rubricated numerals. This method is straightforward but serviceable to any reader of the text, and the fact that such a table of contents is found in every extant edition of the *Old English Herbarium* testifies to the importance of usability and organisation to both its compiler and later scribal copyists and readers.

Another fairly common change in the English version of the sample passage, and elsewhere in the collection, involves syntactically reordering the Latin source text. As mentioned above, one of the features distinguishing the translation style of the *Old English Herbarium* from the *Medicina de Quadrupedibus* is that the *Herbarium* renders Latin phrases more idiomatically, whereas the *Medicina de Quadrupedibus* more frequently attempts to imitate Latin syntax. Thus, the translator of the *Herbarium* regularly renders Latin non-finite clauses into a more intuitive finite clause in Old English (as can be seen both in the directions for the remedies *ad lunaticos* and *ad cicatrices nigras* given above). However, although the translation is made more idiomatic, the translator normally still follows the ordering of the Latin instructions closely. Consider, for example, the second remedy, for black scars. Here, the Old English instructions follow the Latin step-for-step: take the herb (with its roots) and pound it, mix it with vinegar, lay it on the scars. This example is reflective of a general tendency of the Old English translator to render the Latin, if not word for word, then phrase by phrase into Old English. Major changes to the syntactic structure of a remedy generally only occur in two instances: where the Latin syntax is confusing or unclear, or when explanatory clauses are added in the Old English. The addition of alternative instructions or ingredients also sometimes affects the syntax of the remedy, but this will be dealt with later in this section.

The first type of change, simplifying cumbersome passages, can be seen in the remedy against black scars cited above. The Latin text *inponis qui habent cicatrices nigras* ('you lay [it] on those who have black scars'), while intelligible, is certainly more unwieldy than the Old English *lege to ðam dolchum* ('lay [it] on the scars'). In another example, from Chapter 30, the somewhat cumbersome title of the Latin remedy: *ad vitia quae in ore nascuntur* ('for pains which are found in the mouth') has been rendered more simply by the translator as: *wið muðes sare* ('for sore of the mouth').[29] The second type of change, the addition of explanatory phrases, occurs with some frequency in the *Herbarium*. One example can be found in a remedy given under the herb *æscþrote* (L. *hierabotana*). The beginning of the Latin remedy reads: *ad eos qui induratas venas habent et cibos non recipiunt* ('for

---

[29] *OEH*, 30.1 (MSS Vo and V).

those who have hardened veins and those who do not take food').[30] The Old English, clarifying the perhaps obscure *induratas venas*, renders the sentence as: *wið ða þe habbað ætstandene ædran swa þæt þæt blod ne mæg hys gecyndelican ryne habban ond heora þigne gehealdan ne magon* ('for those that have stopped veins, so that the blood may not have its natural run, and for those who are not able to hold down their food').[31] An example of another similar type of change can be seen in Chapter 13, the second chapter on herbs known in Old English as *mugwyrt*.[32] The Anglo-Saxon translator, no doubt aware of this potential for confusion, expands upon the Latin source text, adding after *genim þyssæ wyrte seaw* ('take the juice of this herb') the phrase *þe man eac mugwyrt nemneð, seo ys swaþeah oþres cynnes* ('which some call *mugwyrt* but is another type').[33] In each of these instances mentioned above, the Old English version has taken potentially confusing sections of the Latin text and clarified them. These changes emphasise the understanding and skill of the translator and result in a vernacular text that is overall more usable and clear than its Latin source text.

A final change in the translation of the entry for *clufwort* occurs in the first remedy where the astrological references are switched for Latin month names. In the first remedy, the Latin text suggests that the remedy should be done *cum erit signum tauri vel scorpionis parte prima* ('when it is the sign of Taurus or the first part of Scorpio'), which is rendered in Old English as *on þam monþe ðe man Aprelis nemneð ond on Octobre foreweardum* ('in the month called April and in the beginning of October'). The translator here changes the astrological signs for the Latin month names, which he or she apparently saw as more comprehensible. However, this change comes at the expense of accuracy, as the months and signs do not directly correspond.

Considering these changes helps frame the overall status of this translation, which promotes clarity and usability but probably should not be called 'nativising'. Although some passages from the Alfredian translations substitute English traditions for classical ones – most famously the substitution of Weland for Fabricius in the *Boethius* – the *Herbarium* translation

---

[30] *OEH*, 4.3 (MS Vo).
[31] *OEH*, 4.3 (MS V). In this example, the translator has also altered symptoms involved. Where the Latin text implies that the patient cannot eat food, the Old English seems to imply that food eaten is vomited up. It is hard to know what might have motivated this more fundamental type of change.
[32] *OEH*, 12.1 (MSS V and Vo).
[33] *OEH*, 12.1 (MS V). This change appears to be a response in part to a mistake made in the copying of the exemplar where Chapter XI *Herba Artemisia Tagantes* of the *Pseudo-Apuleius Herbarium* was combined with Chapter XII *Herba Artemisia Leptofillos*. The need for extra clarity in this situation is logical. For discussion of this error, see *OEH*, 12, explanatory notes; D'Aronco, 'The Transmission of Medical Knowledge in Anglo-Saxon England', pp. 40–41. For other examples of these types of changes, see *OEH*, 23.1, 35, 34.1.

clearly asserts itself within the Latin tradition of the text. I would suggest that this can also be seen in the treatment of herb names at the beginning of entries. Generally in the Latin tradition of the *Herbarium* the name of each herb is given not only in Latin but also in Greek, Mediterranean vernaculars, or in other tongues, perhaps with the intention that the usability of the text could transcend the language and culture of its author. The Old English version typically simplifies these lists, giving the name in Latin (and occasionally the Greek) in addition to the Old English designation but omitting other languages. We can see a (somewhat extreme) example of this process in the entry of the herb *proserpinace*:

> A Graecis dicitur poligonos, alii cinocalce, alii poligonatos, alii aspaltion, alii policarpon, alii carcinetron, alii echinopodion, alii mirtopetalon, Aegyptii zeclias, alii thepin, alii setempin, profetae gonos eroos, alii onix mios, Romani sanguinaria, Itali proserpinaca, alii statunaria, alii serutum, alii scorpinacem.[34]

In the Old English version this is much reduced, reading:

> [[This herb] is called *poligonos* by the Greeks, others [call it] *cinocalce*, others *poligonatos*, others *aspaltion*, others *policarpon*, others *carcinetron*, others *echinopodion*, others *mirtopetalon*, Egyptians [call it] *zeclias*, others *thepin*, others *setempin*, the Magi (?) [call it] *gonos eroos*, others *onix mios*, the Romans *sanguinaria*, the Italians *proserpinaca*, others *statunaria*, others *serutum*, others *scorpinacem*.]

> Ðeos wyrt ðe man proserpinacam ond oðrum naman unfortredde nemneð […].[35]

> [This herb which one calls *proserpinaca* and by another name *unfortredde*].

Although the universality of the text is stressed more strongly in the Latin tradition, the parallelism in the English entry serves to emphasise the equal significance of the English name of the herb with the Latin. This basic structure is common throughout the collection and can also be seen in the description of *clufwyrt* given above: *Ðeos wyrt þe man batracion ond oþrum naman clufwyrt nemneð*. By retaining the Latin herb names alongside the Old English, the translator presents his or her work as part of the wider tradition of the text (we could compare this to the other medical texts where herb names are typically given just in Old English). Rather than subsuming or subverting the continental tradition, the translation of the *Herbarium* (and the project implied in its creation) makes a claim to the

---

[34] Howald and Sigerist, 18; references to remedies in Howald and Sigerist are given by chapter. In the Latin tradition this information is given at the end of the remedy.
[35] *OEH*, 19 (MS V).

The Old English Herbarium: Changes in Content

Among the most common changes to the content of the *Old English Herbarium* are instances where either specifically Mediterranean or overly precise ingredients are replaced with more easily accessible ones. This is of course not to suggest that there are no ingredients sourced from outside England, as several remedies call for the use of pepper, for instance. Commonly known spices and herbs are not replaced in the text even when of exotic origin – only when ingredients are overly specific (or assumedly difficult to locate) are they replaced in the translation.[36] This can be seen, for example, in a remedy whose Latin rendering calls for *amineo vino*. In the Old English version, this highly specific ingredient (*amineo* refers to a particular region in Italy, no longer identifiable) is replaced with *ealdum wine* ('old wine').[37] Another example of this type of change occurs in Chapter 17. The Latin version describes the herb as *nascitur gemellis montibus* ('grow[ing] in the twin hills').[38] Although this original remedy likely refers to a particular pair of mountains located in central Italy, in the Old English the herb is simply described as *bið cenned on dunum* ('found on hills'). In both cases, the translation appears aimed at making these ingredients easier to source for an Anglo-Saxon audience, although of course items like wine would still have been considered extremely expensive.

There is also some simplification (and sometimes inconsistency) in the translator's handling of the various alcoholic beverages used in the source text. Both *mero* ('undiluted wine') and *mulsum* (either meaning 'sweetened wine' or 'mead') are often rendered more simply as *win* in the Old English version.[39] However, *beor* also appears as a translation of *mulsum* in a remedy from the *De herba vettonica liber* (treated as the first chapter in the *Old English Herbarium*).[40] Similarly, *aqua mulsa* ('honey

---

[36] For general discussion of the portrayal of the Mediterranean region in the medical corpus, see D. Banham, 'Arestolobius, the Patriarch of Jerusalem and the bark that comes from Paradise: What did the Orient mean to the compilers of Old English medical collections?', in *Proceedings of the 38th International Congress on the History of Medicine*, ed. N. Sari et al., International Society for the History of Medicine (Ankara, 2005), pp. 459–68.
[37] *OEH*, 1.10 (MS V).
[38] *OEH*, 17 (MSS V and Vo).
[39] *OEH*, 2.7, *OEH*, 4.5 (MSS Vo and V). Cf. 30.5 where *vini meri optimi* ('the best undiluted wine') is translated as *on wine* ('in wine').
[40] *OEH*, 1.27 (MS V). In this instance, what is generally one remedy in the Latin version of the text has become two in the English.

water') in another remedy is also replaced with *niwe beor* ('new *beor*').[41] For the Anglo-Saxons, *beor* seems to have indicated a honey-sweetened fruit-based drink rather than the malt-based drink we now commonly refer to as 'beer', so this would have been more similar to *mulsum* or *aqua mulsa* than the modern equivalent but probably was not exactly the beverage the source text intended.[42] *Ealu* (a malted beverage probably somewhat similar to modern beer) is also added to some remedies in the Old English translation or listed as an alternative to wine.[43] Although these remedies are being handled in different ways, the changes made appear to support practicality – whether through the simplification of overly precise requirements or the replacement of more difficult to locate ingredients with simpler ones.

The Anglo-Saxon translator also appears to have found rose oil (L. *oleum rosacium*) to be an unnecessarily specific ingredient, because most often it is rendered simply as oil (OE *ele*).[44] This does not seem to be the case of an unknown ingredient being switched for a known one, as rose oil (OE *gerosod ele*, or *rosen ele*) appears in a later recipe in the *Herbarium* as well as in two instances in *Bald's Leechbook*, and a recipe for making it is also found in the *Lacnunga*.[45] It seems instead that the translator of the *Herbarium*, although obviously aware of rose oil, thought that another oil would work just as well (and, indeed, getting hold of any oil in Anglo-Saxon England may have been difficult).[46] A similar argument might be made about the wine since *merum* and *mulsum* are both fairly common Latin words with which he or she would likely have been acquainted. In replacing *merum* and *mulsum* with *win* or *beor*, and *oleum rosacium* with *ele*, the translator was making the text more versatile and better fitted for everyday use by employing ingredients that were seen as having the same function as in the Latin instructions but were perhaps easier to obtain in England.

A more significant type of deviation from the source text occurs where the translator omits whole Latin cures. In general, throughout the *Old English Herbarium* this practice is fairly rare; the translation is a close one and the vast majority of cures in the Latin recensions of the *Herbarium* are retained in the Old English version. Yet because of this generally inclusive tendency in the translation, the instances of individual remedies being omitted suggest that in each instance there may be a particular reason for not including a remedy.[47] Sometimes the nature of the cures omitted

---

[41] *OEH*, 2.15 (MSS Vo and V).
[42] For a discussion of the meaning of *beor, ealu, win,* and *medu* in Anglo-Saxon England, see C. Fell, 'Old English *Beor*', *Leeds Studies in English* 8 (1975), 76–95.
[43] *OEH*, 2.15, 36.3 (MSS Vo and V).
[44] See, for instance, *OEH*, 12.5, 13.2, 19.2.
[45] *OEH*, 171.1; *BLB*, II 34, 38; *LAC*, vol. I, XX.
[46] D. Banham, *Food and Drink in Anglo-Saxon England* (Stroud, 2004), p. 60.
[47] Of course, it is always possible that in any given instance the Latin exemplar was at fault. Because of this, I have excluded from my analysis any remedies

appears to indicate the translator's lack of confidence with a given Latin medical term. For instance, the Latin terms for jaundice (*aurigino*) and jaundiced (*auriginosus*) seem to have puzzled the translator. His or her general approach is to skip remedies involving this word and in a remedy where it occurs which is included, it is mistranslated.[48] There might be a similar reason behind the omission of several other cures also containing obscure terminology, such as a cure for dislocation (*ad luxum*) and remedies involving an *encanthisma* ('medicinal bath').[49]

Other types of rationale for omitting certain remedies are also in play. For instance, amongst the remedies omitted by the Anglo-Saxon translator there appears an unusually high proportion of cures related to women. Of 25 remedies omitted out of the first 100 chapters of the *Herbarium*, at least four pertain to specifically feminine complaints.[50] This count far exceeds the normal proportion of remedies specifically related to women in the *Old English Herbarium*, whose first 100 chapters, divided into approximately 350 individual remedies, contain only eight cures specifically related to women. The final chapters of the *Old English Herbarium* are harder to systematically compare to their source text as many of them are taken from the *Curae herbarium*, of which there is no modern edition. Yet when considering those entries from the *Ex herbis femininis*, this tendency becomes even clearer. Chapters 135, 136, 138, and 139, are all missing either whole remedies or particular phrases related to female complaints.[51] The translator, then, appears to have had a proclivity for skipping remedies related to the female sex, although he or she by no means did so in every case.

Several of the skipped entries are remedies related to abnormalities in the menstrual cycle or miscarriage. The appearance of these remedies in the Latin text is not unusual, as a significant portion of medieval gynaecological remedies in the Middle Ages dealt with menstrual disorders, and disruptions in the menstrual cycle were seen to be the cause of a whole variety of illnesses and conditions.[52] Alongside a remedy for miscarriage, the Old English also omits several emmenagogic remedies (an

---

apparently skipped in the Old English but also missing from any popular recension of the Latin text. For this information I have referred to Howald and Sigerist's critical edition of the Latin text.

[48] The remedy is omitted entirely in *OEH*, 1, 4, 75. It is mistranslated in 36.4 where the translator has rendered *ad auriginem* as *wið sina togunge* ('for strained tendons').

[49] Cf. *OEH*, 32, 39 with Howald and Sigerist, 31, 38. The translator of the Old English text also skips a sentence featuring the word *encanthisma* in 41, cf. Howald and Sigerist, 40.

[50] Cf. *OEH*, 16, 82, 94, 39 with Howald and Sigerist, 15, 81, 93, 38.

[51] Cf. *OEH*, 135, 136, 138, 139 with H. F. Kästner, 'Pseudo–Dioscorides *De herbis femininis*', ch. XXXII, LXIV, LXIX, LXX.

[52] M. Green, 'Flowers, Poisons and Men: Menstruation in Medieval Western Europe', in *Menstruation: A Cultural History*, ed. A. Shail and G. Howie (Basingstoke, 2005), pp. 51–75, at 54–57.

emmenagogue is a substance that brings on menstruation).[53] John Riddle has argued that emmenagogues may have been frequently used in the ancient world and Middle Ages as abortifacients.[54] If the translator of the *Herbarium* was of this opinion, this might help explain why some of these types of remedies were omitted. However, more typically emmenagogic remedies would have been used in the Middle Ages to promote fertility in accordance with the belief that menstruation was part of the process of bodily purification necessary for conception.[55] Thus it is possible that the omission of a number of these remedies may simply relate to distaste for sex on the part of the translator, as he has also omitted a remedy for men who are not able to perform sexually and a remedy explicitly aimed at promoting female fertility.[56] Nevertheless, some of the women's remedies omitted lack any sexual element and might simply indicate the influence of a male monastic environment.

This comparison of the *Old English Herbarium* with its Latin source texts has not been exhaustive; many aspects of this skilful work of translation could receive still greater attention. However, even without a comprehensive study, certain aspects regarding the translation seem self-evident. The translator himself or herself was by all appearances very careful with the source text. Unlike some other works of translation into Old English, the *Herbarium* could hardly be considered a 'transformation'. Yet, though the translator tended to follow the Latin exemplars quite closely, he or she was not subservient to them and in some cases appears willing to practise the art of *emendatio* upon the text. Through changes which were often small, such as the substitution of a rare ingredient for one more easily obtainable, but occasionally as significant as the omission of remedies he or she found unhelpful, the Anglo-Saxon translator subtly altered the text to promote the clarity and usability of the text.

These changes reveal the hand of a confident and learned translator. This was clearly not an amateur work but required considerable skill, as well as knowledge of medical terminology in both Latin and Old English. The final result of this translator's work was a text that was reliable and useful – and of a quality to match continental practice. The translated collection must have been valuable enough to its English readers that it

---

[53] These are the remedies omitted from Chapters 84, 135, 136.

[54] For the use of emmenagogues as abortifacients, see J. Riddle, *Contraception and Abortion in the Ancient World to the Renaissance* (London, 1992), p. 27. However, see also M. Green, Review of Riddle, *Eve's Herbs: A History of Contraception and Abortion in the West*, *Bulletin of the History of Medicine* 73 (1999), 308–11.

[55] Green, 'Flowers, Poisons and Men', p. 53. See also *The Trotula: An English Translation of the Medieval Compendium of Women's Medicine*, ed. and trans. M. Green (Philadelphia, 2002), p. 182; M. Green, 'Menstruation', in *Women and Gender in Medieval Europe: An Encyclopedia*, ed. M. Schaus (Abingdon, 2006), pp. 557–58.

[56] Cf. *OEH*, 16, 138 and Howald and Sigerist 15 and Kästner LXIX.

The Old English Herbarium *as a Product of the Benedictine Reform*

As we have seen in this chapter, the translation of the *Herbarium* is a skilful and careful one. Such a translation project would have required not only the availability of the several Latin treatises (perhaps even in multiple copies) but probably also glossaries and other reference texts. As D'Aronco comments: *chi ideò e/o eseguì la traduzione dovette aver a disposizione un notevole numero di testi, e forse anche edizioni differenti appartenenti a tradizioni diverse, almeno per quanto si può dedurre dalle testimonianze che ci sono pervenute* ('whoever conceived of and/or produced the translation must have had at his disposal a notable number of texts, and perhaps even different editions belonging to different [textual] traditions, at least in so far as it is possible to deduce from the testimonies that are preserved').[57] It seems nearly certain that a project of this scale must have been undertaken at a major centre of learning. If this translation was made in the tenth century, as seems likely, there are probably only a handful of centres at which it could have been produced. As Lapidge has illustrated, the number of centres that achieved a high level of Latin scholarship was 'surprisingly small' in this period, to the extent that we can often trace which master taught whom.[58] Given this, Maria D'Aronco's suggestion that the *Old English Herbarium* was most likely produced at Æthelwold's school in Winchester deserves further consideration.

Reading the *Old English Herbarium* as a product of the reform movement in England would make sense given the ultimately continental nature of the project. The treatises comprising the larger Herbarium Complex represented current medical practice on the continent in the Early Middle Ages, and it is likely that the high quality exemplars used in the creation of the translation would have come from a continental (very possibly Carolingian) source.[59] D'Aronco has emphasised the similarities between the Old English translation of the *Herbarium* and a Latin version found in Montecassino Biblioteca della Badia MS 97. The illustrations in the

---

[57] M. A. D'Aronco, 'Le conoscenze mediche nell'Inghilterra anglosassone: Il ruolo del mondo carolingio', in *International Scandinavian and Medieval Studies in Memory of Gerd Wolfgang Weber*, ed. M. Dallapiazza, O. Hansen, P. Sorensen, and Y. Bonnetain (Trieste, 2000), pp. 129–46, at 144.

[58] Lapidge, 'Schools, Learning and Literature in Tenth-Century England', p. 3.

[59] Glaze lists Pseudo-Apuleius as among the medical authors popular in Carolingian catalogues, and the *Herbarium* shows up several times in her table of 'Early Medieval Ownership of Medical Books Through the Twelfth Century': Glaze, 'The Perforated Wall', p. 73 and Table 1.

Montecassino manuscript are similar to those found in the Cotton version of the *Herbarium*, with the herbs for instance generally sharing the same shape and number of leaves (although the Montecassino rendition is more simplified than that found in the Cotton manuscript). Additionally, both manuscripts contain the α tradition of the *Pseudo-Apuleius* Herbal, exceptionally paired with *Ex herbis femininis* and *Liber medicinae ex animalibus* of class B (whereas otherwise in the Latin tradition *Pseudo-Apuleius*-α is paired with *Curae herbarum* and *Liber medicinae ex animalibus*-A).[60] The relationship between these manuscripts seems to indicate the role of Benedictine continental houses in the transmission of the treatises of the Herbarium Complex to England. It is likely that one of the main aims of this translation project was to bring England up to date with, and in line with, current continental medical practice.

The leaders of the reform movement in England were influenced by contemporary continental trends and often looked to Carolingian practice, which may well have inspired a renewed study of medicine in the later tenth century. The Carolingian period was characterised by a notable revival in the study and production of medical texts. This can be seen most clearly in the fact that more than half of the surviving medical manuscripts from the ninth to eleventh century had been copied in the ninth century in Frankish and German monastic centres.[61] The renewal in interest in medicine likely also reflects the incorporation of medicine as part of the didactic programme of study within the monasteries in some cases. The importance of studying medicine was stressed by Alcuin, a central figure in the Carolingian *renovatio*, who saw it as belonging to the seven liberal arts (falling under the larger category of *physica*).[62] This view is also repeated in the writings of his student Hrabanus Maurus and in the anonymous *Arzneibuch* from Lorsch.[63] The idea that medicine should be a part of the study of any well-rounded scholar of the liberal arts almost certainly increased interest in the subject during the Carolingian period. Contreni has argued that this may have led to medicine largely being considered as a non-specialist subject.[64] Scholars such as Walafrid Strabo, Lupus of Ferrieres and Grimoald of St Gall all studied medical texts, but this was probably pursued at least partially because of literary interests in

---

[60] See D'Aronco, 'Le conoscenze mediche nell'Inghilterra anglosassone', pp. 37–39; M. A. D'Aronco, 'Gardens on Vellum: Plants and Herbs in Anglo-Saxon Manuscripts', in *Health and Healing from the Medieval Garden*, ed. P. Dendle and A. Touwaide (Woodbridge, 2008), pp. 101–27, at 114–16.

[61] Contreni, 'Masters and Medicine', p. 269; Glaze, 'The Perforated Wall', pp. 70–71.

[62] Alcuin, *Didascalia III*, 'Dialogus de rhetorica et virtutibus', PL vol. 101, col. 947–48; cited in Glaze, 'The Perforated Wall', p. 85.

[63] Glaze, 'The Perforated Wall', pp. 84–89.

[64] Contreni, 'Masters and Medicine', p. 268. Contreni records only one reference to a named 'medicus' from ninth-century French sources.

Greek words and concepts.[65] In all likelihood, the study of medicine at this time tended to combine both the literary and the practical, but in any case it was on the rise during the Carolingian period.

Aside from literary interests, the ninth and tenth-century revival of medicine may also reflect the increased influence of Benedictine monasticism during this period. More so than any other monastic rule practised in the Early Middle Ages, the *Benedictine Rule* emphasises care for the sick, a responsibility that is ultimately held by the abbot himself. Chapter 36 of the *Rule* details what type of care is to be given to sick monks, who are, for instance, to be given a room apart and to be allowed to take baths and eat meat. The chapter begins with the reminder: *infirmorum cura ante omnia et super omnia adhibenda est, ut sicut reuera Christo, ita eis seruiatur: quia ipse dixit: Infirmus fui et uisitastis me* ('the care of the sick must be provided before all and above all; they must be served like Christ, in fact, because he himself said: "I was sick and you visited me"') and concludes: *curam autem maximam habeat abbas ne a cellarariis aut a seruitoribus neglegantur infirmi; et ipsum respicit, quidquid a discipulis delinquitur* ('let the abbot take the greatest care, lest the sick be neglected by the servants, and he similarly should look to see if anything has been forgotten by his followers').[66] A supreme example of the ideal of a medically-minded abbot can be seen in Baldwin, the abbot of Bury St Edmunds in the late eleventh century. Baldwin was a skilled doctor who had previously served as a physician to English kings before becoming abbot.[67]

The Benedictine aim of promoting health received further refinement from the sixth-century monastic founder Cassiodorus, who stressed the importance of monasteries having a well-stocked medical library. He even gave specific instructions on which books to have (his list included the *Herbarium* of Dioscorides, which perhaps refers to Pseudo-Dioscorides's *Liber medicinae ex herbis femininis*).[68] The significance of providing good care for the sick in Benedictine monasteries during the Carolingian period can be seen for instance in the elaborate provisions for the sick in the ninth-century monastic plan found in St Gall. The (apparently never actu-

---

[65] Glaze, 'The Perforated Wall', pp. 158–59: 'The peculiar nature of early medical literature, which combined intellectually challenging materials with practically useful guides and recipe collections, might in fact have contributed to the appeal of these anthologised medical books.'

[66] *Regula Benedicti*, ed. R. Hanslik, Corpus Scriptorum Ecclesiasticorum Latinorum 75 (Vienna, 1960), ch. XXXVI, pp. 95–96.

[67] For a discussion of Baldwin's impact upon the study of medicine at Bury St Edmunds, see Banham, 'Medicine at Bury in the Time of Abbot Baldwin'.

[68] *Cassiodorus senatoris institutiones*, ed. R. A. B. Mynors (Oxford, 1937), bk. I, ch. 31, pp. 78–79; see also Glaze, 'The Perforated Wall', p. 62. For the impact of Cassiodorus's recommendations in Carolingian libraries, see R. McKitterick, *The Carolingians and the Written Word* (Cambridge, 1989), p. 194. It is also worth noting that Cassiodorus's *Institutes* exists in multiple manuscript copies from the Anglo-Saxon period (Lapidge, *The Anglo-Saxon Library*, p. 296).

alised) monastery depicted in this plan designates over one-tenth of the total establishment towards buildings dedicated to the care of the sick. The location for which this plan was made has been the subject of some debate, but some scholars suggest it may well have been in England.[69] It seems likely that increasing pressure on monastic houses in England to conform to the *Benedictine Rule* in the tenth century would have encouraged an impulse towards medical study and training.

It is possible that the emphasis on medical care in Benedictine practice may have encouraged a reform-minded Anglo-Saxon bishop or abbot to commission a work such as the *Herbarium*. One also wonders if the masculine bias of the translation might possibly reflect the desires of a male monastic house. Although not every cure related to feminine disorders is omitted, the fact that a percentage are at least suggests that the translator saw his (or her) audience as principally masculine. A monastic setting may also help explain why remedies with a sexual element could have been seen as unnecessary. Certainly these criteria could describe a number of monastic institutions in tenth-century England. Beyond Winchester, the other important scholarly centres of the reform – Canterbury under Dunstan or Worcester under Oswald – are clear candidates, as one assumes that such a centre would need to be well-connected to the continent in order to have access to the manuscripts necessary for such an elaborate project of translation.

The existing manuscript record suggests that Æthelwold's school at Winchester was the most productive scholarly centre of his time. We also know *Bald's Leechbook* was very likely revisited and recopied in Winchester a generation (or two) earlier, which may indicate the presence of some sort of medical library or interest. There is evidence that some translations were being produced at Winchester under Æthelwold's supervision. The *Vita S. Aethelwoldi* records that *dulce namque erat ei adolescentes et iuuenes semper docere, et Latinos libros Anglice eis soluere* ('and, indeed, it was always a sweet thing for him to teach the youths, changing Latin books into English for them'), and we can count the most prolific author of English prose, Ælfric, among his students.[70]

Æthelwold himself translated the *Regula S. Benedicti* for Queen Ælfthryth. Unlike the verbose hermeneutic style popular in Latin composition in the tenth century, Æthelwold's translation appears to be driven by a desire for clarity and comprehensibility. The most extensive study of the Old English *Regula S. Benedicti* has been done by Mechthild Gretsch,

---

[69] M. D'Aronco, 'The Benedictine Rule and the Care of the Sick: The Plan of St Gall and Anglo-Saxon England', in *The Medieval Hospital and Medical Practice*, ed. B. Bowers (Aldershot, 2007), pp. 235–51.

[70] *The Life of St. Æthelwold*, ed. M. Lapidge and M. Winterbottom (Oxford, 1991), pp. 46–49. See also H. Gneuss 'Origin of Standard Old English and Æthelwold's School at Winchester', *ASE* 1 (1972), 63–83.

who describes Æthelwold's aim as being 'to write clear and fluent English prose', noting also that 'he keeps closely to the original as long as he can fulfil this purpose by means of a literal translation'.[71] As we have seen, these aims are also shared by the translator of the *Old English Herbarium*. This is not to suggest that the two works are in exactly the same style or share an authorship, as they have some stylistic differences. Most notably, Æthelwold frequently coins his own terminology in his translation of the *Regula S. Benedicti* – something that does not appear to happen in the *Old English Herbarium*. Also, Æthelwold has a tendency to render one Latin word into a pair of Old English words, something I have not observed in the translation of the *Herbarium*.[72] However, it is perhaps not difficult to imagine these two works as belonging to the same school or tradition, one which emphasised clear, practical, and faithful prose.

There is also some palaeographical evidence, which, although inconclusive, may point towards Winchester as the locus of this translation.[73] D'Aronco has shown conclusively that the manuscripts V, B, and H (the Cotton manuscript, the Bodleian Library manuscript, and the Hatton manuscript also containing the *Lacnunga*) all share numerous traits and must have been copied from closely related illustrated exemplar(s).[74] B contains notations in the tremulous hand and was most likely copied at Worcester. V, the Cotton manuscript, on the other hand, shares numerous stylistic traits with London, BL, MS Cotton Tiberius B. v, part 1 (containing, among other texts, an illustrated copy of the *Wonders of the East*). The Tiberius manuscript is often considered a quintessential example of the illustrative style associated with the scriptorium of St Augustine's Canterbury in the early eleventh century. The close similarity between these two pieces indicates that the Cotton copy of the *Herbarium* may also have been copied in Canterbury, but this manuscript contains other features associated with a

---

[71] M. Gretsch, 'Æthelwold's Translation of the *Regula Sancti Benedicti* and its Latin Exemplar', *ASE* 3 (1974), 125–51, at 148; Æthelwold's style is also discussed by D'Aronco in 'La traduzione in inglese antico della *Regula Sancti Benedicti*: Neologismi e prestiti nel lessico monastico', *Filologia Germanica* 24 (1981), 105–46, at 128–32.

[72] For discussion of Æthelwold's style in comparison to the *Herbarium*, see D'Aronco, 'L'erbario anglosassone', pp. 348–49. For more general discussions of Æthelwold's style, see M. Lapidge, 'Æthelwold as Scholar and Teacher', in *Bishop Æthelwold: His Career and Influence*, pp. 89–118, esp. 101–02; Gretsch, 'Æthelwold's Translation of the *Regula Sancti Benedicti*', pp. 143–48; D. A. Bullough, 'The Educational Tradition in England from Alfred to Ælfric: Teaching *utriusque linguae*', in *La scuola nell'occidente latino dell alto medioevo*, Settimane di studio sull'alto medioevo 19 (Spoleto, 1972), pp. 453–94, at 480–81.

[73] This argument following is outlined by D'Aronco, 'L'erbario anglosassone', pp. 354–55; 'The Transmission of Medical Knowledge in Anglo-Saxon England', pp. 45–46.

[74] D'Aronco, 'The Transmission of Medical Knowledge in Anglo-Saxon England', pp. 41–45.

Winchester style, including the frames surrounding the two initial pages. This suggests that V was copied at Canterbury but that its exemplar may have been originally from Winchester. It is entirely possible, although not necessary, that this could have been the original autograph (or a clean copy) produced in Winchester.

The series of connections seen in the production of these manuscripts between Winchester, Canterbury, and Worcester reinforces the connections between the creation of this translation and the Benedictine reform movement in England. This translation clearly did not originate as an insignificant venture in an intellectual backwater, but instead was a large-scale project that once completed became a necessary part of the libraries at the foremost scholarly centres in England at that time.

When Æthelwold initiated a new monastic foundation at Peterborough, he donated 21 books to the minster. Michael Lapidge has described these items as 'a sort of start-up collection' for the monastery, and, among the varied lexicographical texts and hagiography, it is also recorded that he gave them a *Medicinalis*.[75] It is unclear from this list if this medical text was in English or Latin, or indeed which text it might have been. However, it does suggest that a dependable medical text was something deemed essential by Æthelwold for an up-to-date monastic house. This idea would have been in keeping with the practice of Benedictine monasticism on the continent at this time. The fact that this type of attitude was also held by one of the leaders of the reform movement in England might help explain why the translation of the *Old English Herbarium* was undertaken at precisely this time.

The scale of this project and the skilful nature of the translation produced (along with its accompanying illuminations) suggest that it must have been undertaken at a major centre with continental ties. Such a house would almost certainly have been part of the larger reform movement. The wide reach of the reform in England also provides an explanation as to why this text is still preserved in four copies today, when so many other texts from the Anglo-Saxon period have been lost.

---

[75] Lapidge, 'Booklists', list IV. Bullough remarks that the list 'is a mixed bag indeed, with some very odd features [...] Taken as a whole, however, it seems to offer the basis of a wide-ranging, even encyclopedic, although not very profound education to those who had already mastered the Latin language': 'The Educational Tradition in England', p. 482.

5

Medicine in Anglo-Saxon England

In the early Anglo-Saxon period, Bede describes one of the most illustrious Anglo-Saxon saints being treated by a physician. In his description of Æthelthryth's death, Bede writes that a certain doctor, Cynifrid, was consulted about her illness and death: *sed certiori notitia medicus Cynifrid, qui et morienti illi et eleuatae de tumulo adfuit; qui referre erat solitus quod illa infirmata habuerit tumorem maximum sub maxilla* ('but with more certain knowledge, the doctor Cynifrid, who was present both during her death and during her exhumation, used to say how she, the sick one, had a great tumour under her jaw').[1] After this description, Cynifrid continues to provide further details about her condition and death. In this account of Æthelthryth's illness, Bede treats Cynifrid with respect, relying on him as a person whose testimony was trustworthy and of particular value because of his expertise. Æthelthryth herself had received his medical care, and although in this case the medical treatment was unsuccessful (and probably also superfluous in light of the saint's prophetic vision of her death), there is no suggestion that the abbess was wrong in seeking professional medical attention.

Bede's account provides a contrast to St Bernard of Clairvaux's notorious remark in the twelfth century, when he discouraged his monks from seeking doctors or purchasing medicines, writing that this *religioni indecens est et contrarium puritati* ('is unseemly for religion and contrary to purity of life').[2] Bernard's outlook is sometimes taken as typical of patristic and medieval theologians, but, in fact, attitudes towards the appropriate use of medicine (perhaps unsurprisingly) varied considerably during the classical and Late Antique periods. While traditionally scholarship has tried to paint the Church Fathers as uniformly suspicious of the medical arts, in the last two decades several scholars have argued that medicine was much more widely approved in the early Church than has generally been assumed.[3] Nevertheless, although some Church Fathers (such as

---

[1] *Bede's Ecclesiastical History of the English People*, bk. 4.17.
[2] Bernard of Clairvaux, *Lettres*, ed. H. Rochais and others (Paris, 1997), ep. 345.
[3] See D. W. Amundsen, 'Medicine and Faith in Early Christianity', *Bulletin of the History of Medicine* 56 (1982), 326–50; D. W. Amundsen, *Medicine, Society, and Faith in the Ancient and Medieval Worlds* (London, 1996); G. B. Ferngren, *Medicine & Health Care in Early Christianity* (Baltimore, 2009).

Clement and Augustine) were generally approving of the practice of medicine, others held more restrictive views. Origen, for instance, suggests that medicine is unacceptable for those aiming for a godly way of life:

Ἀλλὰ χρὴ τὴν θεραπείαν τῶν σωμάτων, εἰ μὲν ἁπλούστερον βούλοιτό τις ζῆν καὶ κοινότερον, ἐφόδῳ ἰατρικῇ θεραπεύειν, εἰ δὲ βέλτιον παρὰ τοὺς πολλούς, εὐσεβείᾳ τῇ εἰς τὸν ἐπὶ πᾶσι θεὸν καὶ ταῖς πρὸς ἐκεῖνον εὐχαῖς.[4]

[A man ought to use medical means to heal his body if he aims to live in the simple and ordinary way. If he wishes to live in a way superior to that of the multitude, he should do this by devotion to the supreme God and by praying to him.]

Through the patristic and classical tradition the Anglo-Saxons would have inherited a variety of often conflicting views concerning the acceptability of medicine.

Against this diverse background of inherited opinions, Anglo-Saxon authors generally defended the practice of medicine. Although it would be impossible to say there was a single, comprehensive theology of medicine in Anglo-Saxon England, the idea that the use of medicine was in opposition to faith (or at least that its use was inappropriate to life in holy orders) does not appear to be at all characteristic of Anglo-Saxon attitudes. Instead Anglo-Saxon sources (whether poetic or practical) on the whole reflect widespread respect and appreciation for the practice of medicine. This may perhaps at least partially reflect the influence of Carolingian sources, where medicine was widely respected and sometimes given the status of a liberal art.

Even against this background, however, the Old English medical collections continue to occupy a central place in discussions of suspect practices in Anglo-Saxon England. It is not uncommon, even in current scholarship, to see the suggestion that these works were unorthodox, backwards, or represent popular folk practice rather than more learned traditions. Certainly the contents of these collections are diverse and entries range in form. Nonetheless, as has been seen in this book, each of the four extant collections continuously displays connections with an elite and literate intellectual culture. While previous chapters have been mostly occupied with internal analysis of these collections, this final chapter will turn instead to the broader question of how these texts may have been understood within Anglo-Saxon monastic and intellectual circles. This will be accomplished primarily through an exploration of how medicine and medical practitioners are treated in literary and ecclesiastical works

---

[4] Origen, *Contre Celse*, ed. Marcel Borret (Paris, 1969), vol. IV, 8.60; trans. H. Chadwick, *Contra Celsum* (Cambridge, 1953), p. 498. Cf. Amundsen, 'Medicine and Faith in Early Christianity', p. 338.

from the period. I will suggest that comparisons between forbidden practices known as *drycræft* or *galdru* (most frequently translated as 'magic' and 'charms' respectively) and the learned and literate material found in the medical corpus are generally inaccurate in a culture where the medical art was held in high esteem.

The Practice of Medicine

Any information about the treatment of medicine in literary sources must first be considered in light of the fact that there is very little evidence concerning the historical reality of medical practice in Anglo-Saxon England. It has been generally assumed in scholarship of the period that monastic houses provided some type of medical care for their members. However, there is little concrete evidence of this, especially in the early part of the period when practices may have varied considerably from house to house. In a colloquy by Ælfric Bata, written around the year one thousand, there is a mention of a monastic *medicus* who also tends the herb garden:

> Fratres mei, dicite mihi nunc, habetis aliquod uiridiarium, aut habetis herbas
> aliquas in uiridiario uestro?
> Etiam, domine, habemus.
> Quis exercet eas?
> Hortulanus monasterii et medicus senioris nostri, qui eas omni anno plantat   ac circumfodit et rigat.
> Estne bonus medicus ille?
> Sic dicunt.[5]

> [My brothers, tell me now, do you have a garden? Do you have any herbs in your garden?/ Yes we do sir./ Who tends them?/ The gardener of the monastery, our abbot's doctor. He plants, cultivates and waters them all year round./ Is he a good doctor?/ They say he is.]

This text was meant for teaching Latin grammar and should not be taken to perfectly reflect real conditions in the monastery. However, to be an effective aid for learning its general contents must have been familiar to students, which suggests that the idea of both a doctor and a herb garden within the monastery must not have been too unusual by this time (even if in the colloquy itself the doctor is described as Frankish (*francigena*)). It seems likely that the richest monastic houses would have had an infirmary and probably, by extension, an infirmerer of some sort, even in the early

---

[5] *Anglo-Saxon Conversations: Colloquies of Ælfric Bata*, ed. S. Gwara and trans. D. W. Porter (Woodbridge, 1997), pp. 156–57 (trans. Porter); cf. Bolotina, 'Medicine and Society in Anglo-Saxon England', p. 37.

Anglo-Saxon period, although it is difficult to know what sort of training these people would have received. It is even more difficult to discern how laypeople received medical aid.[6]

It is likely that most medical care in Anglo-Saxon England would have been carried out by practitioners with no knowledge of medical texts, whether in Latin or English. Little evidence remains of these persons, but it is easy to imagine that nurses and caregivers within homes and local healers provided the majority of treatment during the period, although it has also been suggested that secular clerics performed some role.[7] As has been emphasised throughout this book, the Old English medical texts are products of a literate intellectual culture and must therefore represent only a certain elite facet of medical care. These collections are not textbooks for beginners, as they do not contain basic information such as how to gather and preserve herbs or other medical materials. In most cases, remedies assume a skilled practitioner who was able to form a diagnosis, correctly prepare ingredients, and identify the quantities needed of different plants.[8] Beyond this, many remedies call for ecclesiastical training, such as remedies requiring knowledge of specific prayers and psalms or for the giving of masses. The survival of a large corpus of medical texts (both in Old English and in Latin) provides in itself some of the strongest evidence for the existence of some form of educated medical class in Anglo-Saxon England. Debby Banham has suggested that the lack of attributions to famous physicians in the Old English medical texts, and the inclusion of references to two apparently Anglo-Saxon practitioners (Oxa and Dun), may suggest some form of self-sufficient medical community literate in the vernacular.[9] Such a class of doctors would almost certainly have formed part of a major ecclesiastical centre or perhaps a royal court, and very likely would not have represented the mainstream practice of medicine throughout smaller towns and in more remote places. How many healers would have been educated at the level required to make use of these texts remains unknown. Nevertheless, despite the obscurity of the evidence concerning what it may have meant to be a medical practitioner at this time, it is clear that doctors were a part of the mental and literary landscape of the period.

---

[6] For an in-depth discussion of this question, see Bolotina, 'Medicine and Society in Anglo-Saxon England'.
[7] Bolotina, 'Medicine and Society in Anglo-Saxon England', pp. 20–22.
[8] For a discussion of the tacit knowledge required to use these texts, see Van Arsdall, 'Medical Training in Anglo-Saxon England', pp. 415–36; Bolotina, 'Medicine and Society in Anglo-Saxon England', pp. 46–55.
[9] D. Banham, 'Dun, Oxa, and Pliny the Great Physician: Attribution and Authority in Old English Medical Texts', *Social History of Medicine* 24 (2011), 57–73.

The Heavenly Doctor and Medical Metaphors

It is noteworthy that the majority of references to doctors in the Old English poetic corpus refer to the Lord or occur in analogies related to priests. In the *Lord's Prayer II*, God is not only the *heah casere* ('high emperor') but also a *halig læce* ('holy doctor'); in *Solomon and Saturn I*, he is *lamena* [...] *læce* ('doctor of the lame'); in *Judgement Day II*, he is *uplicum læce* ('heavenly doctor').[10] In most cases, the references to the Lord as a doctor are simply appellations made in passing, but sometimes the metaphor is further developed, with salvation for instance sometimes being described as *læcedom* ('medicine').[11] The art of medicine and its practitioners are also favoured metaphors for many aspects of the religious life in prose homiletic texts. In particular, the language of medicine and remedies is commonly used to convey the necessity of confession and repentance for sin.[12] Daily sins do not grow better except though daily medicines (*læcedomas*), warns the anonymous author of Vercelli XI.[13] Elsewhere, in Ælfric's writings on penitence, we read that prayers, belief, the giving of alms, and true love of God *gehælað and gelacniað ure synna, gif we ða læcedomas geornlice begað* ('heal and cure our sins, if we earnestly turn to those medicines').[14] This metaphoric use of the language of physicians and remedies is also applied to God: *se soða læce* ('the true doctor').[15]

The portrayal of Christ as a physician in Anglo-Saxon texts draws upon a rich tradition. In the gospels, Jesus compares himself with a physician, saying: *non necesse habent sani medicum sed qui male habent non enim veni vocare iustos sed peccatores* ('they that are well have no need of a doctor, but those who are sick: truly, I came not to call the righteous but sinners').[16] This metaphor was exploited in the patristic period, with the

---

[10] See Old English Corpus, 'læce' and 'læcedom'. See 'The Judgement Day II', *ASPR*, vol. VI, ll. 43, 65, 80; 'The Lord's Prayer II', *ASPR*, vol. VI, l. 58; 'Christ', *ASPR*, vol. III, l. 1571; 'Christ and Satan', *ASPR*, vol. I, l. 588; 'Solomon and Saturn I', *ASPR*, vol. VI, l. 77.

[11] See 'Christ and Satan', l. 588; 'Christ', l. 1571; 'Judgement Day II' l. 80. See also 'Resignation', where the Lord sends 'bot' to the sick at heart; 'Resignation', *ASPR*, vol. III, ll. 108–12. This is likely inspired by the Latin tradition, as *salus* can mean 'health' or 'safety' as well as 'salvation'.

[12] *The Blickling Homilies of the Tenth Century from the Marquis of Lothian's Unique MS. A.D. 971*, ed. R. Morris, EETS o.s. 58, 63, 73 (London, 1880), p. 107; Frantzen, *The Literature of Penance*, p. 182; *The Vercelli Homilies and Related Texts*, ed. D. Scragg, EETS o.s. 300 (Oxford, 1992), p. 222; Clemoes, p. 448; Ælfric, *The Homilies of the Anglo-Saxon Church: The First Part, Containing the Sermones Catholici, Or Homilies of Ælfric*, ed. B. Thorpe (London, 1844), vol. II, p. 603 (hereafter referred to as Thorpe in the footnotes).

[13] *The Vercelli Homilies*, p. 222.

[14] Thorpe p. 603.

[15] Clemoes, p. 448.

[16] Mark 2:17 (cf. Mt. 9:12 and Lk. 5:31); text taken from R. Weber, *Biblia Sacra Iuxta Vulgatam Versionem* (Stuttgart, 2007).

theme of *Christus medicus* being particularly pronounced in the works of St Augustine of Hippo.[17] According to Augustine, the wisdom of God can act as both physician and medicine (*ipsa medicus, ipsa medicina*).[18] And in some instances, he compares the suffering of Christ in the passion to a bitter medicine: *calix passionis amarus est, sed omnes morbos paenitus curat; calix passionis amarus est, sed prior eum bibit medicus, ne bibere dubitaret aegrotus* ('the cup of the passion is bitter, but it completely cures every illness; the cup of the passion is bitter but the doctor drank it first, lest the diseased waver over drinking').[19] In this example, Christ is the doctor and his suffering the medicine needed by sinners.

Another avid employer of various forms of medical metaphors was Gregory the Great. Gregory was a heavily influential figure in the Anglo-Saxon period, as is testified to by the many manuscript copies of his works in Anglo-Saxon libraries.[20] His frequent use of medical metaphors can be clearly seen in the fact that, aside from works of Ælfric and the Old English medical texts, the translations of Gregory's *Pastoral Care* and *Dialogues* contain the highest frequency of the words *læce* and *læcedom* in the Old English corpus.[21] In both Gregory's Latin text and in the Old English translation of the *Pastoral Care*, these words most frequently occur in passages emphasising the skill of doctors. This theme is introduced in the first chapter of the work where Gregory laments the lack of shame among ill-trained priests:

> Nulla ars doceri praesumitur, nisi intenta prius meditatione discatur. Ab imperitis ergo pastorale magisterium qua temeritate suscipitur, quando ars est artium regimen animarum. Quis autem cogitationum uulnera occultiora esse nesciat uulneribus uiscerum? Et tamen saepe qui nequaquam spiritalia praecepta cognouerunt, cordis se medicos profiteri non metuunt, dum qui pigmentorum uim nesciunt, uideri medici carnis erubescunt.[22]

---

[17] R. Arbesmann, 'The Concept of "Christus Medicus" in St. Augustine', *Traditio* 10 (1954), 1–28, at 2.

[18] Augustine of Hippo, *De doctrina christiana*, ed. R. P. H. Green (Oxford: 1995), 1.14.13; cited in Arbesmann, 'The Concept of "Christus Medicus" in St. Augustine', p. 13.

[19] Augustine, *Miscellanea Agostiniana: Testi e Studi* (Roma, 1930–31), serm. 310; cited in Arbesmann, 'The Concept of "Christus Medicus" in St. Augustine', p. 15.

[20] See Lapidge, *The Anglo-Saxon Library*, 'Catalogue of Classical and Patristic Authors and Works Composed before AD 700 and Known in Anglo–Saxon England', 'Gregory the Great'.

[21] This estimation is based on the Old English web corpus: *Dictionary of the Old English Web Corpus*, ed. A. diP. Healey, J. P. Wilkin, and X. Xiang, *Dictionary of Old English Web Corpus* (Toronto, 2009), consulted at <http://tapor.library.utoronto.ca/doecorpus/> (accessed 7 March 2016).

[22] Gregory the Great, *Regula pastoralis*, ed. F. Rommel and R. W. Clement, Clavis no. 1712 (Turnhout, 1953), I ch. 1, ll. 1–6. See also Gregory the Great, *King*

[No art is presumed to be taught, unless it is first learnt through attentive study. With what rashness therefore is pastoral teaching undertaken by the inexperienced, when the governance of souls is the art of arts. Moreover, who cannot know that the wounds of the thoughts are more hidden than the wounds of the bowels? And yet often those who know nothing at all of spiritual precepts do not fear to proclaim themselves to be doctors of the heart, when those who do not know the power of drugs blush to be seen to be doctors of the flesh.]

Although Gregory clearly views the priest's role of being 'doctor' to the soul as the higher and more difficult art, physical doctors come off well in this exchange – they too practise a complex trade, one requiring training and skill. The frequency of references to doctors throughout his prose suggests that Gregory saw the medical profession as the closest metaphor for careful practice in clerical life. In the *Pastoral Care*, Gregory is never critical of medical doctors, unless they are amiss in their practice in some way. Generally, the priest is urged to be as skilful and well trained in his art as the physical doctor and to learn from his approach, whether in sweetening the bitter draughts of medicine, or traversing the country to treat patients, or hiding the knife lest the patient fear to be cut.[23] These metaphors rely on the assumption of a prominent and useful medical class.

The doctor-patient relationship was also used by the Church Fathers as a metaphor for priests and their flock; it is within this tradition that Anglo-Saxon penitentials employ the figure of the doctor as their favoured metaphor for the confessor. The analogy of the confessor as a 'doctor of sins' occurs in many places throughout the penitential handbooks extant from Anglo-Saxon England. However, it finds its most elaborate rendition in the *Old English Handbook* (also known as the *Pseudo-Egbert Confessional*):

Se læca þe sceal sare wunda wel gehælan. he mot habban gode sealfe to. Ne syndon nane swa yfele wunda swa sindon synwunda. forðam. þurh þa forwyrð se man ecan deaðe. buton he þurh andetnesse. & þurh geswicenesse. & þurh dædbote gehæled wurðe. þonne mot se læca beon. wis & wær. þe ða wunda hælan sceal. Ðurh gode lare man sceal ærest hi lacnian. & mid þam gedon. þæt man aspiwe þæt attor ut þæt him on innan bið. þæt is þæt he geclænsige hine silfne ærost. þurh andetnesse. Eal man sceal aspiwan synna. þurh gode lare. mid andetnesse. ealswa man unlibban deð ðurh godne drenc. Ne mæg æni læce wel lacnian. ær ðæt attor ute sy. ne æni man eac dædbote wel tæcan þam ðe andettan nele. ne æni man ne mæg synna buton andetnesse næ gebetan · þe ma þe se mæg. wel hal wurðan. þe unlibban gedruncen hæfð. buton he þæt attor swiðe

---

Alfred's West Saxon Version of Gregory's Pastoral Care, ed. Henry Sweet, EETS o.s. 45, 50 (Oxford, 1871), ch. 1, p. 24.
[23] See *King Alfred's West Saxon Version of Gregory's Pastoral Care*, ch. 9, p. 58; ch. 41, p. 302; ch. 26, p. 186.

aspiwe. Æfter andetnesse man mæg mid dædbote. godes mildheortnesse
raðe geearnian. gif he mid inneweardre heortan heofe. þæt bereowsað.
þæt he þurh deofles scyfe ær gefremode to unrihte. On wisum scrifte bið
eac swiðe forðgelang. wislic dædbot. ealswa on godum læce bið.[24]

[If the doctor shall heal painful wounds well, he must have a good salve
for that. Nor are there any wounds as evil as those that are the wounds
of sin, because through these one will perish in eternal death, unless
he is healed through confession and cessation [from sin] and through
repentance. Then must the doctor be wise and on guard, if he will heal
the wounds. They must first be treated with good teaching, and thus
make the person vomit out the poison (*attor*) that is inside them – that
is, that he cleanses himself first, through confession. All men must vomit
up [their] sins through good teaching with confession as one does poison
(*unlibban*) by a good drink. As no doctor may heal completely before the
poison (*attor*) is out, neither may any person offer also penance to those
who do not want to confess. Neither can any person heal his sins without
confession, no more so than one can become well that has drunken poison
(*unlibban*) without having vomited up the poison (*attor*). After confession one may, through penance, quickly earn God's mercy, if he with
inward sorrow of the heart laments what he previously did unrighteously
through the devil's prompting. Wise penance is very much dependent on
a wise confessor, just as [a good remedy] is on a good doctor.]

Although this description has an analogical purpose, the analogy is one that
casts a positive light on trained physicians. It is the wise physician who is
able to provide a good remedy for his patient and cure him of his wounds.
Of course, the priest is styled as the superior doctor, one who can heal the
very worst type of disease: sin. However, in the case of physical ailment, the
passage suggests a good remedy is *dependent upon* a good doctor.

The analogy of the priest (or confessor) as a type of doctor employed
here is clearly not a new one and it echoes Gregory and other patristic authors, as well as Irish sources.[25] However, this particular example
is striking for the length and detail of its description. The procedures
applied, the salve and in particular the emetic drink, are examples of real,
contemporary medical remedies in use in Anglo-Saxon England. Recipes
for salves and emetic solutions known as *spiwdrencas* are common in the
Old English medical corpus. *Spiwdrencas* could be made in many different
ways and were used for treating a variety of illnesses. The description in
the penitential of the use of a *spiwdrenc* to purge poison is similar to the
description in Book I of *Bald's Leechbook*: *gif þonne se seoca man þurh spiwedrenc aspiwð þone yfelan bitendan wætan on weg. þonne forstent se geohsa* ('if

---

[24] A. Frantzen, 'Anglo-Saxon Penitentials: A Cultural Database', consulted at
<www.anglo-saxon.net/penance> (Accessed 23 June 2014), CCCC MS 201, f. 121.
[25] Cf. Frantzen, *The Literature of Penance*, pp. 30–31.

then the sick man throws up the evil biting liquids with an emetic drink (*spiwedrenc*) then the spasm goes away').[26] Although the passage in the pentiential is primarily concerned with conveying a spiritual message, the use of specialised medical language suggests that it was not an entirely theoretical and metaphorical whimsy. It might imply that the author had some familiarity with Anglo-Saxon medical practice, whether as patient or practitioner, and that, when thinking of a priest and his duties, the image that naturally arose was not only the traditional, symbolic vision of a faceless 'doctor', but of a flesh-and-blood Anglo-Saxon physician.

Of course, in these types of texts earthly doctors (OE *læca*) were acknowledged to exist in a firmly secondary role to the power of God and his saints. In homiletic texts, it is a common theme to stress the superiority of the spiritual powers of a saint over the earthly power of doctors. In cases where disease is a direct punishment from God, it is a common trope to stress that even the best doctor can avail nothing; an example of this can be seen when *godcundlice wracu* (divine vengeance) strikes Herod with a terrible and disgusting disease in Ælfric's homily on the 'Nativity of the Innocents'.[27] In the story of Herod and his disease (which has patristic roots), Ælfric stresses that although Herod consulted many doctors, none were of any use. Such stories do not imply that medical help was never useful; indeed, the fact that it cannot help in such examples is meant to illuminate the unusual (and divine) nature of these illnesses.

There is no evidence that the *læce* held a preeminent role in Anglo-Saxon theological thought, and, as far as I am aware, there are no examples where doctors are portrayed as miracle workers. Nevertheless, the idea popular in some medieval and patristic contexts that seeking professional medical attention was somehow in opposition to piety and faith does not seem to have been common in Anglo-Saxon England. Instead, doctors appear as a class to be consulted and respected: the model of skilful training and rationally applied art.

---

[26] Cockayne, vol. II, 1.18. The passage containing this description has its source in Oribasius; this particular sentence, however, is not contained in the Latin source, cf. Appendix 1–A.
[27] Clemoes, pp. 221–22. This is a common story in medieval tradition; cf. Ælfric, *Ælfric's Catholic Homilies: Introduction, Commentary and Glossary*, ed. M. Godden (Oxford, 2000), pp. 44–45.

The Doctor in Literature: Old English Poetry

The most complex and sustained treatment of medical themes in an Old English poetic text is found in *Judgement Day II*. This poem is an imaginative translation of Bede's *De die iudicii*.[28] Like its Latin source, the poem's didactic message is the necessity of confession and repentance of sin in order to avoid the horrors of hell. This premise is explored partly through the use of the metaphor of the Lord as the *uplicum læce* ('heavenly doctor') who offers health and healing to the diseased. This theme is particularly pronounced in the first part of the poem, beginning in line 42:

> Ðis is an hæl earmre sauwle
> and þam sorgiendum selest hihta,
> þæt he wunda her wope gecyðe
> uplicum læce, se ana mæg
> aglidene mod gode gehælan
> and ræplingas recene onbindan.[29]

> [This is one cure for a wretched soul
> and the best hope for those sorrowing,
> that here he speaks with weeping of his wounds
> to the heavenly doctor, He who alone can
> heal the suffering spirit with goodness
> and the prisoners quickly unbind]

This section plays on the double meaning of *hæl* as both 'health' and 'salvation'. This word-play continues in lines 63–74, where we are first told that the Lord will give *hæl* and *help* to those that confess to him, and asks why *þæt þu ðe læce ne cyþst* ('do you not tell the doctor')? The idea of asking the Lord for healing is elaborated in 80–81: *hwi ne bidst þu þe beþunga and plaster/ lifes læcedomes æt lifes frea?* ('why do you not ask for baths and plaster, life's medicine, from the Lord of life?'). The theme resurfaces again at the end of the poem when *adl* ('sickness') is included among the terrors of hell in line 229 and *gesyntum* ('health') among the fruits of heaven in line 249:

---

[28] For an introduction to the manuscript context and discussion of the Old English poem's treatment of its Latin source, see the introduction to G. D. Caie's edition, *The Old English Poem* Judgement Day II: *A Critical Edition with editions of* De die iudicii *and the Hatton 113 Homily* Be Domes Dæge (Cambridge, 2000), pp. 1–45. See also G. D. Caie, 'Doomsday and Nature in the Old English Poem *Judgement Day II*', in *Aspects of Anglo-Saxon and Medieval England*, ed. M. Ogura (Frankfurt, 2014), pp. 93–104; J. Steen, *Verse and Virtuosity: The Adaptation of Latin Rhetoric in Old English Poetry* (Toronto, 2008), pp. 71–88.

[29] 'Judgement Day II', ll. 43–48.

Eala, se bið gesælig   and ofersælig
and on worulda woruld   wihta gesæligost,
se þe mid gesyntum   swylce cwyldas
and witu mæg   wel forbugon.³⁰

[Oh! He will be blessed and exceedingly fortunate
and in all worlds be the most blessed creature,
he who with health such pestilences
and punishments may well avoid]

In these passages, holiness and health are closely intertwined and it is God, the highest doctor, who can provide both.

The only full version of *Judgement Day II* occurs in Cambridge Corpus Christi College MS 201; this is the same manuscript that contains the *Old English Handbook*, referenced above.³¹ Graham Caie has pointed out the similarity in theme between the two works, yet *Judgement Day II*'s description of *beþunga* and *plaster* in line 80 provides a contrast with the pragmatic description of medicine found in the penitential text.³² Prescription of *beþunga*, a medicinal bath or lotion, occurs only seven times in the entire medical corpus (normally with the spelling *beþinge*); *plaster* is even more rare, occurring only twice in the corpus – both instances occurring in the *Old English Herbarium*.³³ The word *plaster* in *Judgement Day II* may be evoked by Bede's *placidae fomenta medelae* ('comfort of a soothing poultice') in the source text; it is possible that *plaster* might have been more familiar to the author than foment but salve (*sealf*) would be a much more typical rendering. The word *plaster* is not necessary for alliterative purposes in line 80, so it is difficult to know what would have encouraged the author of *Judgement Day II* to use this particular Latinate word; there is also nothing in the source to suggest the use of the *beþinge*. The other medical references within the poem similarly share no overlap with terminology associated with Old English medical collections. In my view this suggests that whoever wrote the poem was probably unfamiliar with the vernacular medical tradition and was possibly relying on glossaries. This provides a contrast to the practical vocabulary employed in the *Handbook*. Nevertheless, the poem's evocation of the doctor as a positive force, the knowledgeable and well-intentioned provider of medicine and wellness, is concordant with the other appearances of doctors and medicine across the Old English literary and homiletic corpus.

The majority of references to doctors and medicine (outside of the medical texts) within the Old English corpus occur in a theological context.

---

³⁰ 'Judgement Day II', ll. 247–50.
³¹ Ker no. 49; G&L no. 65.
³² Caie, *The Old English Poem* Judgement Day II, pp. 19–21.
³³ *OEH*, 168.1, 169.1.

There are exceptions to this, most notably within the corpus of saints' lives and in texts such as *Maxims I*, where real medical doctors are clearly indicated.[34] However, in most cases doctors are used metaphorically or for comparison with other positions, such as priests. Even given the established patristic precedent for this type of usage (and in some cases source texts), this raises the question why real medical doctors and physical medicine are so little discussed, especially given the large corpus of medical material preserved in Anglo-Saxon manuscripts. It is possible that this is reflective of circumstances similar to Carolingian Francia, where medicine was typically studied by intellectuals and amateurs as part of a general course of study rather than by trained doctors. If this were the case, few persons might have had the title of *læc*, even if they were practised in the art of medicine. However, even if references to actual doctors are scant, the poetic record testifies to a positive perception of doctors and their role in society. The fact that the doctor is considered an apt metaphor for the Lord and the ordained probably helped to encourage a favourable view of medicine in intellectual circles.

Disease and Sin in Ælfric's Homilies

Ælfric of Eynsham was a prolific writer, the author of, among other things, a voluminous corpus of homilies, saints' lives, and biblical commentaries both in Old English and in Latin. Ælfric's ideas should not be taken as representative for the entirety of Christian culture at his time, yet he was an exceedingly influential author and thinker. As Hugh Magennis writes, Ælfric was: 'the most prolific Old English writer. He is also the most wide-ranging writer, the one whose works survive in the most manuscripts, and the most influential in the post-Conquest period.'[35] Ælfric's writings provide valuable insights on many subjects, and, in this case, they offer some of the most extended thoughts available from the period on the topics of medicine and methods of healing.

Ælfric began his writing career in the late tenth century and continued writing into the first half of the eleventh century. These dates probably put him slightly later than the translation of the *Herbarium* and the compilation of *Bald's Leechbook*. However, his dates are roughly concurrent with those suggested for the only extant manuscript of the *Lacnunga*. It is difficult

---

[34] See, for instance, Ælfric, *Ælfric's Lives of Saints: Being a Set of Sermons on Saints' Days Formerly Observed by the English Church*, ed. W. Skeat, EETS o.s. 76, 82, 94 (London, 1966), 'Saint Basil', ll. 570–94; 'Saint Agatha', l. 134; 'Æthelthryth', ll. 61–93; *The Old English Life of Saint Pantaleon*, ll. 99–213; Krapp and Dobbie, *The Old English Exeter Book*, 'Maxims I', l. 45; 'Riddle 5', l. 10.

[35] H. Magennis, 'Ælfric Scholarship', in *A Companion to Ælfric*, ed. H. Magennis and M. Swan (Leiden, 2009), pp. 5–34, at 7.

to date the Anglo-Saxon medical collections (and more difficult still to date the origin of the individual entries found within), but we can guess that Ælfric's writings are probably somewhat later than many individual components found in the *Lacnunga*; nevertheless he was writing at a time when the entries found in the collection were deemed significant enough to warrant reproduction.

The most thorough treatment of health and medicine in Ælfric's homilies comes in his sermon on the passion of St Bartholomew. This homily tells the story of Bartholomew, a missionary saint who leads the heathen Indians to Christ. When Bartholomew arrives, the Indian natives are used to worshipping an idol (*deofolgylde*) named Astaroð. This idol, or more aptly the demon dwelling within it, was able to cure the inhabitants of their diseases. However, Ælfric is quick to point out that the diseases healed by the demon were the very diseases inflicted by it:

> Nu deð se deofol mid his lotwrencum þæt ða earman men geuntrumiað; ond tiht hi þæt hi sceolon gelyfan on deofolgyldum. Þonne geswicð he þære gedrecednysse ond hæfð heora sawla on his anwealde þonne hi cweðað to þære deofollican anlicnysse þu eart min god.[36]

> [Now the devil through his craftiness (*lotwrenc*) makes wretched men to become ill, and draws them in so that they should believe in idols. Then he withdraws their torment from them and has their souls in his power when they say to the devilish likeness, you are my God.]

This treatment of demonic healing is in keeping with Ælfric's declaration in the preface to his homiletic collection that the Antichrist normally weakens the healthy, but has the power to heal those diseases that he himself inflicts.[37]

The *vita* concludes after Bartholomew binds several demons and converts the peoples of India to the true God. This story of Bartholomew is a fairly close rendering of the anonymous Latin *Passio Bartholomaei*. After the *passio* finishes, however, Ælfric uses the narrative as an opportunity to discuss illness and medicine more generally. This concluding part of the homily is not modelled directly after any classical source; instead it appears to represent Ælfric's own thoughts, drawing loosely on a variety of sources including works by Gregory, Augustine, Caesarius, and the Bible.[38] In this section, Ælfric emphasises that although the figures in the

---

[36] Clemoes, pp. 442–43.

[37] Clemoes, 'praefatio', p. 175.

[38] Godden has assembled the known sources in his commentary to the text. These include: Augustine, *De doctrina christiana*; Augustine, *Sermones*; Caesarius of Arles, *Sermones*; Gregory the Great, *Moralia siue Expositio in Iob* (*Ælfric's Catholic Homilies: Introduction, Commentary and Glossary*, p. 257; see also *Fontes*, Ælfric, *Catholic Homilies* 1. 31).

story are afflicted with disease through the work of a demon, this is by no means the source of all disease. Christian men also often encounter physical maladies and these can occur for a variety of reasons: *hwilon for heora synnum. hwilon for fandunge; hwilon for godes wundrum. hwilon for gehealdsumnysse goddra drohtnunga; þæt hi þy eadmodran beon* ('sometimes for their sins, sometimes as a trial, sometimes for the miracles of God, sometimes for the perseverance of good conduct in life, that they might be more humble').[39] He further elaborates on these categories by giving examples of each situation. During this discourse, it becomes evident that in many cases a man's sickness is not a sign of his sin but of his holiness. Ælfric reminds his readers of the scripture *þa ðe ic lufie ða ic ðreage ond beswinge* ('those whom I love, I discipline and thrash').[40] To illustrate this, he offers the example of St Paul, whose affliction fostered his humility before God, but we might also think of King Alfred who, in his portrayal by Asser, is plagued by recurring sickness yet serves as a model of godly devotion.

Reluctance to link disease directly to sin is not particular to Ælfric. It appears that this was in fact a common position in Anglo-Saxon society. For instance, Victoria Thompson argues that in Anglo-Saxon times leprosy was likely not linked to sinfulness or a spiritual uncleanliness. She offers two examples where leprous persons were found prominently buried in the churchyard, suggesting that they were seen as fully communicant within the Church.[41] Likewise, she suggests that there is no evidence that they were institutionalised and that instead they probably continued to live as part of society. These facts are consistent with the theory that leprosy, like other ailments, was generally seen as originating from a number of causes, of which punishment for sin was only a single possibility.

Aside from simply recognising a number of possible causes for disease, Ælfric appears almost to stress the blessedness of it. This attitude undergirds an analogy offered by Ælfric, similar to that seen in the penitential handbook, where the Lord is compared to a medical practitioner:

> God is se soða læce, þe ðurh mislice swingla his folces synna gehælð. Nis se woruld-læce wælhreow, ðeah ðe he þone gewundodan mid bærnette, oððe mid ceorfsexe gelacnige. Se læce cyrfð oððe bærnð, and se untruma hrymð, þeah-hwæðere ne miltsað he þæs oðres wanunge, forðan gif

---

[39] Clemoes, p. 448.
[40] Clemoes. p. 448; cf. Heb. 12:6.
[41] V. Thompson, *Dying and Death in Later Anglo-Saxon England* (Woodbridge, 2004), p. 98. This point is qualified, however, by Christina Lee, who has suggested that by the end of the Anglo-Saxon period, lepers (and other people with contagious diseases) were often buried away from the other part of the population, although still in common ground: C. Lee, 'Changing Faces: Leprosy in Anglo-Saxon England', in *Conversion and Colonization in Anglo-Saxon England*, ed. C. Karkov and N. Howe (Tempe, 2006), pp. 59–81, at 67–69.

se læce geswicð his cræftes, þonne losað se forwundoda. Swa eac God gelacnað his gecorenra gyltas mid mislicum brocum; and þeah ðe hit hefigtyme sy ðam ðrowigendum, þeah-hwæðere wyle se goda Læce to ecere hælðe hine gelacnigan. Witodlice se ðe nane brocunge for ðisum life ne ðrowað, he færð to ðrowunge.[42]

[God is the true doctor, who through various scourges heals the sins of his people. Nor is the worldly doctor cruel, though he treats the wounded with burning or with the knife. The doctor cuts or burns and the patient wails, nevertheless he does not take pity on account of the lamentation, because if the doctor turns from his art, then he loses the wounded one. So also God heals his chosen ones' sins through various afflictions, and though it may be wearisome to the sufferer, nonetheless the good doctor will bring him to eternal health. Truly, he who suffers no miseries in this life goes to suffering [in the next].]

The first part of the passage has its source in a sermon of St Augustine.[43] Yet in its Augustinian context the metaphor has a quite different meaning. It occurs in a discussion of Matthew 18:22, in which Jesus declares that you must forgive your brother seventy times seven times. Augustine uses the analogy to warn that, while you must forgive your brother, you must still punish his sins, lest they grow worse and destroy him. In his version of the metaphor, Ælfric has changed the roles of the characters. In Ælfric's homily, now it is the Lord who is the *soða læce* ('true doctor'). However, in a startling inversion of the role of bodily doctors, Ælfric uses the analogy to underline why the Lord actually imparts physical illness in order to promote spiritual health.

A different manifestation of this attitude might be present in other passages where Ælfric stresses the spiritual dimension of our healing in Christ; for instance, when he recounts the etymology of *Hælend*, an Old English designation for Jesus. *Hælend* means 'healing', Ælfric writes, a

---

[42] Clemoes, p. 448. Interestingly, there are few references to surgical practices within the Old English medical corpus. However, Debby Banham and Christine Voth have shown that there is evidence for surgical practice in Anglo-Saxon England and have suggested that this type of treatment was considered 'too familiar to need writing down' and was instead learned by practical experience (Banham and Voth, 'The Diagnosis and Treatment of Wounds in the Old English Medical Collections', p. 173).

[43] Augustine of Hippo, *Sancti Augustini Sermones Post Maurinos Reperti: Probatae Dumtaxat Auctoritatis*, PL 38 (Roma, 1930), Serm. 83, 518. *Ælfric's Catholic Homilies: Introduction, Commentary and Glossary*, 265. *Quid enim tam pium quam medicus ferens ferramentum? Plorat secandus, et secatur: plorat urendus, et uritur. Non est illa crudelitas; absit ut saevitia medici dicatur. Saevit in vulnus, ut homo sanetur: quia si vulnus palpetur, homo perditur* ('who is more pious than the doctor who bears the knife? He who must be cut cries, and [yet] is cut: he who must be burned cries and [yet] is burned. That is not cruelty; it is far from seeming to be ferocity in the doctor. He is violent against the wound, so that the man may be healed – because if the wound is [just] caressed, the man is lost').

title that is appropriate *for ðan ðe he gehælð his folc fram heora synnum. and gelæt to ðam ecan earde heofenan rices* ('because [Jesus] heals his people from their sins and leads them to the eternal place of the heavenly kingdom').[44] Elsewhere, when St Simeon calls Jesus by the title *Halwendan* ('the healing one'), Ælfric relates *se halwenda þe he embe spræc is ure hælend crist. se ðe com to gehælenne ure wunda. þæt sindon ure synna* ('the healing one [or 'saviour'] of which he spoke is our Lord Christ, who came to heal our wounds, that is, our sins').[45] Although he would admit both as possible, Ælfric is forceful in stressing that it is *spiritual* healing rather than *physical* healing we should expect from the Lord. This emphasis seems perhaps exaggerated when we consider that the majority of miracles worked by Christ and his apostles were the healing of physical ailments. One wonders if Ælfric himself perhaps suffered from chronic illness, one which he would rather equate with God's blessing than his judgment. In any case, Ælfric's view of sickness and healing is nuanced and complex. Disease can arise from many sources, and we should be careful not to be too hasty in equating sickness with sin. Ælfric's broadminded perspective on disease ultimately helps support a favourable (or at least neutral) position towards the use of medical remedies.

The Place of Medicine in Ælfric's Homilies

Following his discussion of the diverse purposes and causes of sickness, Ælfric uses the final part of his homily on St Bartholomew to caution against the use of forbidden forms of medicine. He warns that the consequences will be dire for those who seek healing from illicit sources:

> se cristena man þe on ænire þyssere gelicnysse bið gebrocod ond he þonne his hælðe secan wile æt unalyfedum tilungum oððe æt awyrigedum galdrum, oþþe æt ænigum wiccecræfte þonne bið he þam hæðenum mannum gelic þe ðam deofolgylde geofrodon for heora lichaman hælðe ond swa heora sawla amyrdon.[46]

> [The Christian man, who suffers anything like this and then seeks health through forbidden practices, or through cursed *galdru*, or through any witchcraft, then he is like the heathen men who offered to the idol for the healing of their bodies and so murdered their souls.]

The intention in this passage is clear: good Christians are not to seek healing through the practice of witchcraft, and if they do, they will undoubtedly reap God's displeasure. However, the prohibitions are not

---

[44] Godden, p. 122.
[45] Godden, p. 253.
[46] Clemoes, pp. 449–50.

specific and leave aside questions about what exactly Ælfric considered to be 'forbidden practices' or 'accursed charms'.

Ælfric makes it clear that he is not talking about medicine generally. Ultimately the power of healing belongs to God, yet Ælfric defends the practice of medicine. Drawing on biblical example, he writes: *we habbað hwæðere þa bysene on halgum bocum þæt mot se ðe wyle mid soþum læcecræfte his lichaman getemprian, swa swa dyde se witega isaias þe worhte þam cyninge ezechie cliðan to his dolge ond hine gelacnode* ('we have, however, the model in holy books, that one might try to cure his body with true medicines, as did the prophet Isaiah who made for King Hezekiah a poultice for his wound and cured him').[47] He follows this by paraphrasing a passage from Augustine's *De doctrina christiana* which outlines the difference between taking a herb as a medicine and using it as an amulet.[48] Ælfric then concludes the Augustinian precept with his own words:

> ðeahhwæðere ne sceole we urne hiht on læcewyrtum besettan, ac on ðam ælmihtigum scyppende þe ðam wyrtum þone cræft forgeaf. Ne sceal nan man mid galdre wyrte besingan ac mid godes wordum hi gebletsian ond swa þicgan.[49]
>
> [Yet we should not set our hope on medical herbs, but on the Almighty Lord, who gave the herbs their power. Nor should any person sing charms over herbs, but with God's words bless them and thus eat [them].]

This passage has drawn some attention because of its references to *galdru* ('charms'), and I will explore the question of *galdru* more closely below. However, for the moment, it is useful to consider what the quotation reveals about licit forms of medicine. Although Ælfric is clearly worried about forbidden and unchristian forms of healing, he defends the legitimate use of medicine and the power of medicinal herbs. Interestingly, Ælfric makes no explicit reference to doctors, though the word *læcecræft* (used in reference to Isaiah) perhaps suggests an educated medical procedure.

Similarly, in his homily 'On Auguries', Ælfric adamantly opposes all forms of witchcraft and heathendom (*hæðengyld*) but makes provision for medicine: *læcedom is alyfed fram lichamena tyddernysse and halige gebedu mid godes bletsunge and ealla oðre tilunga syndon andsæte gode* ('medical remedies are permitted for all infirmity of the body and holy prayers with God's blessings and all other practices are abominable to God').[50] This provision for the appropriate use of medicine is not found in his source and appears

---

[47] Clemoes, p. 450.
[48] Augustine, *De doctrina christiana*, bk II, ch. 29.
[49] Clemoes, p. 450.
[50] *Ælfric's Lives of Saints*, 'On Auguries', p. 378, ll. 213–15.

to be a personal addition by Ælfric.[51] The repeated emphasis on medicine in these passages as something valid – and, indeed, entirely separate from forbidden forms of healing – suggests again a monastic and ecclesiastical culture where doctors and the learned tradition of medicine were valued.

This perspective may perhaps owe something to the influence of Carolingian authors. As discussed in Chapter 4, during the Carolingian period medicine became frequently recognised as belonging to the liberal arts and its practice was promoted by Benedictine monasteries, in accordance with the Benedictine rule. Both of these factors contributed to the positive assessment of medicine as a godly and acceptable art. A strong defence of the orthodoxy of medicine is found in the anonymous *Lorscher Arzneibuch*, which cites numerous examples of the compatibility of medicine and faith from biblical and patristic authors.[52] Like Ælfric's works, this collection also references the book of Isaiah. Alcuin and his student Hrabanus Maurus (the works of both of whom Ælfric knew) also laud the practice of medicine and the use of healing herbs in their works.[53] It is likely that this tradition was influential on Ælfric's positive view of medicine.

Yet although the practice of medicine is clearly defended in Ælfric's works, the fact that it is mentioned so frequently in the context of forbidden practices suggests that there was an inherent tension between these subjects. The potential for confusion between these two spheres clearly made Ælfric uneasy; it seems that he could hardly mention medicine without needing to warn against its false cousin. This suggests that in Anglo-Saxon England healing was not only the domain of trained physicians but that it competed with those who practised doctrinally unacceptable forms of healing. A question long lingering over the study of the medical collections has been how they relate to this other, forbidden form of healing. This subject is best addressed by examining which practices best defined this category of illicit healing.

---

[51] A. Meaney, 'Ælfric's use of His Sources in His Homily on Auguries', *English Studies* 66 (1985), 477–95, at 493.
[52] U. Stoll, *Das 'Lorscher Arzneibuch': Ein medizinisches Kompendium des 8. Jahrhunderts: Text, Übersetzung and Fachglossar* (Stuttgart, 1992). See also M. Leja, 'The Sacred Art: Medicine in the Carolingian Renaissance', *Viator* 47 (2016), 1–34; Glaze, 'The Perforated Wall', pp. 79–86.
[53] F. S. Paxton, 'Curing Bodies—Curing Souls: Hrabanus Maurus, Medical Education, and the Clergy in Ninth-Century Francia', *Journal of the History of Medicine* 50 (1995), pp. 230–52; Glaze, 'The Perforated Wall', pp. 86–90. For Ælfric's sources, see *Fontes Anglo-Saxonici Project* (University of Oxford, 2002), consulted at <http://fontes.english.ox.ac.uk/> (accessed 10 August 2016).

Drycræft in Late Anglo-Saxon England

In discussing unacceptable forms of healing, it is worth spending a moment trying to understand what terms such as *drycræft* and *galdor*, the two terms most frequently used in connection with forbidden practices, would have meant to Ælfric and other late Anglo-Saxon authors. *Drycræft* has normally been translated by the modern term 'magic'. Yet this term carries a different set of connotations from what it would have in the Early Middle Ages. The term 'magic' is an old one, dating back at least to Pliny the Elder in his *Naturalis historia*, where he describes the *vanitates magicae* ('delusions of the magi') as destroying the public faith in true medicine in his day.[54] However, in the Christianised context of the Early Middle Ages, 'magic' lost this clear connection to the magi and instead carried an explicitly demonic connotation in the West. Anglo-Saxon intellectuals were likely to have followed Isidore of Seville in seeing all magic as operating ultimately through demonic power.[55] Yet in popular usage today the term 'magic' can be used to indicate not only the demonic but also simply elements of the fantastic or the supernatural. In keeping with this, Meaney writes: 'there does not seem to have been one comprehensive Old English word which expressed our [modern] idea of "magic" but many, for different aspects.'[56] Therefore, although many of the practices discussed in this chapter fall within the modern concept of 'magic', I have chosen to use the Old English term *drycræft* to prevent confusion between modern and medieval paradigms (although even with this choice there is still the possibility of confusing various Anglo-Saxon categories).

Similar problems arise around the use of the word 'charm' in discussions of the medical texts. Scholars have tended to use the word 'charm' when discussing certain entries of the Old English medical collections. There are several collections of charm texts available from the Anglo-Saxon period. For his 'Anglo-Saxon Charms', Felix Grendon edited and translated 62 separate charms, and also included a reference to 87 additional charms not included in his edition. The other major collection and edition of charms in Old English is Gottfried Storms's *Anglo-Saxon Magic*, which lists 86 charms as well as 16 'prayers used as charm formulas' from Anglo-Saxon England.[57] A good proportion of the 'charm' texts used by both authors are taken from the Old English medical collections, although some come from other types of manuscripts.

---

[54] *Naturalis historia*, xxvi, 9.
[55] *The Etymologies of Isidore of Seville*, VIII.9; cf. R. Kieckhefer, *Magic in the Middle Ages* (Cambridge, 1990), pp. 10–12.
[56] A. Meaney, 'Magic', in *The Wiley-Blackwell Encyclopedia of Anglo-Saxon England*, ed. M. Lapidge *et al.*, 2nd ed. (Chichester, 2014), p. 304.
[57] Storms, *Anglo-Saxon* Magic, pp. vi–ix.

Although the use of the term is widespread in discussion of the Old English medical corpus, definitions of charm vary from scholar to scholar. Grendon, for instance, distinguished between 'incantations' and 'remedies depending for efficacy on the superstitious beliefs of the sufferers'. Pettit defines charms slightly more narrowly as 'incantations and amulets' and Karen Jolly suggests the definition: 'words and actions spoken or performed in a ritual manner with herbs.'[58] In general, most modern scholarly definitions attempt to maintain a sense of objectivity, defining a charm by its inherent qualities rather than by its social or theological acceptability. According to such definitions most prayers could constitute charms (especially if spoken aloud). Employing this type of definition may be a reasonable choice, especially when the term is used for analysing and grouping remedies without particular emphasis on cultural context. Nevertheless, these scholarly definitions also differ from common modern usage in which 'charm' has the connotation of a practice existing outside the accepted realm of established religion. As popularly understood today, prayers and charms (in theory, if not always in practice) are in opposition to each other. These competing definitions of 'charm' allow for confusion in the reading of the Old English medical collections, as well as for understanding the Old English term *galdor* which has almost universally been translated as 'charm' by scholars.

When the term *galdor* is used by late Anglo-Saxon authors such as Ælfric or Wulfstan it has an exclusively negative connotation. Ciaran Arthur has argued there was a shift in the way *galdor* was understood after the Benedictine reform. Prior to the reform, there are several examples where the word has the broader meaning of any powerful utterance and could be used in an ecclesiastical or liturgical context, for instance.[59] Although there is some evidence of the word being used occasionally in a negative sense prior to the reform, it is in the late Anglo-Saxon period that the negative meaning appears to have become fixed. Several remedies in the medical corpus refer to certain utterances as *galdru*, which are normally to be sung, for example: *sing þæt galdor on ælcre þara wyrta* ('sing that *galdor* on each of the herbs').[60] These examples clearly reflect the earlier usage of the word and do not exist in opposition to prayers. In *Bald's Leechbook*, one remedy directs the practitioner to *sing þriwa þæs halgan Sancte Iohannes gebed ond galdor* ('sing three times the prayer and *galdor* of Saint John'). This direction is followed by a Latin prayer against poison and it seems that both *gebed* and *galdor* refer to this same passage. The same Latin passage is paralleled in the *Lacnunga*, where it is given context explicitly

---

[58] Grendon, 'The Anglo-Saxon Charms', p. 110; *LAC*, vol. I, xxvii; Jolly, 'Anglo-Saxon Charms in the Context of a Christian World View', p. 284.

[59] For a discussion of all the non-condemnatory usages of term, see Arthur, *'Charms', Liturgies, and Secret Rites*, pp. 24–44.

[60] *LAC*, vol. I, XXVI.

linking it with St John and is listed among several *gebedu* ('prayers'). The close equation of *gebed* and *galdor* can be seen elsewhere in the *Lacnunga* where essentially the same Irish-derived incantation is referred to as both *galdor* and *gebed* in two separate entries.[61] Thus the use of this word alone is not enough to justify relating the contents of the medical collections with the practices forbidden by Ælfric and other late authors, as they apparently rely on two different senses of the same word. Instead, a closer examination of these prohibitive passages is called for in order to understand what types of practices were most concerning.

The words *drycræft* and *galdor* by themselves are not particularly revealing when used prohibitively as they occur most frequently in general lists of forbidden practices rather than in descriptive passages. Yet by looking at them in the context of other less ambiguous practices it is possible to determine at least their general connotations. A good place to begin considering occurrences of these terms is within the genre of texts known as penitentials. Penitentials are handbooks for priests; they include lists of potential offences, which are followed by the corresponding penance to be imposed by the priest. There are four major penitential collections written in Old English: the *Old English Handbook*, the *Old English Penitential* (also sometimes known as the *Penitential of Pseudo-Egbert*), the *Canons of Theodore*, and the *Scriftboc* (also sometimes known as the *Confessional of Pseudo-Egbert*).[62] Penitentials cover wide varieties of different types of offences, such as sexual sins, sins against the clergy or the sacraments, or acts of violence. The organisation of these penitential texts tends to be broadly topical, which allows the reader to see some relationship between various offences. This makes them useful tools for understanding what types of practices would have been associated with broad categories of error such as *drycræft*. With this aim, I have compiled the passages from these sources related to *drycræft* and listed them below. I have only included those references that are specific enough to mention particular activities; additionally, for clarity and space, I have listed only the transgressions and omitted the penance prescribed. I have not listed passages from the *Old English Handbook* (the latest penitential written in Old English) because it reproduces the passage given from the *Old English Penitential* with only minor deviations.[63]

---

[61] BLB, II XLV. 3; LAC, vol. I, LXIV, XXV, LXIII, LXXXIII.

[62] There is some confusion around the titles of these collections. Throughout, I will use the names given by Frantzen in his book and database: Frantzen, *The Literature of Penance*, pp. 132–33; Frantzen, 'Anglo-Saxon Penitentials: A Cultural Database', 'user guide'. It is difficult to date the penitentials precisely. The *Scriftboc*, *Canons of Theodore*, and the *Old English Penitential* all likely date to sometime in the tenth century and the *Old English Handbook* to sometime in the eleventh (Frantzen, *The Literature of Penance*, pp. 134–41).

[63] A discussion of the Latin penitential sources of some of these passages is found in A. Meaney, 'Old English Legal and Penitential Penalties for "Heathenism"',

From the *Old English Penitential*:

Gif ænig man oðerne mid wiccecræfte fordo [...]. Gif hwa drife stacan on ænigne man [...]. Gif hwa wiccige ymbe æniges mannes lufe. & him on æte sylle. oððe on drence. oððe on æniges cynnes galdor cræfte þæt heora lufe forþam þe mare beon sceole [...]. Gif hwa hlytas oððe hwatunga bega oððe his wæccan æt ænigum wylle hæbbe. oððe æt ænigre oðre ge sceafte butan æt godes cyrcean [...]. Wif beo þæs ylcan wyrðe gif heo tilað hire cilde mid ænigum wiccecræfte. oððe æt wega gelætan þurh eorðan tyhð. forþam hit is mycel hæðenscipe. Gif hwylc wif hire bearn mid drenc on hire sylfre fordo hire agenes willes. oððe mid ænigum þingum hit amyrre [...].[64]

[If any one murders another with witchcraft [...]. If someone drives a stake into any person [...]. If someone enchants the love of any person and gives him [something] to eat or to drink, or with *galdor cræft* of any kind that his love shall be greater [...]. If anyone cast lots (*hlytas*) or practise divination (*hwatunga*) or keeps watch at any well or at any other created thing other than at God's church [...]. Let the same befall a woman if she cures her child with any *wiccecræfte* or drags [him or her] through the earth at a crossroads, because this is great heathendom. If some woman kills the child inside her with a drink by her own will, or by anything murders it [...].]

Gif hwylc man his ælmessan gehate oððe bringe to hwylcum wylle. oððe to stane. oððe to treowe. oððe to ænigum oðrum gesceaftum butan on godes naman to godes cyrcean [...] & þeah he geþristlæce þæt he æt swylcum stowum ete oððe drince. & nane lac ne bringe [...]. Nis na soðlice nanum cristenum men alyfed þæt he idela hwatunga bega[65]† swa hæðene men doð þæt is þæt hi gelyfen on sunnan & on monan & on steorrena ryne & secen tida hwatunga hiara þing to beginnene ne wyrta gade runga mid nanum galdre butan mid pater noster & mid credo. oððe mid sumon gebede þe gode belimpe [...].[66]

[If any person vows or brings alms to any well or stone or tree or to any other created thing except in God's name to God's church [...] and though he dares to eat and drink at any place but does not bring any gift [...]. Nor is it allowed that any true Christian man practise vain things

---

in *Anglo-Saxons: Studies Presented to Cyril Roy Hart*, pp. 127–58, at 139–54. Meaney also discusses relevant passages from law codes in this article.

[64] Frantzen, 'Anglo-Saxon Penitentials: A Cultural Database', Oxford, Bodleian Library, MS Laud Misc. 482, f. 15v–16v.

[65] † *Idela hwatunga bega* read according to Raith's edition: *Die altenglische Version des Halitgar'schen Bussbuches*, Bibliothek der angelsächsischen Prosa 13 (Hamburg, 1933), p. 30.

[66] Frantzen, 'Anglo-Saxon Penitentials: A Cultural Database', MS Laud Misc. 482, f. 9r–9v.

(*idela hwatunga*) as heathen men do, that is that they believe in the sun and the moon, and motion of the stars, and seek time-auguries (*tida hwatunga*) [for when to] to begin their deeds, nor shall herbs be gathered with any *galdru*, only with the Pater Noster and with the Creed or some prayer that belongs to God [...].]

From the *Canons of Theodore*:

Gyf hwylc wif wiccunga bega. & þa deofollican galdorsangas [...]. Ða wif ðe doð aworpennysse hyra bearna [...]. Gyf se leaweda man his agen cild ofþrycce. & acwelle [...].[67]

[If any woman goes about witchcraft and devilish *galdor*-songs [...] a woman who casts away (aborts) her child [...]. If a layman restrain his own child forcibly and kills it [...].]

Seo ðe acwelleð hire cild butan fulluhte [...]. Ða ðe onsæcgeað deoflum & þam leasestum þingum [...]. Gyf hwylc wif seteð hire bearn ofer rof. oððe on ofen. for hwilcere untrymðe hælo [...]. Se ðe corn bærneð for lifigendra hælo ðær deade men beoð bebyrgde [...]. On canone hit cwið. se ðe halsunga. & galdorcreaftas. & swefnhrace behealdað. þa beoð on hæðenra manna gerime. And eac swylce þa þe oðre men on ðam drycræft gebringað. gif hy on mynstre syn hy syn ut aworpene. gif hy on folce syn. betan fulre bote.[68]

[She that kills her child before baptism [...]. Those who offer the smallest things to devils [...]. If any woman sets her child on the roof or in the oven to heal it from any sickness [...]. If one burns grains for the health of the living where dead men are buried [...]. In the canon it is written: he who practises auguries (*halsunga*) and *galdor*-crafts, and interpretations of dreams that is the calculations of heathen men. And likewise also those who lead other people into *drycræft*, if they are in a minster let them be thrown out, if they are lay-persons atone with full penance.]

From the *Scriftboc*:

Gif wif drycræft. & galdorcræft. & unlibban wyrce. & swylc bega [...]. Gif heo mid hire unlibban man acwelleð [...]. Wif þæt ðe gæð in cyrcan ærðon heo clæne sy hire blode [...]. Wif seo ðe mencgð weres sæd in hire mete. & ðone þigeð. þæt be þam wæpnedmen sy beo ðe leofre [...]. Wif seo æwyrpe gedo hire geeacnunga in hire hrife. & cwelle [...].[69]

---

[67] Frantzen, 'Anglo-Saxon Penitentials: A Cultural Database', Brussels, Bibl. MS Royale 8558–8563, f. 148v–149r.
[68] Frantzen, 'Anglo-Saxon Penitentials: A Cultural Database', MS Royale 8558–8563, f. 152v–153r.
[69] Frantzen, 'Anglo-Saxon Penitentials: A Cultural Database', Oxford, Bodleian Library, MS Junius 121, f. 93v.

[If a woman goes about *drycræft* and *galdor*-craft, and *unlibban* (poisoning) and such [...]. If she kill someone through her *unlibban* [...]. A woman that enters in the church before she is clean of her blood [...]. A woman who mixes the seed of a man in her food and then eats it, in order that she be more loved by the man [...]. A woman who casts away her fetus in her womb and kills it [...].]

Gif man medlices hwæthwegu deoflum onsægð [...]. Gif he myceles hwæt on secge deoflum [...]. Wif gif heo set hyre dohtor ofer hus. oððe on ofen. forðam þe heo wille feferadle men gehælan [...]. Swa hwylc man swa corn bærne in ðære stowe. þær man dead wære lifigendum mannum to hæle. & in his huse [...]. Swa hwylc man swa feondum gesenodne mete þigeð [...].[70]

[If one offers some small thing to devils [...]. If he offers something large to devils [...]. If a woman sets her daughter on top of the house, or in the oven, in order to heal her fever [...]. So also if anyone burns grains in the place where the dead are to for bringing health to living men and to the house [...]. Thus anyone who eats food that was given to devils [...].]

One of the first things that can be noticed in these passages is the pronounced tendency to link women with the practice of *drycræft*: five of the six passages above mention women in the context of forbidden practices associated with *drycræft*. Some of the passages explicitly describe *drycræft* as a feminine art: in the *Old English Penitential* it is women who practise healing *wiccecræfte*; in the *Canons of Theodore* it is women who use *wiccunga* ('witchcraft'), *halsunga* ('divination'), and devilish *galdorsangas*; in the *Scriftboc* it is women who practise *drycræft*, *galdorcræft*, *unlibban* ('making poisons'), and *hwatung* ('divination') and can kill others with these crafts. Furthermore, although not explicitly labelled as such, the conventionally female act of producing an abortion is the most frequently mentioned crime associated with *drycræft*.

There also appears to have been an unspoken connection between forbidden practices and women in Ælfric's writings. He clearly thought it was possible for either sex to engage in *drycræft*, as can be seen, for instance, in classical examples such as the Egyptian *dry-men* who strove against Moses.[71] However, in his discussion of forbidden medical practices in his homily 'On Auguries', Ælfric comments: *ne sceal se cristena befrinan þa fulan wiccan be his gesundfulnysse þeahðe heo secgan cunne sum ðincg þurh deofol* ('nor shall the Christian ask the foul witch concerning his

---

[70] Frantzen, 'Anglo-Saxon Penitentials: A Cultural Database', MS Junius 121, f. 94r–v.
[71] *Ælfric's Lives of Saints*, p. 372.

health, though she might be able to tell him something by the devil').[72] Earlier in the same homily he writes *ungeswenlica deofol [...] geswutelað þæra wiccan hwæt heo secge mannum þæt þa beon fordone þe ðæne dry-cræft secað* ('the unseen devil [...] makes clear to the witch what she can say to men that they will be undone, those who seek *drycræft*').[73] The use of the female pronoun rather than the neutral *man* in these clauses is noteworthy and suggests that when Ælfric considered healing magic as something actually being practised in his own time, he envisioned a female practitioner. This tendency exhibited in the penitentials and in some passages by Ælfric does not appear to be unusual: Audrey Meaney has gathered a number of additional sources that suggest the active tendency in Anglo-Saxon culture to associate women (in particular) with witchcraft.[74]

The mention of female practitioners of *drycræft* conforms to the larger emphasis on popular practices within these portions of the penitentials. These practices are often associated with heathenism in these texts. Heathenism is mentioned by name in three of the passages cited above, and all of the rituals related to health or healing that are specifically forbidden appear to have their origins in popular practice; these include dragging a child through the dirt at crossroads, burning grains for health, and setting a child upon a roof to cure a fever. There is no indication that these were ever part of learned or ecclesiastical culture and instead appear to represent native tradition. As we have seen, the *Old English Penitential* also mentions *galdru* as a heathen practice and associates it with pagan forms of belief including worshipping the sun and the moon.

Ælfric himself explicitly links the use of *galdru* with heathenism. In his homily for St Bartholomew's day, Ælfric compares those who use *galdru* or *wiccecræft* in pursuit of health to *hæðenum mannum gelic þe ðam deofolgylde geofrodon for heora lichaman hælðe ond swa heora sawla amyrdon* ('heathen men, who offered to an idol for their bodies' health and so destroyed their souls').[75] In a similar vein, in 'On Auguries' he warns not to seek *galdras* for *se ðe þys deð se forlysð his cristen-dom ond bið þam hæðenum gelic* ('whoever does this forsakes his Christianity and is like the heathens').[76] The noun *galdras* (sg. *galdere*) is unusual; it is otherwise only found in glosses for *aruspex* ('diviner') and *marsus* (a term derived from the name of a region in Italy associated with witchcraft); presumably the connotation is one who uses *galdru*.[77] This association between *drycræft* and heathendom is also

---

[72] *Ælfric's Lives of Saints*, p. 372.
[73] *Ælfric's Lives of Saints*, p. 372.
[74] See A. Meaney, *Anglo-Saxon Amulets and Curing Stones* (Oxford, 1981), pp. 255–59; Meaney, 'Women, Witchcraft and Magic in Anglo-Saxon England'.
[75] Clemoes, pp. 449–50.
[76] *Ælfric's Lives of Saints*, 'On Auguries', ll. 78–80.
[77] DOE, s.v. 'galdere, galdre'.

clear in the works of Ælfric's contemporary, Wulfstan. For example, the *Canons of Edgar*, a legal code authored by Wulfstan, reads:

> And we lærað þæt preosta gehwilc cristendom geornlice arære and ælcne hæþendom mid ealle adwæsce and forbeode wilweorþunga and licwiglunga and hwata and galdra and manweorðunga and þa gemearr, þe man drifð on mistlicum gewiglungum and on friðsplottum and on ellenum and eac on oðrum mistlicum treowum and on stanum and on manegum mistlicum gedwimerum, þe men on dreogað fela þæs, þe hi na ne scoldan.[78]

> [And we teach that priests should earnestly exalt Christianity, and extinguish entirely every heathen practice, and forbid spring-worship, and necromancy, and divination, and *galdru*, and man-worship, and error that is practised in many types of sorcery (*gewiglungum*) and in sanctuaries and at elder trees or other various trees and at stones and in many various fallacies, that people perform many of those which they should not.]

Although it is still difficult to know exactly what some of these words mean, this extensive list gives an idea of the types of practices with which Wulfstan was most concerned, among them most notably worship at pagan sites, auguries, and *drycræft* practised at places associated with paganism including trees and stones. For Wulfstan, these acts fall under the larger category of 'heathen practices'. Similar practices are condemned elsewhere by Ælfric, who, like Wulfstan, condemns those who seek healing (or anything else) from holy wells, trees, or stones.[79] Ælfric used the *Old English Penitential* as a source in some of his homilies, and repeats the penitential's condemnation of eating at gravesites, taking love potions or abortifacients, and dragging one's child through the dirt at crossroads.[80]

In some cases, the use of the words *hæþendom* or *hæþenscip* in Old English sources does not imply non-Christian belief or practice but can simply refer to a variety of behaviours. Both Meaney and Thompson have argued that Wulfstan's concept of *hæþenscip* is not static, but, depending upon context, could range in meaning from actual paganism to the conduct of misbehaving Christians, with an emphasis in particular on

---

[78] Wulfstan, *Wulfstan's Canons of Edgar*, ed. R. Fowler (London, 1972), p. 4; cf. Meaney, 'Wulfstan and Late Anglo-Saxon and Norse "Heathenism"', p. 477.

[79] *Ælfric's Lives of Saints*, p. 372. See further Clemoes, p. 450.

[80] *Ælfric's Lives of Saints*, pp. 374, 460, Ælfric's Pastoral Letter for Wulfsige in Ælfric, *Die Hirtenbriefe Ælfrics*, p. 25; cf. Meaney in 'Ælfric and Idolatry', pp. 132–33; *Homilies of Ælfric: A Supplementary Collection*, ed. E. Pope (London, 1967), EETS o.s. 259, 260, p. 796. Meaney discusses Ælfric's use of this source as well as a sermon by Caesarius of Arles. She stresses that Ælfric draws on these sources very freely, emphasising what he thought was significant, and ultimately creating his own independent piece: Meaney, 'Ælfric's Use of his Sources in his Homily on Auguries', pp. 478, 491–93.

those actions associated with superstitious or unorthodox relationship to nature.[81] This second meaning seems clearly present in some of the passages discussed above. However, there is also the possibility that some of these prohibitions may have been linked to active pagan practice.

Ælfric and Wulfstan were living in a time of increased interaction with Scandinavian peoples. This was particularly true in the north, where, in the wake of the first wave of Viking attacks and the arrival of the Great Army in 865, large areas of land had come under Danish control and were settled by the (largely still un-Christianised) Scandinavians. However, by the reign of Æthelred the population in these areas had become to a large extent mixed. The ascension of the Danish leader Cnut to the English throne in 1016 brought with it new waves of settlers.[82] Although Cnut himself is recorded as being, at least officially, a Christian, many of the settlers would not have been when they arrived. The conversion of these settlers, in what later became the 'Danelaw', has traditionally been portrayed as rapid and thorough. However, Lesley Abrams has suggested that their conversion may not have been as immediate as previously imagined and that parts of the Danelaw may not have become Christian until the late tenth century.[83] This could well indicate that Wulfstan especially, whose episcopal see was in the north, may have encountered active heathen practice. Prohibitions against paganism occur in the law code of 'Edward and Guthrum' (authored by Wulfstan):

Prologue:

1. Ðis is ærest, þæt hig gecwædon, þæt hi ænne God lufian woldan ond ælcne hæþendom georne aworpen.
2. ond gif hwa Cristendom wyrde oððe hæþendom weorþige wordes oððe weorces, gylde swa wer swa wite swa lahslitte, be þam þe syo dæd sy.[84]

---

[81] A. Meaney, 'Women, Witchcraft and Magic in Anglo-Saxon England'; A. Meaney, '"And we forbeodað eornostlice ælcne hæðenscipe": Wulfstan and Late Anglo-Saxon and Norse "Heathenism"', in *Wulfstan, Archbishop of York: Proceedings of the Second Alcuin Conference*, ed. M. Townend (Turnhout, 2004), pp. 461–500, at 471; Thompson, *Dying and Death*, p. 36.
[82] J. Jesch, 'Scandinavians and "Cultural Paganism" in Late Anglo-Saxon England', in *The Christian Tradition in Anglo-Saxon England: Approaches to Current Scholarship and Teaching*, ed. P. Cavill (Cambridge, 2004), pp. 55–68, at 57.
[83] L. Abrams, 'The Conversion of the Danelaw', in *Vikings and the Danelaw*, ed. J. Graham-Campbell, R. Hall, J. Jesch, and D. N. Parsons (Oxford, 2001), pp. 31–44, at 40.
[84] *Councils and Synods with other Documents Relating to the English Church*, ed. D. Whitelock, M. Brett, and C. N. L. Brooke (Oxford, 1981), vol. I, pp. 304–06; cf. Jesch, 'Scandinavians and "Cultural Paganism"', pp. 63–64. For the attribution of this law code to Wulfstan, see *Councils and Synods*, vol. I, p. 302.

> [1. This is first, that they said that they would love one God and would earnestly put aside every heathen practice.
> 2. And if anyone injures Christendom or venerates heathendom with words or deeds, [he must] pay *wergild* or a punishment or *lahslit*, according to the deed done.]

The second injunction is noteworthy for its inclusion of the Scandinavian legal term *lahslit*, which indicates that it was directed towards Scandinavian settlers in the Danelaw.[85] This would at least suggest that in this case 'honouring heathendom by word or deed' was to have been meant literally and not simply as a shorthand for any type of inappropriate behaviour.

Both Ælfric and Wulfstan make mention of Englishmen joining the Viking cause. Wulfstan gives the examples of serfs who *hlaforde ætleape and of cristendom to wicinge wurðe* ('abandon their lord and leave Christianity to become Vikings').[86] In his *Natale Quadraginta militum*, Ælfric also reflects on the possibility of apostasy to the Viking cause:

> Swa fela manna gebugað mid ðam gecorenum, to Cristes geleafan on his Gelaðunge, þæt hy sume yfele eft ut abrecað, and hy on gedwyldum adreogað heora lif, swa swa þa Engliscan men doð þe to ðam Deniscum gebugað, and mearciað hy deofle to his mannrædene, and his weorc wyrcað, hym sylfum to forwyrde, and heora agene leode belæwað to deaðe.[87]

> [So many men submit with the chosen to belief in Christ and in his Church, [then] some through evil again break away, and they offer their lives to error, as Englishmen do who submit to the Danes and submit themselves to pay homage to the devil and perform his work. [In doing this] they destroy themselves and betray their own people to death.]

This same anxiety about English persons defecting to the Danish cause can also be seen in the anonymous 'Letter to Brother Edward', presumed to have been written by Ælfric. The author berates his brother for having taken up the customs of *hæðenra manna* ('heathen people'), which apparently included dressing in the Danish fashion.[88] These references suggest

---

[85] Jesch, 'Scandinavians and "Cultural Paganism"', p. 64. The term *lahslit* also occurs in injunctions against heathenism in the 'Law of the Northumbrian Priests', a code probably written by a successor of Wulfstan to the archbishopric.

[86] *The Homilies of Wulfstan*, ed. D. Bethurum (Oxford, 1957), xx (c), ll. 98–103, cited in M. Godden, 'Apocalypse and Invasion in Late Anglo-Saxon England', in *From Anglo-Saxon to Early Middle English: Studies Presented to E. G. Stanley*, ed. M. Godden, D. Gray, and T. Hoad (New York, 1994), pp. 130–62, at 148.

[87] *Homilies of Ælfric: A Supplementary Collection*, no. xiv, ll. 128–35, cited in Godden, 'Apocalypse and Invasion in Late Anglo-Saxon England', p. 139.

[88] M. Clayton, 'An Edition of Ælfric's Letter to Brother Edward', in *Early Medieval English Texts and Interpretations: Studies Presented to Donald G. Scragg*, ed. E. Treharne and S. Rosser (Temple, 2002), pp. 263–83, at 280–83; cf. S. Keynes, 'An

that both Ælfric and Wulfstan were plagued by a degree of fear that some might be tempted away from English political and religious customs to embrace those of the new Scandinavian settlers. This fear of apostasy, or backsliding into prior pagan practices, may underlie some of the prohibitions against heathenism in these texts. John Blair has suggested the influx of Scandinavian settlers might help explain the rise of prohibitions against worshiping stones, trees, and springs, which he contrasts with the earlier period where such observances appear to have been viewed as sufficiently integrated into Christianity (principally through assigning of such sites to local saints).[89] Perhaps the paganism that worried these authors was Norse rather than traditionally Anglo-Saxon. In this case, it might not be a stretch to suggest that *drycræft*, intimately connected with *hæthendom*, could have also in some cases referred to Norse practices.

Whether Ælfric and Wulfstan were primarily concerned about Norse paganism or residual folk practices in Christianised England, the emphasis in all these texts seems to be on suppressing public practices, rather than on condemning anything learned. This can be particularly seen in the repeated references to the worship of natural sites and prohibitions against the bringing of offerings or eating and drinking there, as well as in the suggestion that *drycræft* was seen as a traditionally feminine art. The penitential texts alongside the writings of Ælfric and Wulfstan offer a fairly uniform picture and probably give a reliable indication of what *drycraeft* would have meant in the late Anglo-Saxon period. This 'popular' depiction of *drycræft* can be contrasted with the learned type of 'magic' that was indeed a phenomenon in the Late Antique period and Early Middle Ages on the continent. This is the variety that Peter Brown invokes when he describes sorcery as 'an occult skill to which anyone can resort'. He writes: 'Late Roman sorcery was an "art". It was an art consigned to great books. To possess or transcribe such books might jeopardise the owner, but their destruction was accepted as sufficient guarantee of the change of heart of the sorcerer.'[90] Discussion of this type of forbidden learned practice concentrated in books is seemingly entirely absent in Old English descriptions of *drycræft* and *galdru*. It is unlikely that a learned author such as Ælfric could have been completely unaware of this tradition, and it finds a place in some of his source authors. However, this type of practice does not seem to have been his concern when it came to practically admonishing his readers.

  Abbot, an Archbishop, and the Viking Raids of 1006–7 and 1009–12', *ASE* 37 (2007), 151–220.
[89] J. Blair, *The Church in Anglo-Saxon Society* (Oxford, 2005), pp. 481–82.
[90] P. Brown, 'Sorcery, Demons, and the Rise of Christianity: From Late Antiquity into the Middle Ages', in *Religion and Society in the Age of Saint Augustine* (London, 1972), pp. 119–46, at 139.

The Old English Medical Collections and the Question of Galdru

Many of the remedies already discussed in this book are found in various collections of 'charms' or Anglo-Saxon 'magical' texts. The remedies examined in the chapter on the *Lacnunga*, in particular, are likely to be considered to be charms. The most prominent medical remedies occurring in charm-related discussions are the metrical charms in Old English. However, the 'gibberish' remedies with (sometimes unintelligible) words in exotic tongues such as Old Irish, Greek, and Hebrew are considered to be charms by both Grendon and Storms. Additionally, remedies containing ritualistic elements (such as the call for Latin prayers) are often considered to be Christian charms. The prohibitions made against *galdru* by Ælfric and other late Anglo-Saxon authors are routinely evoked in discussions of remedies of these types.

However, although some entries from the medical texts are often considered 'magical' by critics, it is worth observing that they look nothing like most of the practices explicitly condemned in the theology of late Anglo-Saxon England. As we have seen, those practices include: the worship of springs, wells, stones, or trees; building sanctuaries or eating at these places; offering sacrifices to the devil; eating food sacrificed to devils; divination; murdering through witchcraft; using love potions; using abortifacients; poisoning; dragging one's child through the earth; setting one's child on a roof; cursing one's enemies; and burning grains for health. None of these practices occur in the Old English medical corpus. The only possible exceptions to this are the prohibitions against gathering herbs using *galdru* or wearing amulets, which, depending on one's definitions, may resemble some practices in the medical texts. However, in each case that a text gives such a prohibition, it is softened by suggesting that Christian prayers can be used when gathering herbs, and Christian relics can be used as amulets.

In fact, it is striking how little the medical texts resemble these forbidden activities. In the entire corpus of medical literature, we find not a single recipe for a love potion, an abortifacient, poison, or for cursing enemies. There are some remedies that may have worked as abortifacients but there is no clear evidence that this was their intention.[91] In all of Ælfric's homilies and saints' lives there is no mention of practices (most typical of the *Lacnunga*) such as the use of communion wafers or the use of holy water in several remedies that have been sometimes singled out as unorthodox by critics. Additionally, there is no mention of clerics or learned individuals as the purveyors of forbidden forms of medicine.

---

[91] Certain remedies from the *Old English Herbarium* appear to be emmenagogic in nature and could possibly have been used to produce abortions. However, it is more likely that these remedies would have been understood as regulating the menstrual cycle and promoting fertility (see Chapter 4, p. 146).

Instead, ecclesiastical works from the period stress that it is *ill-learned* persons who both provide and desire illicit healing. As we have seen, the figures most often associated with forbidden forms of healing are not priests but women. Indeed, in her comparison of 'On Auguries' with its source material, Meaney finds that Ælfric chooses to emphasise the foolishness of those who seek medical aid from illicit healers, describing them scornfully as *ablende* ('blinded') and *stuntlice* ('foolish') men and *gewitlease* ('witless') women.[92]

I would argue that the image being fostered in the penitentials (and echoed in the writings of Ælfric and Wulfstan) is of lay healers engaged in popular superstitious practices and the 'foolish' folk that frequent them. This image is contrary to the generally learned traditions found within the Old English medical collections. As we have seen, a great part of the 'charms' found within the medical collections come from a literate textual tradition and recent scholarship has emphasised the closeness of these practices and ecclesiastical rites. Certainly, the *galdru* involving tongues other than Old English are products of an educated textual tradition and would only have been available to the smallest section of Anglo-Saxon society – most likely those in monastic orders or secular clerics. It is possible that some of the metrical cures in Old English derive from popular oral traditions. However, by the time the medical collections were compiled and copied by scribes even these pieces had become textual artefacts.

In all the passages related to *galdru* there is no hint that Ælfric is worried about learned error infecting his flock. In other passages in his homilies it is clear that he was concerned by the spread of heresies in England, including the reading of apocryphal texts, yet he never uses the term *galdor* or *drycræft* in association with these dangers.[93] It seems that when these late Anglo-Saxon authors envisioned the practice of *drycræft* it was as something popular, rather than learned. As Ciaran Arthur has also argued, it is very likely then that when Ælfric and these other late Anglo-Saxon authors discuss *galdru* they are using the term in a different sense from how we find it used in the medical texts.[94] If Ælfric was suspicious of exotic incantations or poetic pieces recorded in books, it is surprising that he fails to mention them even once. It could be suggested that this could be partly a question of the audience of his works. The intended

---

[92] *Ælfric's Lives of Saints*, pp. 372, 374, cited in Meaney, 'Ælfric's use of His Sources in His Homily on Auguries', p. 495.

[93] Ælfric generally uses the words *gedwola* ('error') or *lease gesetnysse* ('false writings') to refer to what he considered either apocryphal works or heresy. For more on Ælfric's use of these terms, see F. Biggs, 'An Introduction and Overview of Recent Work', in *Apocryphal Texts and Traditions in Anglo-Saxon England*, ed. K. Powell and D. Scragg (Cambridge, 2003), pp. 18–21. See also T. Hall, 'Ælfric and the Epistle to the Laodicians', in *Apocryphal Texts and Traditions in Anglo-Saxon England*, pp. 65–84.

[94] Cf. Arthur, *'Charms', Liturgies, and Secret Rites*, pp. 12–17.

audience of Ælfric's homilies has been a much-debated question. The fact that they are written in Old English vernacular perhaps indicates an ill-educated, non-Latin reading audience, and the introduction to the first volume makes this explicit, where Ælfric writes that he has translated this text because *ungelærede menn* have so little access to books containing correct doctrine.[95] However, in the introduction to his more recent edition of the homilies, Godden suggests a more mixed audience, writing: 'if the primary target audience was the laity and their ill-educated preachers, there is also much in the Catholic Homilies that reflects the specialist concerns of monks, the clergy and the more learned.'[96] In this setting, counsel against dangerous reading, or improper learning, would not have seemed out of place.

It is difficult to imagine that Ælfric did not know that collections similar to the extant Old English medical texts existed. Ælfric was bishop in Winchester, where the Royal manuscript containing *Bald's Leechbook* and *Leechbook III* was very likely located and the *Old English Pharmacopeia* may well have been first translated, which is of course not to mention the source texts that underlie these works, some of which would almost certainly have been found in Winchester as well. It seems untenable that a learned man like Ælfric would have been unfamiliar with material found in his own library.

The emphasis on *drycræft* as a traditional rather than learned threat is found not only in Ælfric's writings but, as we have seen, also in other late Anglo-Saxon sources including Wulfstan's writings and the Old English penitential tradition. The penitential texts were certainly intended to cover the crimes of all of society and include penance recommendations for the laity, but also for clerics and those in monastic orders. In this setting, counsel against dangerous reading, or improper learning, would not have been out of place. Yet in none of these texts is there any mention of forbidden books, dangerous reading, written charms, or statements against religious rituals being used the way they are in some medical remedies. This seems to suggest that these types of practices were not their concern.

Medicine and Faith

In this book I would like to suggest that the Old English medical collections formed an intimate part of the wider intellectual culture of the Anglo-Saxon period. Each of the extant collections was likely compiled at a monastic house of some size and importance. In some cases, as with *Bald's Leechbook* and the *Old English Herbarium*, these were likely among the most prominent

---

[95] Clemoes, p. 174.
[96] *Ælfric's Catholic Homilies: Introduction, Commentary and Glossary*, p. xxvi.

houses in England. All four collections, however, contain contents drawing on multiple source texts, whether from Latin medical treatises, liturgical books, hermeneutic poems in Anglo-Latin, or vernacular medicine and poetry. Whether or not they represent practices typical across wide segments of society, these texts are the best examples of learned and academic medicine from the period. These collections also provide the best evidence for what may have characterised the practices envisioned by literary authors who wrote of doctors, as these authors in most cases would have shared a similar learned milieu to the compilers of the medical texts.

Although the Old English medical collections have sometimes been depicted as fringe texts, representing popular belief and lingering on the edges of orthodoxy, they should instead be viewed alongside literary depictions of medicine from the period. It is of course difficult to know the social position of various types of medical practitioners throughout Anglo-Saxon England or how they may have been viewed by the general population. However, within the learned sphere it is clear that the medical art was highly respected. In both poetry and didactic works from Anglo-Saxon England the *læce* is a figure granted approbation and respect – they are depicted as learned figures, employing an important art.

While it is clear that medicine was an accepted (even acclaimed) art, it shared a sometimes uncomfortable boundary with less theologically acceptable forms of healing. However, as has been seen, the predominance of evidence suggests that the term *drycræft* (and by extension *galdru*) reflects types of popular folk traditions, rather than any type of learned magical art, at least when used by the reformers in the late Anglo-Saxon period. Although the medical texts are always brought into discussions about magic or charms in Anglo-Saxon England, there is remarkably little similarity between these texts and the actual practices associated with *drycræft*.

We can observe in this period, in particular during the late-tenth and eleventh centuries, instead an increased concern with popular and pagan practices. John Blair has suggested that this increased anxiety (which is manifest during the period not only in penitentials and homilies but also in law codes) arose partially in response to the recent influx of pagan and recently pagan Danes in the North, but may also reflect concerns over the imminent arrival of the Antichrist, at which time there would be *mare [...] wracu ond gedrecednes þonne æfre ær wære ahwar on worulde* ('more [...] suffering and tribulation than there was anywhere in the world ever before').[97] This background may help to contextualise the strong prohibitions against popular practices found in the sources from this period,

---

[97] *The Homilies of Wulfstan*, III, 11–12. See also: Blair, *The Church in Anglo-Saxon Society*, pp. 481–82; P. Wormald, *The Making of English Law: King Alfred to the Twelfth Century* (Oxford, 1999), pp. 451–60.

but should not affect our reading of the generally learned and accepted materials found within the Old English medical corpus.

Indeed, authors from this period offer instead a very favourable reading of the study and practice of medicine. Ælfric and Wulfstan have both been frequently characterised as exceptionally strict on issues such as the use of charms or magic, yet their positive stance on medical treatment has never been emphasised. While there could have been precedent for rejecting the practice of medicine, the use of medicinal herbs and prayers is fully accepted and approved of in Ælfric's writings. Indeed, Ælfric's multi-faceted approach towards both sickness and healing allowed for many alternatives when it came to both cause and cure of disease. Sickness could be a result of sin, but it also could be a sign of divine favour. All healing ultimately came from God, but it could come miraculously or through a doctor's poultice. Even when it comes to forbidding certain types of healing, I would suggest that Ælfric's position is not an extreme one. It is clear that he perceived popular paganism (or the remnants of paganism) as a problem during his time. Yet although Ælfric clearly condemned certain types of popular practices, there is substantially less evidence that he had the same concern about the learned medical practices of his day, even if these may seem unorthodox to some modern readers.

The number and variety of vernacular medical collections extant from Anglo-Saxon England is unparalleled in Europe during the Early Middle Ages, a fact that itself suggests that the formal study of medicine was held in high esteem. This may have been particularly true within the monastic houses or cathedral sites where these various collections were most likely compiled and copied. For these monks and members of the clergy, the figure of Christ as the 'good physician' or the priest as the idealised 'doctor of souls' would be familiar concepts, not least through the writings of Gregory, often considered to be the father of the English Church.

A favourable view of medical learning likely helped to give rise to the importation into England of Latin texts on medical topics, probably in much larger numbers than testified to by the manuscript record, but also to the production of a group of texts in the vernacular language, which preserved Latin remedies alongside prayers, liturgical material, and native medical traditions. The creation of such texts was unique in the period. These texts did not arrive by chance but represent the result of considerable effort, skill, and resources. The Old English medical collections should be viewed as not only an important stage in the development of vernacular medical traditions but also as one of the intellectual and literary achievements of England in the Early Middle Ages.

Appendices

Extended Quotations

Appendix A: Bald's Leechbook *and its Latin Source Material*

This appendix shows remedies from Bald's Leechbook *in parallel with their probable Latin sources (those portions directly incorporated into the Old English text are given in bold). More information on these texts can be found in the introduction. Citations follow those used in the body of the text, except the passages from the* Latin Alexander, *which are taken from Angers, Bibliothèque Municipale MS 457. For these transcriptions I am indebted to David Langslow, who very kindly shared them with me at an early stage of his work towards the first critical edition of the* Latin Alexander; *the translations are my own. For more information on the Greek original of this text and its manuscript tradition, see Langslow,* The Latin Alexander.

Bald's Leechbook II, Chapter 21

Old English	Latin Sources
1 Her sint tacn aheardodre lifre ge on þam læppum ond healocum ond filmenum. Sio aheardung is on twa wisan gerad. Oþer biþ on fruman ær þon þe ænig oþer earfeþe on lifre becume. oþeru æfter oþrum earfeþum þære lifre cymð. sio biþ butan sare.	Liber tertius 43.1 a Incipit curatio scleriae, ex qua incipit causa epatis. Nam ideo intelligitur et discernitur inter scleriam et scirrosin, quod **duritia a se incipiat et nulla fuit ante eparis causa[s]**. Scirrosis autem, quamuis et ipsa duritia dicatur et <similia habeat et> nomina et signa, tamen inde agnoscitur atque discernitur ab scleria, quod ante scirrosin multae eparis causae fuerint. Nam scirrosis esse non potest, nisi fuerit phlegmone iecoris aut dolor. Ergo cum haec cognoueris, scleriae congrua auxilia sunt adhibenda.

2 ond þonne se man mete þigð þonne awyrpð he eft ond onwendeþ his hiw ond hæfð ungewealdene wambe ond þa micgean. ond þonne þu ðine handa setst ufan on þa lifre þonne beoð swa hefige swa stan ond ne biþ sar. gif þæt lange swa biþ þonne gehæfþ hit on uneþelicne wæterbollan.	<u>Liber tertius 48.1</u> b Incipit \<de\> scirrosi id est duritia iecoris. Signa habent haec: Duritia est in iecore grandis, sine dolore. **Cum escam acceperint, eam reiciunt. Colorem immutant et uentrem non facilem habent \<et\> urinam similiter. Et cum manus imposueris super iecur, sentis quomodo lapidem sic esse, et non eis dolet, et si ista causa in longum tempus protrahi\<tur\>, hydropicum facit, qui hydropicus non curatur.**
3 Ealle þa blawunge ond þa welmas þa þe beoþ gehwær geond þone lichoman. þa cumað of hatum blode ond weallendum. swa bið eac swilce on ðære lifre to ongitanne hwæþer sio hæto ond sio ablawung sie on þære lifre selfre on þam filmenum. ond on þam þingum þe ymbutan þa lifre beoþ. ond hwæþer hio sie on ðam liferbylum ond læppum þe on þam liferholum ond healcum þe on þam dælum bæm. þonne se læce þæt ongit þonne mæg he þone læcedom þe raðor findan.	<u>Latin Alexander II. 57</u> c **Q(uonia)m quidem omnes inflammationes de calido et feruido sanguine in toto corpore generantur sic etiam in epate ab omnibus fieri +-sapientibus -+ dictum est. Quomodo autem oporteat agnoscere aut discernere seu in ipso epate contingat inflammatio siue in tunicis ipsius aut in aliquibus locis sit qui extrinsecus circumposita sunt considerari oportet.** Neque enim mox febris fit nisi aliqua inflammatio sit in epate. Iterum contemplari oportet et p(er)quirere seu circa **(epa)tis patiatur quam nos gibbam dicimus siue sima quam nos concauam epatis partem dicimus aut pariter ambe partes inflammationem patiantur. Si enim hec omnia cognoscuntur uel determinantur, curatio fit citata et sine aliquo impedimento adhibentur adiutoria.**

4 Þis synd þa tacn. gif sio ablawung sio hate biþ on þære lifre ofrum oððe bylum þonne biþ þær micel aþundenes ond fefer mid sweopunga⁺ omena ond stingende sar oþ þa wiþoban oð ða eaxle ond hwosta ond nearones breosta ond mare hefignes þonne sar ond þonne sio ablawung bið on þam filmenum ond on þam ædrum þe on ond ymb þa lifre beoð þonne biþ þæt sar scearpre þonne þæs welmes sar þe on þære lifre selfre beoð ond þu meaht be þon ongitan þæt sio adl biþ þære lifre læppum ond ofrum.	Latin Alexander II. 58 d Signa si in cirta epatis flegmon fuerit, Si ergo in cirta magis quam alibi fiat. facilem autem habet cognitionem et maxime si in magnum uenerit tumorem tunc **etiam febres fiunt causodes cum uomitu colerum et sepius iodis et dolor usque ad iugulum uenit. et tussis mouetur. et coangustantur praecordia et grauatur amplius locus quam dolor consistat. Fit etiam et in tunicis epatis flegmon uel in uenis que circa epatem sunt quibus acutissimi dolores plus quam in ipso epate fiunt. His etiam signis inflammatio epatis certa esse cognoscitur** et uisu uel tactu uel aliis supradictis signis. Quod si non grandem contigerit esse flegmonem sed paruum difficilius cognoscetur. Neque enim mox febris fit nisi aliquo op(er)e p(rae)cio extendatur magnitudine. Neque enim oculis p(er)spicitur neque tactu manifestius poterit sciri sed est eius cognitio ex aliis signis. Si ergo p(er)spiciatur a nobis respirare fortius infirmus et grauitatem in ea sentiat parte cum dolore sciendum est inflammationem aliquantam in ipso aut circa ipsum esse epatem.

5 Gif þonne sio lifre aheardung ond sio adl ond sio ablawung biþ on þære lifre healcum ond holocum gecenned þonne þincþ him sona on fruman þæt sio wæte swiþor niþor gewite þonne hio upstige. ond se mon geswogunga þrowað ond modes geswæþrunga. ne mæg him se lichoma batian ac he bið blac ond þynnne ond acolod ond forþon ætfilð him wæterbolla.	Latin Alexander II. 59 e Signa si in simma epatis inflammatio fuerit. **Si autem in simma epatis fuerit flegmon generatus. hoc modo cognoscetur. Mox enim in principio in inferioribus magis partibus uidetur esse tumor quam in superioribus. Angustias quoque cum defectione animi patitur nec corpus reficitur sed pallidus efficitur et extenuatur corpore infrigdato. Igitur et ydrops subsequitur.** Hoc enim modo in simma epatis inflammationem oportet discernere a cirta epatis.

[1] 'Here are the signs of a hardened liver either in the lobes or the crevices or the membranes. The hardening occurs in two manners: one is from the beginning before there is any other condition in the liver, the second comes after other pains of the liver; it is without soreness.'

[a] 'Here begins the treatment of *scleria*, from which a condition of the liver arises. Indeed, for this reason it is known and distinguished between *scleria* and *scirrosis*, that the **hardening begins by itself and there has been no earlier condition of the liver. But** *scirrosis*, **although it too is called hardness and it has both similar names and symptoms, nevertheless it is recognised and distinguished from** *scleria* **because there have been many conditions of the liver before** *scirrosis*. **For it cannot be** *scirrosis*, **if there has not been inflammation of the liver or pain.** Therefore, when you have recognised this, suitable remedies for *scleria* should be employed.'

[2] ' […] and when the person eats food, then throws it up again and he changes his colour and has lack of control over his stomach and urine, and when you set your hand over the liver it is as heavy as a stone and it is not sore. If it is like that for a long time, then it becomes a dropsy that is difficult to cure.'

[b] 'Here begins [the section] concerning *scirrosis*, which is hardening of the liver. The signs are these: great hardness in the liver, without pain. **When they have taken food, they throw it up. They change color and do not have an easy stomach, and likewise urine. And when you have placed hands over the liver, you feel it to be just like a rock, and it does not hurt them, and if that situation continues for a long time, it creates a dropsy, and this dropsy cannot be cured.'**

[3] 'All the inflammation and swellings that are anywhere throughout the body come from hot and boiling blood, so it is also to be understood of the liver whether the heat or swelling be on the liver itself, or on the membranes, or on the things which are around the liver, and whether they are on the bulges of the liver or on the lobes, or in the hollows or in the crevices or on both of those parts. When the doctor understands this, then he may more quickly find the treatment.'

[c] '**Since, indeed, all inflammations in the whole body are generated from hot and boiling blood, so also it is said by all wise men to be thus also in the liver. How therefore one should know or learn whether the inflammation**

Appendices

happens in the liver itself or in its membranes or if it is in other places which are externally located around it. Neither is there fever soon, unless any sort of inflammation is in the liver. Again, it is necessary to understand and examine whether it is felt around the liver, which we call a lump, or the *sima*, which we call the hollow part of the liver or if both parts equally endure the inflammation. Truly, if all these things are known or figured out, the cure is speeded up and aid is applied without impediment.'

[4] 'These are the signs, if the swelling, the heat, is either on the liver edges or the bulges, then there is great swelling and fever with burning inflammation, and stinging soreness all the way to the collar-bone to the shoulder and cough and distress (tightness) of the chest, and more heaviness than soreness, then the swelling is on the membrane and on the veins which are on and around the liver, then that soreness is more sharp than the soreness of the inflammation which is on the liver itself, and you can understand by this that the illness is on the lobes and edges of the liver.'

[+] Being read as *sweolunga* in keeping with Cockayne's edition.

[d] 'Signs if there is inflammation in the *cyrta* of the liver. If therefore there is more in the *cyrta* than in other places, it is easy to recognise and especially if it comes with a big swelling, the **fevers become extreme fevers with vomiting of dark biles, and more often of violet colour, and the pain extends until the collar bone, and a cough is produced, the chest is constricted, and the area is weighed down more widely than the pain occupies. Also the inflammation happens in the membrane of the liver or in the veins which are around the liver, in which the pains become sharper than in the liver itself. With these signs, it is recognised that inflammation of the liver is certain**: by seeing or touching of the above-mentioned signs. It is more difficult to recognise if the inflamed swelling happens to be not big but small. Indeed, neither will there be fever soon, if it is not extended in size with any significant work, neither can it be seen by the eyes, nor can it be known more clearly by touch, but its knowledge is by other signs. Therefore if the infirm is seen by us breathing more strongly, and if he feels heaviness in that same part with pain we must know that there is some inflammation in or around the liver itself.'

[5] 'If however the hardening of the liver and the sickness and the swelling are produced on the crevices and hollows of the liver, then it seems to him immediately from the beginning that the humour (liquid) goes downward rather than rising up, and the person suffers with fainting and failings of the mind; for him, the body may not heal but he is pale, and thin, and chilled, and therefore dropsy afflicts him.'

[e] 'Signs if inflammation is in the *sima* (bottom) of the liver. If then inflammation is generated in the hollows (bottom) of the liver, this is how it is known: indeed, immediately from the beginning the swelling seems to be greater in the lower part rather than the upper part. Also, [the infirm] suffers constrictions with fainting, neither is the body nourished but it becomes pale, and it becomes thin as the body is chilled. Therefore, dropsy follows. For in this way one should distinguish inflammation in the *sima* of the liver from [one in] the *cyrta* of the liver.'

Bald's Leechbook *I, Chapter 18*

Old English	Latin Sources
1 Hwonan se micla geoxa cume oþþe hu his mon tican scule. Se cymð of þam swiðe acolodan magan. oþþe of þam to swiðe ahatodan. oððe of to micelre fylle. oþþe of to micelre lærnesse. oððe of yfelum wætan. slitendum ond sceorfendum þone magan. gif þonne se seoca man þurh spiwedrenc aspiwð þone yfelan bitendan wætan on weg. þonne forstent se geohsa. spiwe þa deah þam monnum þe for fylle gihsa slihð oððe forþon þe hie INnan scyrfð ond eac se geohsa se þe of þæs yfelan wætan micelnysse cymð hæfð þearfe spiwdrinces. se wyrcð micelne fnoran eac ond se hine bet. Þonne se geohsa of þære idlan wambe cymð ond of þære gelæran ne bet þone se fnora. Gif se geohsa of cile cume þonne sceal mon mid wyrmendum þingum lacnian swile swa pipor is ond oþra wermenda wyrta oþþe rudan gegnide mon owin[+] selle drincan. oþþe merces sæd mid wine oþþe eced selle drincan oððe mintan broð oþþe moran. oððe cymenes oþþe gingifran hwilum anlepig swa gerenode. hwilum þa wyrta togædere gedon on þæt wos selle drincan.	Oribasius V 43 a **Singultus fit aut ex plenitudine, aut de evacuatione, vel inaninate, aut certe ex acros humores mordicationem in stomacho facta, sed mox vomuerit humores, requiescit singultus.** Multi etiam antidotum dia trion pipereon acceptum, si mox biberint vinum, singultum patiuntur. Similiter etiam et piper solus acceptus aliquibus facere solit; nam multis cum corruptus fuerit in ventre cibus, singultum patiuntur; aliqui etiam cum degelaberint, singultiunt. **Curatio: hii ergo qui ex plenitudinem aut mordicationem humorum singultiunt, sufficientem adjutorium per vomitum adjutorium invenitur. Nam si de frigidore efficitur, calefaciendus est;** si autem ex plenitudinem humorum fit singultus, evacuandus est. **Hoc autem et sternutamenta adhibita faciunt. Quod si de evacuatione aut inanitate fiat singultus, sanat si sternutatio ad bibendum ruta cum vino,** aut nitrum in mulsa, **aut apii semen, aut daucu, aut cyminu, aut gingiver,** aut calaminthes, aut nardu Celtices.

[1] 'Where the great spasm comes from and how one ought to attend to it. It comes from a very cold stomach or from one that is very hot, or one that is overly full or one that is very empty, or from harmful humours rending and cutting at the stomach. If then the sick person throws up the harmful biting humours (liquids) with an emetic drink then the spasm goes away. Vomiting then is of use for those persons who are attacked by spasm due to fullness, or also when

Appendices

it cuts at them within, and also the spasm which comes of the abundance of harmful humours (liquids) has need of an emetic drink that produces much sneezing and make him well. When the spasms come from a void(?) or empty stomach sneezing will not cure it. If the spasm comes from chill, then one must treat it with warming things, such as pepper, or other warming herbs or one can give *rudan* rubbed in wine to drink or give to drink *merces* seed with wine or vinegar or *mintan* broth or *moran* or *cymen* or *gingifer*, sometimes separately prepared like this, sometimes give the plants put together in the juice to drink.'

[+] Being read as *on win*, as in Cockayne's edition.

[a] **'Spasm arises from fullness, or from emptying or emptiness, or certainly from sharp humours, biting produced in the stomach, but as soon as one vomits the humours, the spasm will cease.** Many people also suffer from spasm, if they immediately drink wine having taken the antidote of three peppers. Likewise, too, even pepper eaten on its own usually creates spasm in some people. For many when food is corrupted in their stomach suffer spasm; some, even when they are thawed out, spasm. **Remedy: therefore, for those who spasm from excessive fullness or corrosion by humours, help through vomiting has been found to be sufficient aid. If it is caused by cold, let him [the patient] be warmed**, but if the spasm comes from an excess of humours, [he] must be emptied. **They do this too when sternutatory remedies have been offered. Because if the spasm comes from emptiness or emptying, a sternutatory is administered: *ruta* with wine**, or *nitrum* in sweetened wine, **or *apium*, or carrot, or *cyminu*, or *gingiver***, or calaminthes, or Celtic nard.'

Appendix B: Parallel Passages in the Lacnunga and MS CCCC 41

This appendix shows the correspondences between some remedies found in MS Cambridge Corpus Christi College 41 and MS Harley 585. The remedies found in the two manuscripts are presented in parallel, with translations following in footnotes. For the remedies from the Lacnunga I have supplied the translations found in Pettit's edition; the translations of CCCC 41 are my own. In the second entry, I have put the parts paralleled in the two remedies in bold for clarity.

CCCC 41	Harley 585
<u>Marginalia p. 206</u>	<u>Entry CXLIX</u>
1 Þis man sceal cweðon ðonne his ceapa hwilcne man forstolenne. Cwyð ær he ænyg oþer word cweðe:	a Þonne þe mon ærest secge þæt þin ceap sy losod, þonne cweð þu ærest ær þu elles hwæt cweþe:
'Bathlem hattæ seo burh ðe Crist on geboren wes. Seo is gemærsod ofer ealne middangeard; Swa ðeos dæd wyrþe for mannum mære, per crucem Cristi.'	'Bæðleem hatte seo buruh þe Crist on acænned wæs. Seo is gemærsad geond ealne middangeard; Swa þyos dæd for monnum mære gewurþe, Þurh þa haligan Cristes rode. Amen.'
ond gebide þe þonne þriwa east and cweð þriwa: 'Cristi ab oriente reducat'; ond in west ond cweð: 'Crux Cristi ab occidente reducat'; ond in suð ond cweð: 'Crux Cristi a meridie reducant'; ond in norð ond cweð: 'Crux Cristi abscondita sunt & inventa est; Iudeas Crist ahengon, gedidon him dæda þa wyrstan, hælon þæt hi forhelan ne mihton; swa næfre ðeos dæd forholen ne wyrðe; per crucem Cristi.'	Gibide þe þonne þriwa east ond cweþ þonne þriwa: 'Crux Cristi ab oriente reducað'; gebide þe þonne þriwa west ond cweð þonne þriwa: 'Crux Cristi ab occidente reducat'; gebide þe þonne þriwa suð ond cweþ þriwa: 'Crux Cristi ab austro reducat'; gebide þonne þriwa norð ond cweð / þriwa: 'Crux Cristi ab aquilone reducað; Crux Cristi abscondita est et inuenta est; Iudeas Crist ahengon, dydon dæda þa wyrrestan, hælon þæt hy forhelan ne mihtan; swa þeos dæd nænige þinga f[o]rholen ne wurþe, þurh þa haligan Cristes rode. Amen.'

Gif feoh sy undernumen: gif hit sy hors, sing þis on his fetera oððe on his bridel; gif hit si oðer feoh, sing on þæt hofrec and ontend .iii. candella, dryp þriwa weax- ne mag hit nan man forhelan; gif hit sy oþer orf, þonne sing ðu hit on .iiii. healfa ðin.

ond sing ærest uprhite hit: -
ond Petur, Pol, Patric, Pilip, Marie, Brigit, Felic,
in nomine dei, ond Chiric.
Qui queri inuenit.

Christus illum sive elegit in terriis ficarium
qui de gemino captiuos liberet seruitio
plerosque; de seruitute quos redemet hominum innumeros de sabuli obsoluit dominio.

Ymnos cum apocalipsi salmos; cantat dei
cousque; et edificandum dei tractat pupulum quem legem in trinitate sacre credent nominis trib; que personis unam.

Sona domine praecintus diebus; ac noctib;
intermissione deum oret dominum cuius ingentes laboris praecepturis premium cum apostoli regnauit sanctus super israel

Audite omnes amantes deum sacnta merita
uiri in Christo beati Patricii episcopi quomodo bonum ab actum simulatur angelis perfectumque; propter uitam equatur apostolis.

Patricii laudes semper dicamus ut nos cum illo defendat deus. Crux Christi reducat, crux Christi periit et inuenta est. Habracham tibi uias montes siua semitas fluminas Andronas cludat. Isaac tibi tenebras inducat. Crux Iacob te ad iudicium ligatum perducat. Iudei Christum crucifixerunt persimum sibimet ipsum perpetrauerunt. Opus celauerunt quod non potuerunt celare; sic nec hoc furtum celatur nec celare possit. Per dominum nostrum	
Marginalia p. 272	Entry LXIII (excerpt)
2 Wið ealra feonda grimnessum. Dextera domini fecit uirtutem; dextera domini exaltauit me; non moriar, sed uiuam & narrabo opera domini. Dextera glorificata est in uirtute; dextera manus tua confringit inimicos & per multitudinem magestatis tue contreuisti aduersarios meos, misisti iram tuam & commedit eos. Sic per uerba ueritatis amedatio, sic eris inmundissime spiritus, flectus⁺ oculorum tibi gehenna ignis. **Cedite a capite, a capillis, a labiis, a lingua, a collo, a pectoribus, ab uniuersis conpaginibus membrorum eius, ut non habeant potestatem diabulus ab homine isto .N. de capite, de capillis. nec nocendi, nec tangendi, nec dormiendi, nec tangendi, nec insurgendi, nec in meridiano, nec in uisu, nec in risu, nec in fulgendo, ll effuie. Sed in nomine domini nostri ihesu Christi, qui cum patre & spiritu sancto uiuis & regnas in unitate spiritu sancti per omnia secula seculorum.**	b Domine, sancte Pater, omnipotens eterne Deus per inpositionem manum mearum refugiat inimicus diabolus **a capillis, a capite, ab oculis, a naribus, a labis, a linguis, a sublinguis, a collo, a pectore, a pedibus, a calcaneis, ab uniuersis confaginibus membrorum eis, ut non habeat potestatem diabolus, nec lo-/ quendi, nec tacendi, nec dormiendi, nec resurgendi, nec in die, nec in nocte, nec in tangendo, nec in somno, nec in gressu, nec in uisu, nec in risu, nec in legendo;** sed in nomine Domini Ihesu Cristi, qui nos suo sancto sanguine redemit, qui cum Patre uiuit et regnat Deus in secula seculorum. Amen.

Appendices

Marginalia p. 326	Entry CL
3 Wiþ sarum eagum. Domine sancte pater omnipotens aeterne deus sana occulos hominis istius N. sicut sanasti occulos filii Tobi et multorum cecorum, manus aridorum, pes claudorum, sanitas egrorum, resurrectio mortuorum, felicitas martirum et omnium sanctorum. Oro domine ut erigas et inluminas occulos famuli tui. N. in quacumque ualitudine constraitum+ medellis celestibus sanare digneris; tribue famulo tuo. N., ut armis iustitie munitur diabolo resistat et regnum consequatur æternum. Per.	c Domine, sancte Pater, omnipotens aeterne Deus, sana oculos hominis istius N. sicut sanasti oculos filii Tobi et multorum cecorum quos [...]; Domine, tu es oculos caecorum, manus aridorum, pes claudorum, sanitas egrorum, resurrectio mortuorum, felicitas martyrum / et omnium sanctorum; oro, Domine, ut eregas et inlumnas oculos famuli tui N.; in quacumque ualitudine constitutum medelis celestibus sanare digneris, tribuere famulo tuo N., ut armis iustitiae munitus diabolo resistat et regnum consequatur aeternum; per.

[1] Text borrowed from Pettit's edition in *Lacnunga*, vol. II, CXLIX (translation mine). 'This one shall say when his cattle have been stolen by anyone. Before he says any other word, let him say: "The city is called Bethlehem where Christ was born. She is celebrated throughout the whole earth; as this deed may become notorious among men, through the cross of Christ." And pray then three times to the east and say three times "May [the cross] of Christ bring [them] back from the east"; and in the west and say "May the cross of Christ bring [them] back from the west" and in the south and say: "May the cross of Christ bring [them] back from the south", and in the north and say: "the cross of Christ has been hidden, and was found; the Jews hung Christ, they did to him the worst of deeds, that they could not conceal, so may this deed never be concealed, through the cross of Christ."'

[a] *Lacnunga*, vol. I, CXLIX. 'As soon as someone tells you that your cattle are lost, then before you say anything else say: "The city is called Bethlehem in which Christ was born. It is glorified throughout the whole world; so may this deed become notorious in the sight of men, through the holy Cross of Christ. Amen." Pray then thrice eastwards and then say thrice: "May the Cross of Christ bring (them) back from the east"; pray then thrice westwards and then say thrice: "May the Cross of Christ bring (them) back from the west"; pray then thrice southwards and say thrice: "May the Cross of Christ bring (them) back from the south"; pray then thrice northwards and say thrice: "May the Cross of Christ bring (them) back from the north; the Cross of Christ was lost and is found; the Jews hung Christ, did the worst of deeds, hid that which they could not fully conceal; so may this deed not be concealed by any means, through the holy Cross of Christ. Amen."'

[2] Grant, *The Loricas and the Missal*, pp. 15–16, expansions mine. 'Against the cruelty of all enemies, the right hand of Lord created strength, the right hand of the Lord elevated me, I shall not die but live and tell of the works of the Lord.

The right hand was glorified for its valour, your right hand scatters enemies, and through multiplicity of your majesty you tread on my enemies, you sent your anger and it devoured them. And so, through the words of truth *amedatio* [?], thus you will be most filthy spirit, for you [will be] the crying of the eyes [and] the fires of Gehenna. **Leave from the head, from the hair, from the lips, from the tongue, from the neck, from the chest, from the whole structure of his members, that the devil should not have power over this man .N., from the head, from the hair, [power] neither in suffering, nor in touching, nor in sleeping, nor in touching, nor in rising, nor at midday, nor in sight, nor in laughing, nor in gleaming.** *ll* [?] escape! But in the name of the Lord Jesus Christ, who with the Father and Holy Spirit lives and reigns in the unity of the Holy Spirit for all the centuries of centuries.'

⁺ Being read as 'fletus' in my translation.

^b *Lacnunga*, vol. I, LXIII 'Lord, holy Father, omnipotent (and) eternal God, by the application of my hands may the Enemy, the Devil, flee **from the hair, from the head, from the eyes, from the nose, from the lips, from the tongue, from under the tongue, from the neck, from the breast, from the feet, from the heels, from the whole framework of his members, so that the Devil may have no power [over him], neither in speaking, nor in keeping quiet, nor in sleeping, nor in rising, nor by day, nor by night, nor in touching, nor in rest, nor in going, nor in sight, nor in laughter, nor in reading;** but in the name of the Lord Jesus Christ, who redeemed us by his holy blood, who lives and reigns with the Father, God for the centuries of the centuries. Amen.'

³ Text borrowed from Pettit's edition in *Lacnunga*, vol. II, CL (translation mine). 'For sore eyes. Holy Lord, all-powerful Father, eternal God, heal the eyes of this man .N. just as you healed the eyes of the son of Tobit and many blind persons, hands of the crippled, feet of the lame, health for the sick, resurrection of the dead, joy of the martyrs and all the saints. I pray, O Lord, that you will raise and illumine the eyes of your servant. N. in whatever condition of health you may deem it worthy to heal him through your celestial blessings, grant that your servant. N. may resist the devil, defended with the arms of justice, and follow [you] to the eternal kingdom. Through.'

⁺ *constraitum* being read as *constitutum*, as in Pettit's edition.

^c Lacnunga, vol. I, CL 'Lord, holy Father, omnipotent (and) eternal God, heal the eyes of this man, .N., just as you healed the eyes of the son of Tobit and of many blind men who [...]; Lord, you are the eye of the blind, the hand of the crippled, the foot of the lame, the health of the sick, the resurrection of the dead, the joy of the martyrs and of all the saints; I pray, Lord, that you raise up and illumine the eyes of your servant .N.; may you deign to heal him with celestial remedies in whatever state of health he may be, to grant it to your servant, .N., that, fortified with the arms of justice, he may resist the devil and reach the eternal kingdom; through.'

Bibliography

Primary Sources

Aldhelm. *De virginitate.* Aldhelmi Opera, ed. Rudolf Ehwald. Monumenta germaniae historica. Auctores Antiquissimi. Volume 15. Weidmann: Berlin, 1919.

Alexander of Tralles. *Alexandri Practica cum Optimis Declarationibus Jacobi de Partibus et Simonis Januensis.* Venice, 1522.

Ælfric of Eynsham. *Two Ælfric Texts: The Twelve Abuses and the Vices and Virtues, an Edition and Translation of Ælfric's Old English Versions of De duodecim abusivis and De octo vitiis et de duodecim abusivis,* ed. and trans. Mary Clayton. D. S. Brewer: Cambridge, 2013.

—— *Ælfric's Catholic Homilies: The First Series, Text,* ed. Peter Clemoes. EETS s.s. 17. Oxford University Press: Oxford, 1997.

—— *Ælfric's Catholic Homilies: The Second Series, Text,* ed. Malcolm Godden. EETS s.s. 5. Oxford University Press: Oxford, 1979.

—— *The Homilies of the Anglo-Saxon Church: The First Part containing the Sermones Catholici, or Homilies of Ælfric,* ed. Benjamin Thorpe. Ælfric Society: London, 1844–46. Reprinted, Johnson: New York, 1971.

—— *Homilies of Ælfric: A Supplementary Collection,* ed. John C. Pope. EETS o.s. 259, 260. 2 Volumes. Oxford University Press: London, 1967–68.

—— *Die Hirtenbriefe Ælfrics in altenglischer und lateinischer Fassung,* ed. Bernhard Fehr with a Supplement to the Introduction by Peter Clemoes. Wissenschaftliche Buchgesellschaft: Darmstadt, 1966.

—— *Ælfric's Lives of Saints: Being a Set of Sermons on Saints' Days Formerly Observed by the English Church,* ed. Walter Skeat. EETS o.s. 76, 82, 94. 2 Volumes. Oxford University Press: London, 1966.

Anlezark, Daniel (ed.). *The Old English Dialogues of Solomon and Saturn.* D. S. Brewer: Cambridge, 2009.

Asser. *Annales Rerum Gestarum Ælfredi Magni,* ed. Francis Wise. Oxford University Press: Oxford, 1722.

—— *Asser's Life of King Alfred: Together with the Annals of Saint Neots Erroneously Ascribed to Asser,* ed. with an Introduction and Commentary by William Henry Stevenson. Clarendon Press: Oxford, 1904.

Augustine of Hippo. *De doctrina christiana,* ed. and trans. R. P. H. Green. Clarendon Press: Oxford, 1995.

—— *De beata vita,* ed. W. M. Green. CCSL 29. Brepols: Turnhout, 1970.

Reprinted online 2010. *Library of Latin Texts*. Brepols: Turnhout. Consulted at <www.brepols.net>. Accessed 10 June 2016.

Baring-Gould, Sabine and John Fisher (eds). *The Lives of British Saints: The Saints of Wales and Cornwall and such Irish Saints as have Dedications in Britain*. Honourable Society of Cymmrodorion: London, 1907.

Bately, Janet (ed.). *The Old English Orosius*. EETS s.s. 6. Oxford University Press: London, 1980.

Beccaria, Augusto. *I codici presalernitano (secoli IX, X, e XI)*. Edizioni di storia e letteratura: Rome, 1956.

Bede. *On the Nature of Things and On Times*, trans. with Introduction, Notes, and Commentary by Calvin B. Kendall and Faith Wallis. Liverpool University Press: Liverpool, 2010.

—— *Bede's Ecclesiastical History of the English People*, ed. Bertram Colgrave and R. A. B. Mynors. Clarendon Press: Oxford, 1969.

Benedict of Nursia. *Benedicti Regula*, ed. Rudolphus Hanslik. Corpus Scriptorum Ecclesiasticorm Latinorum 75. Hoelder-Pichler-Tempsky: Vienna, 1960.

Bernard of Clairvaux. *Lettres*, ed. J. Leclerq, H. Rochais, and C. H. Talbot, with Introduction and Notes by Monique Duchet-Suchaux. Editions du Cerf: Paris, 1997.

Birch, Walter de Gray (ed.). *An Ancient Manuscript of the Eighth or Ninth Century: Formerly Belonging to St. Mary's Abbey, or Nunnaminster, Winchester*. Simpkin & Marshall: Winchester and London, 1889.

—— *Cartularium Saxonicum: A Collection of Charters Relating to Anglo-Saxon History*. 3 Volumes. Whiting: London, 1885–93.

Bischoff, Bernhard. *Katalog der festländischen Handschriften des neunten Jahrhunderts (mit Ausnahme der wisigotischen)*. 3 Volumes. Harrassowitz Verlag: Wiesbaden, 2014.

Bjork, Robert E. and John D. Niles (eds). *Klaeber's Beowulf and the Fight at Finnsburg*. University of Toronto Press: Toronto, 2008.

Boethius. *The Theological Tractates, The Consolation of Philosophy*, ed. H. F. Stewart, E. K. Rand, and S. J. Tester. Loeb Classical Library. Harvard University Press: Cambridge, MA, 1973.

Byrhtferth of Ramsey. *Byrhtferth's Enchiridion*, ed. Michael Lapidge and Peter Baker. EETS s.s. 15. Oxford University Press: Oxford, 1995.

Caie, Graham D. (ed.). *The Old English Poem* Judgement Day II: *A Critical Edition with Editions of* De die iudicii *and the Hatton 113 Homily* Be domes dæge. D. S. Brewer: Cambridge, 2000.

Campbell, Alistair (ed.). *The Tollemache Orosius*. Early English Manuscripts in Facsimile. Rosenkilde and Bagger: Copenhagen, 1953.

Carnicelli, Thomas A. (ed.). *King Alfred's Version of St. Augustine's Soliloquies*. Harvard University Press: Cambridge, MA, 1969.

Cassiodorus. *Cassiodori senatoris institutiones*. Edited from the Manuscripts of R. A. B. Mynors. Clarendon Press: Oxford, 1937.

Bibliography

Cockayne, Oswald (ed. and trans.). *Leechdoms, Wortcunning, and Starcraft of Early England, Being a Collection of Documents Illustrating the History of Science in this Country Before the Norman Conquest*, with a new Introduction by Charles Singer. 3 Volumes. The Holland Press: London, 1961.

—— (ed. and trans.) *Leechdoms, Wortcunning, and Starcraft of Early England, Being a Collection of Documents Illustrating the History of Science in this Country Before the Norman Conquest*. 3 Volumes. Rolls Series. London, 1864–66. Reprinted as part of the Cambridge Library Collection. Cambridge University Press: Cambridge, 2012.

Colgrave, Bertram (ed. and trans.). *Two Lives of Saint Cuthbert: A Life by an Anonymous Monk of Lindisfarne and Bede's Prose Life*. Cambridge University Press: Cambridge, 1985.

Collectanea pseudo-Bedae, ed. Martha Bayless and Michael Lapidge. Scriptores Latini Hiberniae. Dublin Institute for Advanced Studies: Dublin, 1998.

Correa, Alicia (ed.). *The Durham Collectar*. Henry Bradshaw Society: London, 1992.

Cynewulf. *Cynewulf's Elene*, ed. P. O. E. Gradon. University of Exeter Press: Exeter, 1996.

D'Aronco, Maria Amalia and M. L. Cameron (eds). *The Old English Illustrated Pharmacopoeia*. Rosenkilde and Bagger: Copenhagen, 1998.

Davies, Oliver (ed. and trans.). *Celtic Spirituality*. Paulist Press: New York, 1999.

De Vriend, Hubert Jan (ed.). *The Old English Herbarium and Medicina de Quadrupedibus*. EETS o.s. 286. Oxford University Press: London, 1984.

Dioscorides, Pedanius. *De materia medica*, trans. Lily Beck. Olms-Weidmann: Hildesheim, 2011.

Dobbie, Elliot van Kirk (ed.). *The Anglo-Saxon Minor Poems*. Columbia University Press: New York, 1942.

Doble, G. H. (ed.). *Pontificale lanaletense (Bibliothèque da la ville de Rouen A. 27 cat. 368). A Pontifical Formerly in Use at St. Germans, Cornwall*. Harrison and Sons: London, 1937.

Felix. *Felix's Life of Saint Guthlac*, ed. and trans. Bertram Colgrave. Cambridge University Press: Cambridge, 1985.

Fischer, Klaus-Dietrich. 'Der pseudogalenische *Liber tertius*', in *Galenismo e medicina tardoantica: Fonti greche, latine e arabe: Atti del seminario internazionale di Siena, Certosa di Pontignano, 9–10 settembre 2002*, ed. Ivan Garofalo and Amneris Roselli. Istituto Universitario Orientale: Naples, 2003, pp. 101–32.

Frantzen, Allen (ed.). 'Anglo-Saxon Penitentials: A Cultural Database'. Consulted at <www.anglo-saxon.net/penance>. Accessed 23 June 2014.

Galen. *Galen: On Food and Diet*, ed. and trans. Mark Grant. Routledge:

London, 2000.

—— *Selected Works*, trans. with an Introduction and Notes by P. N. Singer. Oxford University Press: Oxford, 1997.

—— *Scripta minora*, ed. Iwan von Müller. Teubner: Leipzig, 1891.

Gariopontus. *Galeni Pergameni Passionarius, a doctis medicis multum desideratus: Egritudines a capite ad pedes usque*, ed. Barthélemy Trot. Lyon, 1526.

Godden, Malcolm and Susan Irvine (eds). *The Old English Boethius: An Edition of the Old English Versions of Boethius's De Consolatione Philosophiae*. Oxford University Press: Oxford, 2009.

Gregory the Great. *Regula pastoralis*, ed. Floribert Rommel and R. W. Clement. Clavis no. 1712. Brepols: Turnhout, 1953.

Hippocrates. *Nature of Man. Regimen in Health. Humours. Aphorisms. Regimen 1–3. Dreams. Heracletius: On the Universe*, trans. W. H. S. Jones. Loeb Classical Library 150. Harvard University Press: Cambridge, MA, 1931.

—— *Ancient Medicine. Airs, Waters, Places. Epidemics 1 and 3. The Oath. Precepts. Nutriment*, trans. W. H. S. Jones. Loeb Classical Library 147. Harvard University Press: Cambridge, MA, 1923.

The Hisperica Famina: A New Critical Edition with English Translation and Philogical Commentary, ed. and trans. Michael W. Herren. Pontifical Institute of Mediaeval Studies: Toronto, 1987.

The Hisperica Famina II: Related Poems, ed. Michael W. Herren. Pontifical Institute of Mediaeval Studies: Toronto, 1987.

Howald, Ernst and Henry E. Sigerist (eds). *Antonii Musae de herba vettonica liber. Pseudoapulei herbarius. Anonymi de taxone liber. Sexti Placiti liber medicinae ex animalibus etc.* Corpus Medicorum Latinorum, Volume 4. Teubner: Leipzig, 1927.

The Irish Liber Hymnorum, ed. and trans. John Henry Bernard and Robert Atkinson. Henry Bradshaw Society: London, 1898.

Irvine, Susan (ed.). *Old English Homilies from MS Bodley 343*. EETS o.s. 302. Oxford University Press: Oxford, 1993.

Isidore of Seville. *The Etymologies*, ed. and trans. Stephen A. Barney, W. J. Lewis, J. A. Beach, Oliver Berghof. Cambridge University Press: Cambridge, 2006.

Karasawa, Kazutomo (ed. and trans.). *The Old English Metrical Calendar (Menologium)*. D. S. Brewer: Cambridge, 2015.

Kästner, H. F. (ed.). 'Pseudo-Dioscorides *De herbis femininis*'. *Hermes*. 1896, 31, 578–635; 1897, 32, 160.

Kuypers, A. B. (ed.). *The Prayer Book of Aedelwald the Bishop, commonly called the Book of Cerne*. Cambridge University Press: Cambridge, 1902.

The Leofric Missal, ed. Nicholas Orchard. 2 Volumes. Henry Bradshaw Society: London, 2002.

Maion, Danielle (ed.). 'Traduzione e commento del Peri Didaxeon'. Unpublished Ph.D. Dissertation. Università degli Studi Roma Tre, 1998.

Marcellus. *Marcelli De medicamentis liber*, ed. Max Niedermann. Corpus Medicorum Latinorum 5. Leipzig: Teubner, 1916.

Miller, Thomas (ed. and trans.). *The Old English Version of Bede's Ecclesiastical History*. EETS o.s. 95, 96, 110, 111. Oxford University Press: London, 1959–63.

Milo of St Amand. *De sobrietate*, ed. Ludwig Traube. Monumenta germaniae historica, Poetae Latini Carolini. Volume 3. Weidmann: Berlin, 1896.

Morris, Richard (ed. and trans). *The Blickling Homilies of the Tenth Century from the Marquis of Lothian's Unique MS A.D. 971*. EETS o.s. 58, 63, 73. Trübner & Co: London, 1880.

O'Neill, Patrick (ed.). *King Alfred's Old English Prose Translation of the First Fifty Psalms*. Medieval Academy of America: Cambridge, MA, 2001.

Önnersfors, Alf (ed.). *Physica Plinii Bambergensis*. Georg Olms: Hildesheim and New York, 1975.

Orchard, Nicholas (ed.). *The Sacramentary of Ratoldus (Paris, Bibliothèque Nationale de France, lat. 12052)*. Henry Bradshaw Society: Cranbrook, 2005.

Oribasius. *Dieting for an Emperor: A Translation of Books 1 and 4 of Oribasius' Medical Compilations with an Introduction and Commentary*, trans. M. Grant. Brill: Leiden, 1997.

—— *Œuvres d'Oribase*, ed. U. C. Bussemaker, C. Daremberg, and A. Molinier. 6 Volumes. Collection des Medecins Grecs et Latins. Impr. National: Paris, 1856–76.

Origen. *Contra Celsum*, ed. and trans. Henry Chadwick. Cambridge University Press: Cambridge, 1980.

Pettit, Edward (ed. and trans.). *Anglo-Saxon Remedies, Charms, and Prayers from British Library MS Harley 585: The Lacnunga*. Edwin Mellen Press: Lewiston, 2001.

Pliny the Elder. *Natural History: With an English Translation in Ten Volumes*, ed. and trans. W. H. S. Jones. Volumes 6–8. Loeb Classical Library. Harvard University Press: Cambridge, 1975.

Priscianus, Theodorus. *Theodori Prisciani Euporiston libri III, cum physicorum fragmento et additamentis pseudo-Theodoreis*, ed. Valentin Rose. Teubner: Leipzig, 1894.

Scragg, Donald (ed.). *The Vercelli Homilies and Related Texts*. EETS o.s. 300. Oxford University Press: Oxford, 1992.

Stokes, Whitley (ed. and trans.). *The Birth and Life of St. Moling*. Harrison and Sons: London, 1907.

Stoll, Ulrich (ed.). *Das 'Lorscher Arzneibuch': Ein medizinisches Kompendium des 8. Jahrhunderts (Codex Bambergensis Medicinalis 1)*. Franz Steiner: Stuttgart, 1992.

Sweet, Henry (ed.). *King Alfred's West Saxon Version of Gregory's Pastoral Care*. EETS o.s. 45, 50. Oxford University Press: Oxford, 1871.

The Trotula: An English Translation of the Medieval Compendium of Women's Medicine, ed. and trans. Monica Green. University of Pennsylvania Press: Philadelphia, 2002.

Vleeskruyer, R (ed.). *The Life of St. Chad: An Old English Homily*. North-Holland Publishing Co.: Amsterdam, 1953.

Vogel, Cyrille and Reinhard Elze (eds). *Le pontifical romano-germanique du dixième siècle*. 3 Volumes. Studi e Testi 226, 227, 229. Biblioteca Apostolica Vaticana: Vatican City, 1963.

Warren, Frederick E. (ed.). *The Antiphonary of Bangor: An Early Irish Manuscript in the Ambrosian Library of Milan*. 2 Volumes. Henry Bradshaw Soceity 4. Harrison: London, 1893–95.

Winterbottom, Michael and Michael Lapidge (ed. and trans.). *The Early Lives of St Dunstan*. Clarendon Press: Oxford, 2012.

Wright, C. E. (ed.). *Bald's Leechbook: British Museum Royal Manuscript 12 D. xvii*. Early English Manuscripts in Facsimile 5. Rosenkilde and Bagger: Copenhagen, 1955.

Wulfstan of Winchester. *The Life of St. Æthelwold*, ed. Michael Lapidge and Michael Winterbottom. Clarendon Press: Oxford, 1991.

Wulfstan of York. *Wulfstan's Canons of Edgar*, ed. Roger Fowler. EETS s.o. 266. Oxford University Press: London, 1972.

Yerkes, David (ed.). *The Old English Life of Machutus*. University of Toronto Press: Toronto, 1984.

Secondary Sources

Abrams, Lesley. 'The Conversion of the Danelaw'. *Vikings and the Danelaw: Selected Papers from the Proceedings of the Thirteenth Viking Congress*, ed. James Graham-Campbell, R. A. Hall, Judith Jesch, and David Parsons. Oxbow Books: Oxford, 2001, pp. 31–44.

Adams, J. N. and Marilyn Deegan. '*Bald's Leechbook* and the *Physica Plinii*'. *ASE*. 1992, 21, 87–114.

Alexander, Michael. *Old English Literature*. Macmillan: London, 1983.

Amies, Marion. 'The *Journey Charm*: A Lorica for Life's Journey'. *Neophilologus*. 1983, 67.3, 448–62.

Amirav, Hagit. 'The Application of Magical Formulas of Invocation in Christian Contexts'. *Demons and the Devil in Ancient and Medieval Christianity*, ed. Nienke Vos and Willemien Otten. Brill: Leiden, 2011, pp. 117–27.

Amundsen, Darrel W. *Medicine, Society, and Faith in the Ancient and Medieval Worlds*. John Hopkins University Press: Baltimore and London, 1996.

—— 'Medicine and Faith in Early Christianity'. *Bulletin of the History of Medicine*. 56.3, 1982, 326–50.

Anlezark, Daniel. 'The Fall of the Angels in Solomon and Saturn II'.

Apocryphal Texts and Traditions in Anglo-Saxon England, ed. Kathryn Powell and Donald Scragg. D. S. Brewer: Cambridge, 2003, pp. 121–34.

Arbesmann, Rudolph. 'The Concept of "Christus Medicus" in St. Augustine'. *Traditio*, 10, 1954, 1–28.

Arnovick, Leslie K. *Written Reliquaries: The Resonance of Orality in Medieval English Texts*. John Benjamins Publishing Co.: Amsterdam, 2006.

Arthur, Ciaran. *'Charms', Liturgies, and Secret Rites in Early Medieval England*. Boydell Press: Woodbridge, 2018.

—— 'Ex Ecclesia: Salvific Power Beyond Sacred Space in Anglo-Saxon Charms'. *Incantantio*. 2013, 3, 9–32.

Ayoub, Lois. 'Old English Wæta and the Medical Theory of the Humours'. *JEGP*. 1995, 94.3, 332–46.

Banham, Debby. 'Medicine at Bury in the Time of Abbot Baldwin'. *Bury St Edmunds and the Norman Conquest*, ed. Tom Licence. Boydell Press: Woodbridge, 2014, pp. 226–46.

—— 'Dun, Oxa, and Pliny the Great Physician: Attribution and Authority in Old English Medical Texts'. *Social History of Medicine*. 2011, 24, 57–73.

—— 'England Joins the Medical Mainstream: New Texts in Eleventh-Century Manuscripts'. *Anglo-Saxons and the Continent*, ed. Hans Sauer and Joanna Storey. Arizona Center for Medieval and Renaissance Studies: Tempe, AZ, 2011, pp. 341–52.

—— 'The Old English Nine Herbs Charm'. *Medieval Christianity in Practice*, ed. M. Rubin. Princeton University Press: Princeton and Oxford, 2009, pp. 189–93.

—— 'A Millennium in Medicine? New Medicine Texts and Ideas in England in the Eleventh Century'. *Anglo-Saxons: Studies Presented to Cyril Roy Hart*, ed. Simon Keynes and Alfred P. Smyth. Four Courts Press: Dublin, 2006, pp. 230–42.

—— 'Arestolobius, the Patriarch of Jerusalem and Bark that comes from Paradise: What did the Orient mean to the Compilers of Old English Medical Collections?'. *Proceedings of the 38th International Congress on the History of Medicine*, ed. N. Sari, A. H. Bayat, Y. Ulman, M. Isin. 3 Volumes. Türk Tarih Kurumu: Ankara, 2005, pp. 459–68.

—— *Food and Drink in Anglo-Saxon England*. Tempus: Stroud, 2004.

—— 'Investigating the Anglo-Saxon *Materia Medica*: Latin, Old English and Archaeobotany'. *The Archaeology of Medicine: Papers Given at a Session of the Annual Conference of the Theoretical Archaeology Group held at the University of Birmingham on 20 December 1998*, ed. Robert Arnott. BAR International Series 1046. Archaeopress: Oxford, 2002, pp. 95–99.

—— and Conan T. Doyle. 'An Instrument of Confusion: The Mystery of the Anglo-Saxon Syringe'. *Recipes for Disaster*, ed. Jennifer Rampling, Debby Banham, and Nick Jardine. Whipple Museum of the History of Science: Cambridge, 2010, pp. 27–38.

—— and Christine Voth. 'The Diagnosis and Treatment of Wounds in the

Old English Medical Collections: Anglo-Saxon Surgery?'. *Wounds and Wound Repair in Medieval Culture*, ed. Larissa Tracy and Kelly DeVries. Brill: Leiden and Boston, 2015, pp. 153–74.

Barkai, Ron. *A History of Jewish Gynaecological Texts in the Middle Ages*. Brill: Leiden and Boston, 1998.

Barker, Mona and Gabriela Saldanha (eds). *Routledge Encyclopedia of Tranlsation Studies*. 2nd Edition. Routledge: Abingdon, 2009.

Barrow, Julia. 'The Chronology of the Benedictine "Reform"'. *Edgar, King of the English, 959–975*, ed. Donald Scragg. Boydell Press: Woodbridge, 2008, pp. 211–23.

—— 'The Community of Worcester, 961–1100'. *St Oswald of Worcester: Life and Influence*, ed. Nicholas Brooks and Catherine Cubitt. Leicester University Press: London, 1996, pp. 84–99.

—— 'English Cathedral Communities and Reform in the Late Tenth and Eleventh Centuries'. *Anglo-Norman Durham, 1093–1193*, ed. David Rollason, Margaret Harvey, and Michael Prestwich. Boydell Press: Woodbridge, 1994, pp. 25–39.

Bassett, Steven. 'Church and Diocese in the West Midlands: the Transition from British to Anglo-Saxon Control'. *Pastoral Care Before the Parish*, ed. John Blair and Richard Sharpe. Leicester University Press: Leicester, 1992, pp. 13–40.

Bassnett, Susan. *Translation Studies*. 3rd Edition. Routledge: London, 1980.

Bastiaensen, Toon. 'Exorcism: Tackling the Devil by Word of Mouth'. *Demons and the Devil in Ancient and Medieval Christianity*, ed. Nienke Vos and Willemien Otten. Brill: Leiden, 2011, pp. 129–44.

Bately, Janet. 'Did King Alfred Actually Translate Anything? The Integrity of the Alfredian Canon Revisited'. *MÆ*. 2009, 78.2, 189–206.

—— 'Old English Prose Before and During the Reign of Alfred'. *ASE*. 1988, 17, 93–138.

—— *The Literary Prose of King Alfred's Reign: Translation or Transformation*. University of London: London, 1980.

—— 'King Alfred and the Old English Translation of Orosius'. *Anglia*. 1970, 88, 433–60.

—— 'The Relationship Between the MSS of the Old English *Orosius*'. *English Studies: A Journal of English Language and Literature*. 1967, 48, 410–16.

Bayless, Martha. 'The Collectanea and Medieval Dialogues and Riddles'. *Collectanea pseudo-Bedae*, ed. Martha Bayless and Michael Lapidge. Scriptores Latini Hiberniae. Dublin Institute for Advanced Studies: Dublin, 1998, pp. 13–41.

Beagon, Mary. *Roman Nature: The Thought of Pliny the Elder*. Clarendon Press: Oxford, 1992.

Beechy, Tiffany. *The Poetics of Old English*. Ashgate: Burlington, 2010.

Benefiel, Rebecca R. 'Magic Squares, Alphabet Jumbles, Riddles and More:

The Culture of Word-Games among the Graffiti of Pompeii'. *The Muse at Play: Riddles and Wordplay in Greek and Latin Poetry*, ed. Jan Kwapisz, David Petrain, and Mikolaj Szymanski. De Gruyter: Berlin, 2013, pp. 65–79.

Bezzo, Luisa. 'Parallel Remedies: Old English "Paralisin þæt is lyftadl"'. *Form and Content of Instruction in Anglo-Saxon England in the Light of Contemporary Manuscript Evidence: Papers Presented at the International Conference, Udine, 6–8 April 2006*, ed. Patrizia Lendinara, Loredana Lazzari, and Maria Amalia D'Aronco. Brepols: Turnhout, 2007, pp. 435–45.

Bierbaumer, Peter. *Der botanische Wortschatz des Altenglischen*. 3 Volumes. Peter Lang: Frankfurt am Main, 1975–79.

Biggs, Frederick M. 'An Introduction and Overview of Recent Work'. *Apocryphal Texts and Traditions in Anglo-Saxon England*, ed. Kathryn Powell and Donald Scragg. D. S. Brewer: Cambridge, 2003, pp. 1–26.

Birkett, Thomas Eric. 'Rað Rett Runar: Reading the Runes in Old English and Old Norse Poetry'. Unpublished D.Phil. Dissertation. Oxford University, 2011.

Blair, John. *The Church in Anglo-Saxon Society*. Oxford University Press: Oxford and New York, 2005.

Bodden, Mary Catherine. 'Evidence for Knowledge of Greek in Anglo-Saxon England'. *ASE*. 1988, 17, 217–46.

—— 'Detailed Description of Oxford Bodleian Manuscript Auctarium F. 4. 32 Along with a Close Study of its Second Gathering, an 11th Century Old English Homily on the Finding of the True Cross'. Unpublished Ph.D. Dissertation. University of Toronto, 1979.

Bolotina, Julia. 'Medicine and Society in Anglo-Saxon England: The Social and Practical Context of *Bald's Leechbook* and the *Lacnunga*'. Unpublished Ph.D. Dissertation. University of Cambridge, 2016.

—— 'Support for the Sick Poor in Anglo-Saxon England'. *The Reading Medievalist: A Postgraduate Journal*. 2015, 2, 4–28.

Bonser, Wilfrid. *The Medical Background of Anglo-Saxon England: A Study in History, Psychology and Folklore*. Wellcome Historical Medical Library: London, 1963.

—— 'Magical Practices Against Elves'. *Folklore*. 1926, 37.4, 350–63.

—— 'The Dissimilarity of Ancient Irish Magic from that of the Anglo-Saxons'. *Folklore*. 1926, 37.3, 271–88.

Bosworth, Joseph. *An Anglo-Saxon Dictionary: Based on the Manuscript Collections of the Late Joseph Bosworth*. Supplement by Thomas Northcote Toller. Clarendon Press: Oxford, 1908–21.

Bracciotti, A. 'Osservazioni sulla forma del latino *lauer* nell'edizione Wellmann di (pseudo-) Dioscoride e nelle edizioni di alcuni erbari latini'. *Filologia antica e moderna*. 2004, 26, 45–55.

Breen, Aidan. 'The Liturgical Materials in MS Oxford, Bodleian Library,

Auct. F.4/32'. *Archiv für Liturgiewissenchaft*. 1992, 34, 121–53.

Brennessel, Barbara, Michael D. C. Drout, and Robyn Gravel. 'A Reassessment of the Efficacy of Anglo-Saxon Medicine'. *ASE*. 2005, 34, 183–95.

Brown, Michelle. 'Female Book-Ownership and Production in Anglo-Saxon England: The Evidence of the Ninth-Century Prayerbooks'. *Lexis and Texts in Early English: Studies Presented to Jane Roberts*, ed. Christian J. Kay and Louise M. Sylvester. Rodopi: Amsterdam, 2001, pp. 45–67.

—— 'Mercian Manuscripts? The "Tiberius" Group and its Historical Context'. *Mercia: An Anglo-Saxon Kingdom in Europe*, ed. Michelle P. Brown and Carol A. Farr. Leicester University Press: London, 2001, pp. 281–91.

—— *The Book of Cerne: Prayer, Patronage and Power in Ninth-Century England*. The British Library and University of Toronto Press: London, 1996.

Brown, Peter. 'Sorcery, Demons, and the Rise of Christianity: From Late Antiquity into the Middle Ages'. *Witchcraft Confessions and Accusations*, ed. Mary Douglas. Tavistock: London, 1970, pp. 17–45. Reprinted in *Religion and Society in the Age of Saint Augustine*. Faber and Faber: London, 1972, pp. 119–46.

Bullough, Donald A. 'The Educational Tradition in England from Alfred to Ælfric: Teaching *utriusque linguae*'. *La scuola nell' Occidente latino dell' alto medioevo*. Settimane di studio del centro italiano di studi sull' alto medioevo. 1972, 19, 453–94. Reprinted and updated in Donald A. Bullough. *Carolingian Renewal: Sources and Heritage*. Manchester University Press: Manchester, 1991, pp. 297–334.

Bundy, Mildred. 'St Dunstan's Classbook and its Frontispiece: Dunstan's Portrait and Autograph'. *St Dunstan: His Life, Times and Cult*, ed. Nigel Ramsay, Margaret Sparks, and Tim Tatton Brown. Boydell Press: Woodbridge, 1992, pp. 103–42.

Butler, Robert M. 'Glastonbury and the Early History of the Exeter Book'. *Old English Literature in its Manuscript Context*, ed. Joyce Tally Lionarons. West Virginia University Press: Morgantown, 2004, pp. 173–215.

Caciola, Nancy. 'Discerning Spirits: Sanctity and Possession in the Later Middle Ages'. 2 Volumes. Unpublished Ph.D. Dissertation. University of Michigan, 1994.

Caie, Graham D. 'Doomsday and Nature in the Old English Poem *Judgement Day II*'. *Aspects of Anglo-Saxon and Medieval England*, ed. Michiko Ogura. Peter Lang: Frankfurt, 2014, pp. 93–104.

Cameron, M. L. *Anglo-Saxon Medicine*. Cambridge University Press: Cambridge, 1993.

—— '*Bald's Leechbook* and Cultural Interactions in Anglo-Saxon England'. *ASE*. 1990, 19, 5–12.

—— 'On *þeor* and *þeoradl*'. *Anglia*. 1988, 106, 124–29.

—— 'Anglo-Saxon Medicine and Magic'. *ASE*. 1988, 17, 191–215.

—— '*Bald's Leechbook*: Its Sources and Their Use in its Compilation'. *ASE*.

1983, 12, 153–82.

—— 'The Sources of Medical Knowledge in Anglo-Saxon England'. *ASE*. 1982, 11, 135–55.

Carley, James. 'More Pre-Conquest Manuscripts from Glastonbury Abbey'. *ASE*. 1994, 23, 265–81.

—— 'Two Pre-Conquest Manuscripts from Glastonbury Abbey'. *ASE*. 1987, 16, 197–212.

Chardonnens, László Sándor. 'An Arithmetical Crux in the Woden Passage in the Old English *Nine Herbs Charm*'. *Neophilologus*. 2009, 93.4, 691–702.

Chave-Mahir, Florence. 'Medieval Exorcism: Liturgical and Hagiographical Sources'. *Understanding Medieval Liturgy: Essays in Interpretation*, ed. Helen Gittos and Sarah Hamilton. Ashgate: Farnham, 2015, pp. 159–75.

Chibnall, Marjorie. 'Pliny's Natural History and the Middle Ages'. *Empire and Aftermath: Silver Latin II*, ed. T. A. Dorey. Routledge & Kegan Paul: London, 1975, pp. 57–78.

Clark, Cecily. 'Onomastics'. *The Cambridge History of the English Language, Volume 1: The Beginning to 1066*, ed. Richard M. Hogg. Cambridge University Library: Cambridge, 1992, pp. 452–89.

Clayton, Mary. 'An Edition of Ælfric's Letter to Brother Edward'. *Early Medieval English Texts and Interpretations: Studies Presented to Donald G. Scragg*, ed. Elaine Treharne and Susan Rosser. Arizona Center for Medieval and Renaissance Studies: Tempe, 2002, pp. 280–83.

—— 'Homiliaries and Preaching in Anglo-Saxon England'. *Peritia*. 1985, 4, 207–42. Reprinted in *Old English Prose: Basic Readings*, ed. Paul E. Szarmach. Garland Publishing: London, 2000, pp. 115–98.

Collins, Minta. *Medieval Herbals: The Illustrative Traditions*. British Library and University of Toronto: London, 2000.

Colman, Fran. *The Grammar of Names in Anglo-Saxon England: The Linguistics and Culture of the Old English Onomasticon*. Oxford University Press: Oxford, 2014.

Conrad, Lawrence I. *The Western Medical Tradition: 800 BC to AD 1800*. Cambridge University Press: Cambridge, 1995.

Contreni, John J. 'Masters and Medicine in Northern France During the Reign of Charles the Bald'. *Charles the Bald: Court and Kingdom*, ed. Margaret Gibson and Janet Nelson. BAR International Series: Oxford, 1981, pp. 43–54.

Cowen, Alice. 'Byrstas and Bysmeras: The Wounds of Sin in the Sermo Lupi ad Anglos'. *Wulfstan, Archbishop of York: Proceedings of the Second Alcuin Conference*, ed. Matthew Townend. Brepols: Turnhout, 2004, pp. 397–412.

Crawford, Jane. 'Evidences for Witchcraft in Anglo-Saxon England'. *MÆ*. 1963, 32, 99–116.

Cross, James E. 'The Literate Anglo-Saxon: On Sources and Disseminations'. Sir Israel Gollancz Memorial Lecture. Oxford University Press: London,

1972.

Cubitt, Catherine. 'The Tenth-Century Benedictine Reform in England'. *Early Medieval Europe*. 1997, 6.1, 77–94.

D'Aronco, Maria Amalia. 'A Problematic Plant Name: *Elehtre*. A Reconsideration'. *Herbs and Healers from the Ancient Mediterranean through the Medieval West: Essays in Honor of John R. Riddle*, ed. Anne Van Arsdall and Timothy Graham. Ashgate: Farnham, 2012, pp. 187–216.

—— 'Gardens on Vellum: Plants and Herbs in Anglo-Saxon Manuscripts'. *Health and Healing from the Medieval Garden*, ed. Peter Dendle and Alain Touwaide. Boydell Press: Woodbridge, 2008, pp. 101–27.

—— 'The Benedictine Rule and the Care of the Sick: The Plan of St Gall and Anglo-Saxon England'. *The Medieval Hospital and Medical Practice*, ed. Barbara S. Bowers. Ashgate: Aldershot, 2007, pp. 235–51.

—— 'The Transmission of Medical Knowledge in Anglo-Saxon England: The Voices of the Manuscripts'. *Form and Content of Instruction in Anglo-Saxon England in the Light of Contemporary Manuscript Evidence: Papers Presented at the International Conference, Udine, 6–8 April 2006*, ed. Patrizia Lendinara, Loredana Lazzari, and Maria Amalia D'Aronco. Brepols: Turnhout, 2007, pp. 35–58.

—— 'How "English" is Anglo-Saxon Medicine? The Latin Sources for Anglo-Saxon Medical Texts'. *Britannia Latina: Latin in the Culture of Great Britain from the Middle Ages to the Twentieth Century*, ed. Charles Burnett and Nicholas Mann. Warburg Institute: London, 2005, pp. 27–41.

—— 'The Old English Pharmacopoeia: A Proposed Dating for the Translation'. *Avista Forum Journal*. 2003, 13, 9–18.

—— 'Anglo-Saxon Plant Pharmacy and Latin Medical Tradition'. *From Earth to Art. The Many Aspects of the Plant-World in Anglo-Saxon England*. Proceedings of the First ASPNS Symposium, University of Glasgow, 507 April 2000. Rodopi: Amsterdam, 2003, pp. 133–51.

—— 'Le conoscenze mediche nell'Inghilterra anglosassone: Il ruolo del mondo carolingio'. *International Scandinavian and Medieval Studies in Memory of Gerd Wolfgang Weber*, ed. Michael Dallapiazza, Olaf Hansen, Preben Meulengracht Sorensen, and Yvonne Bonnetain. Edizioni Parnaso: Trieste, 2000, pp. 129–46.

—— 'L'erbario anglosassone, un'ipotesi sulla data della traduzione'. *Romanobarbarica*. 1994–95, 13, 325–66.

—— 'The Botanical Lexicon of the Old English Herbarium'. *ASE*. 1988, 17, 15–33.

—— 'La traduzione in inglese antico della *Regula Sancti Benedicti*: Neologismi e prestiti nel lessico monastico'. *Filologia Germanica*. 1981, 24, 105–28.

Debru, Armelle. 'Physiology'. *The Cambridge Companion to Galen*, ed. R. J. Hankinson. Cambridge Univeristy Press: Cambridge, 2008, pp. 263–82.

Deegan, Marilyn. 'Pregnancy and Childbirth in the Anglo-Saxon Medical

Texts: A Preliminary Study'. *Medicine in Early Medieval England: Four Papers*, ed. Marilyn Deegan and Donald Scragg. Centre for Anglo-Saxon Studies, University of Manchester: Manchester, 1989, pp. 17–26.

—— 'A Critical Edition of MS B. L. Royal 12.D. xvii, Bald's "Leechbook"'. Unpublished Ph.D. Dissertation. 2 Volumes. University of Manchester, 1988.

Dendle, Peter. *Demon Possession in Anglo-Saxon England*. Medieval Institute Publications: Kalamazoo, MI, 2014.

—— 'Textual Transmission of the Old English "Loss of Cattle" Charm'. *JEGP*. 2006, 105.4, 514–39.

—— *Satan Unbound: The Devil in Old English Narrative Literature*. University of Toronto Press: London and Toronto, 2001.

Dictionary of Old English: A to G, ed. Angus Cameron, Antonette diPaolo Healey, *et al*. Dictionary of Old English Project: Toronto. Consulted at <www.doe.utoronto.ca>. Accessed 10 August 2016.

Discenza, Nicole Guenther. 'The Old English *Boethius*'. *A Companion to Alfred the Great*, ed. Nicole Guenther Discenza and Paul E. Szarmach. Brill: Leiden and Boston, 2014, pp. 200–26.

—— *The King's English: Strategies of Translation in the Old English Boethius*. State University of New York Press: Albany, 2005.

Dodds, E. R. *Pagan and Christian in an Age of Anxiety: Some Aspects of Religious Experience from Marcus Aurelius to Constantine*. Cambridge University Press: Cambridge, 1965.

Dorey, Thomas Alan. *Empire and Aftermath: Silver Latin II*. Routledge & Kegan Paul: London, 1975.

Doyle, Conan. 'Anglo-Saxon Medicine and Disease: A Semantic Approach'. Unpublished Ph.D. Dissertation. 2 Volumes. University of Cambridge, 2017.

—— '*Dweorg* in Old English: Aspects of Disease Terminology'. *Quaestio Insularis*. 2008, 9, 99–117.

DuBois, Thomas A. *Nordic Religions in the Viking Age*. University of Pennsylvania Press: Philadelphia, 1999.

Dumville, David N. *Wessex and England from Alfred to Edgar: Six Essays on Political, Cultural, and Ecclesiastical Revival*. Boydell Press: Woodbridge, 1992.

Duncan, Ian. 'Epitaphs for Æglæcan: Narrative Strife in *Beowulf*'. *Modern Critical Interpretations: Beowulf*, ed. Harold Bloom. Chelsea House: New York, 1987, pp. 111–30.

Eco, Umberto. *Mouse or Rat? Translation as Negotiation*. Weidfeld & Nicolson: London, 2003.

Edelstein, Ludwig. *Ancient Medicine: Selected Papers of Ludwig Edelstein*, ed. Owsei Temkin and C. Lilian Temkin, trans. C. Lilian Temkin. John Hopkins Press: Baltimore, 1967.

Eijk, Philip J. van der. *Medicine and Philosophy in Classical Antiquity*:

Doctors and Philosophers on Nature, Soul, Health, and Disease. Cambridge University Press: Cambridge, 2005.

Fell, Christine. 'Runes and Semantics'. *Old English Runes and their Continental Background*, ed. Alfred Bammesberger. Carl Winter Universitatsverlag: Heidelberg, 1991, pp. 195–299.

—— 'Old English *Beor*'. *Leeds Studies in English*. 1975, 8, 76–95.

Fera, Rosa Maria. 'Translating the Five Senses in Alfredian Prose'. *Studia Neophilologica*. 2012, 84.2, 189–200.

Ferngren, Gary B. *Medicine & Health Care in Early Christianity*. John Hopkins University Press: Baltimore, 2009.

Finan, Thomas. 'Hiberno-Latin Christian Literature'. *An Introduction to Celtic Christianity*, ed. J. P. Mackey. T & T Clarke: Edinburgh, 1989, pp. 64–100.

Fleming, Damian. '"The Most Exalted Language": Anglo-Saxon Perceptions of Hebrew'. Unpublished Ph.D. Dissertation. University of Toronto, 2006.

Flint, Valerie. *The Rise of Magic in Early Medieval Europe*. Clarendon Press: Oxford, 1991.

Foot, Sarah. '"By Water in the Spirit": The Administration of Baptism in Early Anglo-Saxon England'. *Pastoral Care Before the Parish*, ed. John Blair and Richard Sharpe. Leicester University Press: Leicester, 1992.

Frantzen, Allen. *The Literature of Penance in Anglo-Saxon England*. Rutgers University Press: New Brunswick, 1983.

Franz, Adolph. *Die kirchlichen Benediktionen im Mittelalter*. 2 Volumes. Herder: Freiburg im Breisgau, 1909.

—— *Das Rituale von St Florian aus dem zwölften Jahrhundert*, ed. Adolph Franz. Herder: Freiburg im Breisgau, 1904.

Frazer, William O. 'Introduction: Identities in Early Medieval Britain'. *Social Identity in Early Medieval Britain*, ed. William O. Frazer and Andrew Tyrrell. Leicester University Press: London and New York, 2000.

Garner, Lori Ann. 'Anglo-Saxon Charms in Performance'. *Oral Tradition*. 2004, 19.1, 20–42.

Garrison, Mary. 'The Collectanea and Medieval Florilegia'. *Collectanea pseudo-Bedae*, ed. Martha Bayless and Michael Lapidge. Scriptores Latini Hiberniae. Dublin Institute for Advanced Studies: Dublin, 1998, pp. 42–83.

Gatch, Milton. 'King Alfred's Version of Augustine's Soliloquia: Some Suggestions on its Rationale and Unity'. *Studies in Earlier Old English Prose*, ed. Paul E. Szarmach. State University of New York Press: Albany, 1986, pp. 17–46.

Gilbert, Sarah. 'Anglo-Saxon Medical Fragments: Wellcome Library, Western MS 46 and the Omont Leaf in Context'. Unpublished M.Phil Dissertation. University of Cambridge, 2011.

Gittos, Helen. 'Researching the History of Rites'. *Understanding Medieval Liturgy: Essays in Interpretation*, ed. Helen Gittos and Sarah Hamilton. Ashgate: Farnham, 2016, pp. 13–37.

—— and Sarah Hamilton. 'Introduction'. *Understanding Medieval Liturgy: Essays in Interpretation*, ed. Helen Gittos and Sarah Hamilton. Ashgate: Farnham, 2016, pp. 1–10.

Glaze, Florence Eliza. 'Master-Student Medical Dialogues: The Evidence of London British Library, Sloane 2839'. *Form and Content of Instruction in Anglo-Saxon England in the Light of Contemporary Manuscript Evidence: Papers Presented at the International Conference, Udine, 6–8 April 2006*, ed. Patrizia Lendinara, Loredana Lazzari, and Maria Amalia D'Aronco. Brepols: Turnhout, 2007, pp. 415–34.

—— 'Galen Refashioned: Garioputus in the Later Middle Ages and Renaissance'. *Textual Healing: Essays in Medieval and Early Modern Medicine*, ed. Elizabeth Furdell. Brill: Leiden, 2005, pp. 53–75.

—— 'The Perforated Wall: the Ownership and Circulation of Medical Books in Medieval Europe, ca. 800–1200'. Unpublished Ph.D. Dissertation. Duke University, 1999.

Glosecki, Stephen. '"Blow these Vipers from Me": Mythic Magic in *The Nine Herbs Charm*'. *Essays on Old, Middle, Modern English and Old Icelandic in Honor of Raymond P. Tripp, Jr*, ed. Loren C. Gruber. Edwin Mellen Press: Lewiston, NY, 2000, pp. 117–19.

Gneuss, Helmut and Michael Lapidge. *Anglo-Saxon Manuscripts: A Bibliographical Handlist of Manuscripts and Manuscript Fragments Written or Owned in England up to 1100*. University of Toronto Press: Toronto and London, 2014.

—— 'The Origins of Standard Old English and Æthelwold's School at Winchester'. *ASE*. 1972, 1, 63–83.

Godden, Malcolm. 'Stories From the Court of King Alfred'. *Saints and Scholars: New Perspectives on Anglo-Saxon Literature and Culture*, ed. Stuart McWilliams. D. S. Brewer: Cambridge, 2012, pp. 123–40.

—— 'The Old English Orosius and its Sources'. *Anglia*. 2011, 129, 297–320.

—— 'The Old English *Orosius* and its Context: Who Wrote It, for Whom, and Why?'. *Quaestio Insularis*. 12, 2011, 1–30.

—— 'The Alfred Project and its Aftermath: Rethinking the Literary History of the Ninth and Tenth Centuries'. *Proceedings of the British Academy*. 162, 2009, 93–122.

—— 'Did King Alfred Write Anything?'. *MÆ*. 2007, 76, 1–23.

—— *Ælfric's Catholic Homilies: Introduction, Commentary and Glossary*. EETS s.s. 18. Clarendon Press: Oxford, 2006.

—— *The Translations of Alfred and his Circle, and the Misappropriation of the Past*. H. M. Chadwick Memorial Lecture 14. University of Cambridge, Department of Anglo-Saxon, Norse, and Celtic: Cambridge, 2004.

—— 'The Anglo-Saxons and the Goths: Rewriting the Sack of Rome'. *ASE*.

2002, 31, 47–68.

—— 'King Alfred's Preface and the Teaching of Latin in Anglo-Saxon England'. *English Historical Review*. 2002, 117, 596–604.

—— 'Wærferth and King Alfred: The Fate of the Old English *Dialogues*'. *Alfred the Wise: Studies in Honour of Janet Bately*, ed. Jane Roberts, Janet L. Nelson, Malcolm Godden. D. S. Brewer: Cambridge, 1997, pp. 35–51.

—— 'Apocalypse and Invasion in Late Anglo-Saxon England'. *From Anglo-Saxon to Early Middle English: Studies Presented to E. G. Stanley*, ed. Malcolm Godden, Douglas Gray, and Terry Hoad. Clarendon Press: Oxford, 1994, pp. 130–62.

—— 'Anglo-Saxons on the Mind'. *Learning and Literature in Anglo-Saxon England: Studies Presented to Peter Clemoes on the Occasion of his Sixty-Fifth Birthday*, ed. M. Lapidge and H. Gneuss. Cambridge University Press: Cambridge, 1985, pp. 271–98.

—— 'Ælfric's Changing Vocabulary'. *English Studies*. 1980, 61.3, 206–23.

—— 'An Old English Penitential Motif'. *ASE*. 1973, 2, 221–39.

Godel, Willibrord. 'Irish Prayer in the Early Middle Ages'. *Milltown Studies*. 1979, 4, 60–99.

Grant, Raymond. *Cambridge, Corpus Christi College 41: The Loricas and the Missal*. Rodopi: Amsterdam, 1978.

Grattan, J. H. G. and Charles Singer (eds). *Anglo-Saxon Magic and Medicine, Illustrated specially from the Semi-Pagan Text 'Lacnunga'*. Oxford University Press: Oxford, 1952.

Green, D. H. *Language and History in the Early Germanic World*. Cambridge University Press: Cambridge, 1998.

Green, Monica. 'Contraceptives'. *Women and Gender in Medieval Europe: An Encyclopedia*, ed. Margaret Schaus. Routledge: Abingdon, 2006, pp. 168–69.

—— 'Gynecology'. *Women and Gender in Medieval Europe: An Encyclopedia*, ed. Margaret Schaus. Routledge: Abingdon, 2006, pp. 339–43.

—— 'Menstruation'. *Women and Gender in Medieval Europe: An Encyclopedia*, ed. Margaret Schaus. Routledge: Abingdon, 2006, pp. 557–58.

—— 'Flowers, Poisons and Men: Menstruation in Medieval Western Europe'. *Menstruation: A Cultural History*, ed. Andrew Shail and Gillian Howie. Palgrave Macmillan: Basingstoke, 2005, pp. 51–71.

—— Review of John Riddle. *Eve's Herbs: A History of Contraception and Abortion in the West. Bulletin of the History of Medicine*. 1999, 73, 308–11.

Grendon, Felix. 'The Anglo-Saxon Charms'. *The Journal of American Folklore*. 1909, 22.84, 105–237.

Gretsch, Mechthild. *The Intellectual Foundations of the English Benedictine Reform*. Cambridge University Press: Cambridge, 1999.

—— 'Æthelwold's Translation of the *Regula Sancti Benedicti* and its Latin Exemplar'. *ASE*. 1974, 3, 125–51.

Grmek, Mirko D. (ed.), Antony Shugaar, and Bernardino Fantini (trans).

Western Medical Thought from Antiquity to the Middle Ages. Harvard University Press: Cambridge, MA, 1998.

Gullick, Michael. 'An Eleventh-Century Bury Medical Manuscript'. *Bury St Edmunds and the Norman Conquest*, ed. Tom Licence. Boydell Press: Woodbridge, 2014, pp. 190–225.

Hall, Alaric. 'Elleborus in Anglo-Saxon England, 900–1100: *Tunsingwyrt* and *Wodewistle*'. *Leeds Studies in English*. 2013, New Series 44, 70–93.

—— 'Madness, Medication – and Self-Induced Hallucination? Elleborus (and Woody Nightshade) in Anglo-Saxon England, 700–900'. *Leeds Studies in English*. 2013, New Series 44, 43–69.

—— *Elves in Anglo-Saxon England: Matters of Belief, Health, Gender and Identity*. Boydell Press: Woodbridge, 2009.

—— 'The Evidence for *maran*, the Anglo-Saxon "Nightmares"'. *Neophilologus*. 2007, 91.2, 299–317.

—— 'Calling the Shots: The Old English Remedy *Gif hors ofscoten sie* and Anglo-Saxon "Elf-Shot"'. *Neuphilologische Mitteilungen*. 2005, 106, 195–209.

—— 'The Meaning of Elf and Elves in Medieval England'. Unpublished Ph.D. Dissertation. University of Glasgow, 2004.

Hall, Thomas H. 'Ælfric and the Epistle to the Laodicians'. *Apocryphal Texts and Traditions in Anglo-Saxon England*, ed. Kathryn Powell and Donald Scragg. D. S. Brewer: Cambridge, 2003, pp. 65–84.

Hebing, Rosanne. 'The Textual Tradition of Heavenly Letter Charms in Anglo-Saxon Manuscripts'. *Secular Learning in Anglo-Saxon England*, ed. László Sándor Chardonnens and Bryan Carella. *Amsterdamer Beiträge zur älteren Germanistik* 69. Rodopi: Amsterdam, 2012, pp. 203–22.

Herren, Michael. *Christ in Celtic Christianity*. Boydell Press: Woodbridge, 2002.

—— 'The Authorship, Date of Composition and Provenance of the so-called "Lorica Gildae"'. *Royal Irish Academy*. 1973, 24, 35–51.

Hill, Joyce. 'The Apocrypha in Anglo-Saxon England: the Challenge of Changing Distinctions'. *Apocryphal Texts and Traditions in Anglo-Saxon England*, ed. Kathryn Powell and Donald Scragg. D. S. Brewer: Cambridge, 2003, pp. 165–68.

Hill, Thomas D. 'The Rod of Protection and the Witches' Ride: Christian and Germanic Syncretism in Two Old English Metrical Charms'. *JEGP*. 2012, 111.2, 145–68.

—— 'The "Palmtwigede" Pater Noster: Horticultural Semantics and the Old English *Solomon and Saturn I*'. *MÆ*. 2005, 74.1, 1–9.

—— 'The Devil's Forms and the Pater Noster's Powers: "The Prose Solomon and Saturn 'Pater Noster' Dialogue" and the Motif of the Transformation Combat'. *Studies in Philology*. 1988, 85.2, 164–76.

—— 'Invocation of the Trinity and the Tradition of the *Lorica* in Old English Poetry'. *Speculum*. 1981, 56, 259–67.

—— 'The Æcerbot Charm and its Christian User'. *ASE*. 1977, 6, 213–21.
—— 'Two Notes on *Solomon and Saturn*'. *MÆ*. 1971, 40, 217–20.
Hitch, S. J. 'Alfred's Reading of Augustine's Soliloquies'. *Sentences: Essays Presented to Alan Ward*, ed. D. M. Reeks. Bosphoros: South Hampton, pp. 21–29.
Hofstetter, Walter. 'Winchester and the Standardization of Old English Vocabulary'. *ASE*. 1988, 17, 139–61.
—— *Winchester und der spätaltenglische Sprachgebrauch: Untersuchungen zur geographischen und zeitlichen Verbreitung Altenglischer Synonyme*. Fink: Munich, 1987.
Hohler, Christopher. Review of R. J. S. Grant, *Cambridge, Corpus Christi College 41: The Loricas and the Missal*. *MÆ*. 1980, 49, 275–78.
Hollis, Stephanie. 'The Social Milieu of *Bald's Leechbook*'. *Avista Forum Journal*. 2004, 14.1, 11–16.
—— and Michael Wright. *Old English Prose of Secular Learning*. Annotated Bibliographies of Old and Middle English Literature: Volume 4. D. S. Brewer: Cambridge, 1992.
Horden, Peregrine. 'A Non-natural Environment: Medicine without Doctors and the Medieval European Hospitals'. *The Medieval Hospital and Medical Practice*, ed. Barbara S. Bowers. Ashgate: Aldershot, 2007, pp. 133–46.
—— 'The Millennium Bug: Health and Medicine around the Year 1000'. *The Year 1000: Medical Practice at the End of the First Millennium*, ed. Peregrine Horden and Emilie Savage-Smith. *Social History of Medicine*. 2000, 13.2, 201–20.
Howe, Nicholas. *Migration and Mythmaking in Anglo-Saxon England*. Yale University Press: London and New Haven, 1989.
Howlett, David. '"Tres Linguae Sacrae" and Threefold Play in Insular Latin'. *Peritia*. 2002, 16, 94–115.
—— 'Aldhelm and Irish Learning'. *Bulletin du Cange*. 1994, 52, 50–72.
Hübener, Gustav. '*Beowulf* and Germanic Exorcism'. *The Review of English Studies*. 1935, 11.42, 163–81.
Hull, Eleanor. 'The Ancient Hymn-Charms of Ireland'. *Folklore*. 1910, 21, 417–46.
Hunt, Richard William. *Saint Dunstan's Classbook from Glastonbury: Codex Biblioth. Bodleianae Oxon. Auct. F.4/32*. Umbrae Codicum Occidentalium 4. North Holland Publishing Company: Amsterdam, 1961.
Irvine, Martin. *The Making of Textual Culture: 'Grammatica' and Literary Theory, 350–1100*. Cambridge University Press: Cambridge, 1994.
Jardine, Nick. 'Avoiding Disaster in Translation: On the Advantages of "Old Friends"'. *Recipes for Disaster*, ed. Jennifer Rampling, Debby Banham, and Nick Jardine. Whipple Museum of the History of Science: Cambridge, 2010, pp. 39–46.
Jesch, Judith. 'Scandinavians and "Cultural Paganism" in Late Anglo-

Saxon England'. *The Christian Tradition in Anglo-Saxon England: Approaches to Current Scholarship and Teaching*, ed. Paul Cavill. D. S. Brewer: Cambridge, 2004, pp. 55–68.

Johnson, Richard F. 'Archangel in the Margins: St. Michael in the Homilies of Cambridge, Corpus Christi College 41'. *Traditio*. 1998, 53, 63–91.

Jolly, Karen Louise. 'On the Margins of Orthodoxy: Devotional Formulas and Protective Prayers in Cambridge, Corpus Christi College 41'. *Signs on the Edge: Space, Text and Margins in Medieval Manuscripts*, ed. Sarah Larratt Keefer and Rolf H. Bremmer. Medievalia Groningana Series. Peeters: Leuven, 2007, pp. 135–83.

—— 'Prayers from the Field: Practical Protection and Demonic Defense in Anglo-Saxon England'. *Traditio*. 2006, 61, 95–147.

—— 'Tapping the Power of the Cross: Who and for Whom?'. *The Place of the Cross in Anglo-Saxon England*, ed. Catherine E. Karkov, Sarah Larratt Keefer, and Karen Louise Jolly. Boydell Press: Woodbridge, 2006, pp. 58–79.

—— 'Cross-Referencing Anglo-Saxon Liturgy and Remedies: The Sign of the Cross and Ritual Protection'. *The Liturgy of the Late Anglo-Saxon Church*, ed. Helen Gittos and M. Bradford Bedingfield. Henry Bradshaw Society: London, 2005, pp. 213–43.

—— *Popular Religion in Late Saxon England: Elf Charms in Context*. University of North Carolina Press: Chapel Hill, 1996.

—— 'Anglo-Saxon Charms in the Context of a Christian World View'. *Journal of Medieval History*. 1985, 11, 279–93.

——, Catharina Raudvere, and Edward Peters. *Witchcraft and Magic in Europe: The Middle Ages*. The Athlone Press: London, 2002.

Jonassen, Frederick B. 'The Pater Noster Letters and the Poetic *Solomon and Saturn*'. *Modern Language Review*. 1988, 83, 1–9.

Keefer, Sarah Larrat. 'Ut in omnibus honorificetur Deus: The *Corsnæd* Ordeal in Anglo-Saxon England: What's the Problem with Barley?'. *The Community, the Family, and the Saint: Patterns of Power in Early Medieval Europe: Selected Proceedings of the International Medieval Congress, University of Leeds*. Brepols: Turnhout, 1998, pp. 237–64.

—— 'Margin as Archive: The Liturgical Marginalia of a Manuscript of the Old English Bede'. *Traditio*. 1996, 51, 147–77.

—— 'Manuals'. *The Liturgical Books of Anglo-Saxon England*, ed. Richard W. Pfaff. Medieval Institute Press: Kalamazoo, 1995, pp. 99–110.

Kelly, Henry Ansgar. 'Canon Law and Chaucer on Licit and Illicit Magic'. *Law and the Illicit in Medieval Europe*, ed. Ruth Mazo Karras, Joel Kaye, and E. Ann Matter. University of Pennsylvania Press: Philadelphia, 2008.

Ker, N. R. *Catalogue of Manuscripts Containing Anglo-Saxon*. Clarendon Press: Oxford, 1957.

Kershaw, Paul. 'Illness, Power, and Prayer in Asser's Life of King Alfred'.

Early Medieval Europe. 2001, 10, 201–24.

Keynes, Simon. 'An Abbot, an Archbishop, and the Viking Raids of 1006–7 and 1009–12'. *ASE*. 2007, 36, 151–220.

—— 'Royal Government and the Written Word in Late Anglo-Saxon England'. *The Uses of Literacy in Early Medieval Europe*, ed. Rosamond McKitterick. Cambridge University Press: Cambridge, 1990, pp. 226–57.

Kibre, Pearl and Irving A. Kelter. 'Galen's "Methodus medendi" in the Middle Ages'. *History and Philosophy of the Life Sciences*. 1987, 9, 17–36.

Kieckhefer, Richard. 'The Specific Rationality of Medieval Magic'. *American Historical Review*. 1994, 99.3, 813–36.

—— *Magic in the Middle Ages*. Cambridge University Press: Cambridge, 1990.

Kitson, Peter. 'From Eastern Learning to Western Folklore: The Transmission of Some Medico-Magical Ideas'. *Superstition and Popular Medicine in Anglo-Saxon England*, ed. Donald Scragg. Manchester Centre for Anglo-Saxon Studies: Manchester, 1989, pp. 51–71.

Langslow, David. *The Latin Alexander Trallianus: The Text and Transmission of a Late Latin Medical Book*. Society for the Promotion of Roman Studies, monograph 10. Society for the Promotion of Roman Studies: London, 2006.

—— *Medical Latin in the Roman Empire*. Oxford University Press: Oxford, 2000.

Lapidge, Michael. *The Anglo-Saxon Library*. Oxford University Press: Oxford, 2006.

—— 'The Origin of the Collectanea'. *Collectanea pseudo-Bedae*, ed. Martha Bayless and Michael Lapidge. Scriptores Latini Hiberniae. Dublin Institute for Advanced Studies: Dublin, 1998.

—— 'Æthelwold as Scholar and Teacher'. *Bishop Æthelwold: His Career and Influence*, ed. Barbara Yorke. Boydell Press: Woodbridge, 1997, pp. 13–42.

—— 'Schools, Learning and Literature in Tenth-Century England'. *Settimane di Studio del Centro Italiano di Studi sull'Alto Medioevo*. 1991, 38, 951–1005. Reprinted in *Anglo-Latin Literature*. Hambledon Press: London, 1993, pp. 1–48.

—— 'Surviving Booklists from Anglo-Saxon England'. *Learning and Literature in Anglo-Saxon England: Studies Presented to Peter Clemoes on the Occasion of his Sixty-Fifth Birthday*, ed. Michael Lapidge and Helmut Gneuss. Cambridge University Press: Cambridge, 1985, pp. 35–89.

—— 'Latin Learning in Dark Age Wales: Some Prolegomena'. *Proceedings of the Seventh International Congress of Celtic Studies, Oxford, 1983*, ed. D. Ellis Evans, John G. Griffith, and E. M. Jope. Proceedings of the International Congress of Celtic Studies. Oxbow Books: Oxford, 1983.

—— 'The Cult of St. Indract at Glastonbury'. *Ireland in Early Medieval Europe: Studies in Memory of Kathleen Hughes*, ed. D. Whitelock, R. McKitterick,

and D. Dumville. Cambridge University Press: Cambridge, 1982, pp. 179–212.
—— 'The Hermeneutic Style in Tenth-Century Anglo-Latin Literature'. *ASE*. 1975, 4, 67–111.
Lass, Roger. *Old English: A Historical Linguistic Companion*. Cambridge University Press: Cambridge, 1994.
Law, Vivien. *Grammar and Grammarians in the Early Middle Ages*. Longman: London, 1997.
—— *The Insular Latin Grammarians*. Boydell Press: Woodbridge, 1982.
Lawn, Brian. *The Salernitan Questions: An Introduction to the History of Medieval and Renaissance Problem Literature*. Clarendon Press: Oxford, 1963.
Lee, Christina. 'Changing Faces: Leprosy in Anglo-Saxon England'. *Conversion and Colonization in Anglo-Saxon England*. Arizona Center for Medieval and Renaissance Studies: Tempe, AZ, 2006, pp. 59–81.
Leeper, Elizabeth Ann. 'Exorcism in Early Christianity'. Unpublished Ph.D. Dissertation. Duke University, 1991.
Leja, Meg. 'The Sacred Art: Medicine in the Carolingian Renaissance'. *Viator*. 2016, 47, 1–34.
Lemke, Andreas. *The Old English Translation of Bede's* Historica Ecclesiastica Gentis Anglorum *in its Historical and Cultural Context*. Göttinger Schriften zur Englischen Philologie, Band 8. Universitätsverlag Göttingen: Göttingen, 2015.
Lindsay, Wallace Martin. *Notae Latinae: An Account of Abbreviations in Latin MSS. of the Early Minuscule Period (c. 700–850)*. Cambridge University Press: Cambridge, 1915.
Liuzza, Roy Michael. 'Anglo-Saxon Prognostics in Context: A Survey and Handlist of Manuscripts'. *ASE*. 2001, 30, 181–230.
Lockett, Leslie. *Anglo-Saxon Psychologies in the Vernacular and Latin Traditions*. University of Toronto Press: Toronto, 2011.
Longrigg, James. *Greek Rational Medicine: Philosophy and Medicine from Alcmaeon to the Alexandrians*. Routledge: London, 1993.
Mackey, James P. 'Introduction: Is There a Celtic Christianity?'. *An Introduction to Celtic Christianity*, ed. James Mackey. T&T Clark: Edinburgh, 1989, pp. 1–21.
MacKinney, Loren C. *Early Medieval Medicine with Special Reference to France and Chartres*. Johns Hopkins Press: Baltimore, 1937.
Magennis, Hugh. *Translating Beowulf: Modern Versions in English Verse*. D. S. Brewer: Cambridge, 2011.
Magoun, Francis P. Jr. 'Zu den ae. Zaubersprüchen'. *Archiv für der neueren Sprachen und Literaturen*. 1937, 171, 17–35.
Maion, Danielle. 'The Fortune of the So-called *Practica Petrocelli Salernitani* in England: New Evidence and Some Considerations'. *Form and Content of Instruction in Anglo-Saxon England in the Light of Contemporary*

Manuscript Evidence: Papers Presented at the International Conference, Udine, 6–8 April 2006, ed. Patrizia Lendinara, Loredana Lazzari, and Maria Amalia D'Aronco. Brepols: Turnhout, 2007, pp. 479–96.

Markus, Robert A. Review of V. Flint, *The Rise of Magic in Early Medieval Europe*. *English Historical Review*. 1992, 107, 378–80.

—— 'Gregory the Great and a Papal Missionary Strategy'. *The Mission of the Church and the Propagation of the Faith: Papers Read at the Seventh Summer Meeting and the Eighth Winter Meeting of the Ecclesiastical History Society*, ed. G. J. Cuming. Cambridge University Press: Cambridge, 1970, pp. 29–38.

Marson, Charles Latimer. *Glastonbury: The Historic Guide to the 'English Jerusalem'*. Simpkin, Marshall, Hamilton, Ket & Co.: London, 1909.

McGowan, Joseph. 'Elves, Elf-shot, Epilepsy: OE ælfadl, ælfsiden, ælfsogeþa, bræccoþu, and bræcseoc'. *Studia Neophilologica*. 2009, 81.2, 116–20.

McGrath, Fergal. *Education in Ancient and Medieval Ireland*. Studies Special Publications: Dublin, 1979.

McKitterick, Rosamond. *The Carolingians and the Written Word*. Cambridge University Press: Cambridge, 1989.

McNally, Robert E. 'The "Tres Linguae Sacrae" in Early Irish Bible Exegesis'. *Theological Studies*. 1958, 19, 395–403.

Meaney, Audrey L. 'Magic'. *The Wiley-Blackwell Encyclopedia of Anglo-Saxon England*, ed. Michael Lapidge, John Blair, Simon Keynes, and Donald Scragg. 2nd Edition. John Wiley & Sons: Chichester, 2014, p. 304.

—— 'The Devil Can Seriously Damage your Health: Reflections on Anglo-Saxon Demonology'. *The Devil in Society in Premodern Europe*, ed. Richard Raiswell and Peter Dendle. Centre for Reformation and Renaissance Studies: Toronto, 2012, pp. 69–108.

—— 'Extra-Medical Elements in Anglo-Saxon Medicine'. *Social History of Medicine*. 2011, 24.1, 41–56.

—— 'Old English Legal and Penitential Penalties for "Heathenism"'. *Anglo-Saxons: Studies Presented to Cyril Roy Hart*, ed. Simon Keynes and Alfred P. Smyth. Four Court Press: Dublin and Portland, 2006, pp. 127–58.

—— '"And we forbeodað eornostlice ælcne hæðenscipe": Wulfstan and Late Anglo-Saxon and Norse "Heathenism"'. *Wulfstan, Archbishop of York: Proceedings of the Second Alcuin Conference*, ed. Matthew Townend. Brepols: Turnhout, 2004, pp. 461–500.

—— 'The Practice of Medicine in England about the Year 1000'. *The Year 1000: Medical Practice at the End of the First Millennium*, ed. Peregrine Horden and Emilie Savage-Smith. *Social History of Medicine*, 2000, 13.2, 221–37.

—— 'The Anglo-Saxon View of the Causes of Illness'. *Health, Disease and*

Healing in Medieval Culture, ed. Sheila Campbell, Bert Hall, and David Klausner. Macmillan: Basingstoke, 1992, pp. 12–33.

—— 'Women, Witchcraft and Magic in Anglo-Saxon England'. *Superstition and Popular Medicine in Anglo-Saxon England*, ed. Donald Scragg. Manchester Centre for Anglo-Saxon Studies: Manchester, 1989, pp. 9–40.

—— 'Ælfric's Use of his Sources in his Homily on Auguries'. *English Studies*. 1985, 66.6, 477–95.

—— 'Variant Versions of Old English Medical Remedies and the Compilation of Bald's *Leechbook*'. *ASE*. 1984, 13, 235–68.

—— 'Ælfric and Idolatry'. *Journal of Religious History*. 1984, 13.2, 119–35.

—— *Anglo-Saxon Amulets and Curing Stones*. British Archaeological Reports, British Series: Oxford, 1981.

—— 'Alfred, the Patriarch and the White Stone'. *Aumla: Journal of the Australian Universities Language and Literature Association*. 1978, 49, 65–89.

Meroney, Howard. 'Irish in the Old English Charms'. *Speculum*. 1945, 20, 172–82.

Middle English Dictionary, ed. Hans Kurath. University of Michigan Press: Ann Arbor, 1952–2001. Consulted at <http://quod.lib.umich.edu/m/med/>. Accessed 10 August 2016.

Mize, Britt. 'The Representation of the Mind as an Enclosure in Old English Poetry'. *ASE*. 2006, 35, 57–90.

Morrish, Jennifer. 'King Alfred's Letter as a Source on Learning in England'. *Studies in Earlier Old English Prose*, ed. Paul E. Szarmach. State University of New York Press: Albany, 1986, pp. 87–108.

Motz, Lotte. *The Wise One of the Mountain: Form, Function, and the Significance of the Subterranean Smith: a Study in Folklore*. Kümmerle: Göttingen, 1983.

—— 'Of Elves and Dwarfs'. *Arv: Journal of Scandinavian Folklore*. 1973–74, 29–30, 93–127.

Murray, Alexander. 'Missionaries and Magic in Dark-Age Europe'. *Past and Present*. 1992, 136, 186–205.

Nightingale, John. 'Oswald, Fleury and Continental Reform'. *St Oswald of Worcester: Life and Influence*, ed. Nicholas Brooks and Catherine Cubitt. Leicester University Press: London, 1996, pp. 23–45.

Nokes, Richard Scott. 'The Several Compilers of Bald's *Leechbook*'. *ASE*. 2004, 33, 51–76.

—— 'The Old English Charms and Their Manuscript Context, British Library Royal 12 D. xvii and the British Library Harley 585'. Unpublished Ph.D. Dissertation. Wayne State University, 2002.

North, Richard. *Heathen Gods in Old English Literature*. Cambridge University Press: Cambridge, 1997.

O'Brien O'Keeffe, Katherine. 'Old English Literature and the Negotiations of Tradition'. *A Companion to British Literature, Volume 1: Medieval*

Literature, 700–1450, ed. Robert Demaria, Jr., Heesok Chang, and Samantha Zacher. John Wiley & Sons: Chichester, 2014, pp. 16–29.

—— *Visible Song: Transitional Literacy in Old English Verse*. Cambridge University Press: Cambridge, 1990.

O'Donoghue, Noel D. 'St Patrick's Breastplate'. *An Introduction to Celtic Christianity*, ed. J. P. Mackey. T & T Clark: Edinburgh, 1989, pp. 43–63.

Olds, Barbara M. 'The Anglo-Saxon *Leechbook III*: A Critical Edition and Translation'. Unpublished Ph.D. Dissertation. University of Denver, 1984.

Olsan, Lea. 'Charms and Prayers in Medieval Medical Theory and Practice'. *Social History of Medicine*. 16, 2003, 343–66.

—— 'The Inscription of Charms in Anglo-Saxon Manuscripts'. *Oral Tradition*. 1999, 14, 401–19.

—— 'Latin Charms of Medieval England: Verbal Healing in a Christian Oral Tradition'. *Oral Tradition*. 1992, 7, 116–42.

—— 'The Arcus Charms and Christian Magic'. *Neophilologus*. 1989, 73, 438–47.

Olsen, Karin. 'Thematic Affinities between the Non-Liturgical Marginalia and the Old English Bede in Cambridge, Corpus Christi College 41'. *Practice in Learning: The Transfer of Encyclopaedic Knowledge in the Early Middle Ages*, ed. Rolf H. Bremmer Jr. and Kees Dekker. Mediaevalia Groningana new series 16. Peeters: Paris, 2010, pp. 133–45.

O'Neill, Patrick. 'On the Date, Provence and Relationship of the "Solomon and Saturn" Dialogues'. *ASE*. 1997, 26, 139–68.

Orchard, Andy. 'The Word Made Flesh: Christianity and Oral Culture in Anglo-Saxon Verse'. *Oral Tradition*. 2009, 24, 293–318.

—— 'Looking for an Echo: The Oral Tradition in Anglo-Saxon Literature'. *Oral Tradition*. 2004, 18, 225–27.

—— *Pride and Prodigies: Studies in the Monsters of the Beowulf-Manuscript*. D. S. Brewer: Cambridge, 1995. Reprinted, University of Toronto Press: Toronto, 2003.

—— *Cassell Dictionary of Norse Myth and Legend*. Cassell: London, 1997.

—— '"Audite Omnes Amantes": A Hymn in Patrick's Praise'. *Saint Patrick, A. D. 493–1993*, ed. David N. Dumville and Lesley Abrams. Boydell Press: Woodbridge, 1993, pp. 153–73.

Osborn, Marijane. 'Anglo-Saxon Ethnobotany: Women's Reproductive Medicine'. *Health and Healing from the Medieval Garden*, ed. Peter Dendle and Alain Touwaide. Boydell Press: Woodbridge, 2008, pp. 145–61.

Oxford English Dictionary Online. Oxford University Press. Consulted at <www.oed.com>. Accessed 10 August 2016.

Parker, S. J. 'Skulls, Symbols and Surgery: A Review of the Evidence for Trepanation in Anglo-Saxon England and a Consideration of the Motives Behind the Practice'. *Superstition and Popular Medicine in Anglo-Saxon England*, ed. Donald Scragg. Manchester Centre for Anglo-Saxon

Studies: Manchester, 1989, pp. 73–84.

Parkes, Henry. 'Questioning the Authority of Vogel and Elze's *Pontifical romano-germanique*'. *Understanding Medieval Liturgy: Essays in Interpretation*, ed. Helen Gittos and Sarah Hamilton. Ashgate: Farnham, 2016, pp. 75–101.

Parkes, Malcolm. 'The Palaeography of the Parker Manuscript of the Chronicle, Laws and Sedulius, and Historiography at Winchester in the Late Ninth and Tenth Centuries'. *ASE*. 1976, 5, 149–71.

PASE, *Prosopography of Anglo-Saxon England*. Consulted at <http://www.pase.ac.uk>. Accessed 26 September 2017.

Paxton, Frederick S. 'Curing Bodies – Curing Souls: Hrabanus Maurus, Medical Education, and the Clergy in Ninth-Century Francia'. *Journal of the History of Medicine*. 1995, 50, 230–52.

Payne, Anne. 'The Danes' Prayers to the "Gastbona" in Beowulf'. *Neuphilogische Mitteilungen*. 1979, 80, 308–14.

Payne, Joseph Frank. *The Fitz-Patrick Lectures for 1903: English Medicine in Anglo-Saxon Times*. Clarendon Press: Oxford, 1904.

Pettit, Edward. 'Some Anglo-Saxon Charms'. *Essays on Anglo-Saxon and Related Themes in Memory of Lynne Grundy*, ed. Jane Roberts and Janet Nelson. King's College London, Centre for Late Antique & Medieval Studies: London, 2000, pp. 411–33.

—— 'Anglo-Saxon Charms in Oxford, Bodleian Library MS Barlow 35'. *Nottingham Medieval Studies*. 1999, 43, 33–46.

Pfaff, Richard W. *The Liturgy in Medieval England: A History*. Cambridge University Press: Cambridge, 2009.

Pratt, David. *The Political Thought of Alfred the Great*. Cambridge University Press: Cambridge, 2009.

—— 'Problems of Authorship and Audience in the Writings of King Alfred the Great'. *Lay Intellectuals in the Carolingian World*, ed. Patrick Wormald and Janet L. Nelson. Cambridge University Press: Cambridge, 2007, pp. 162–91.

—— 'Persuasion and Invention at the Court of King Alfred the Great'. *Court Culture in the Early Middle Ages*, ed. C. Cubitt. Brepols: Turnhout, 2003, pp. 189–221.

—— 'The Illnesses of King Alfred the Great'. *ASE*. 2001, 30, 39–90.

Pryce, Huw. 'Pastoral Care in Early Medieval Wales'. *Pastoral Care Before the Parish*, ed. John Blair and Richard Sharpe. Leicester University Press: Leicester, 1992, pp. 41–62.

Raiswell, Richard and Peter Dendle. 'Demon Possession in Anglo-Saxon and Early Modern England: Continuity and Evolution in Social Context'. *Journal of British Studies*. 2008, 47.4, 738–67.

Ramsay, Nigel, Margaret Sparks, and Tim Tatton-Brown (eds). *St Dunstan: His Life, Times, and Cult*. Boydell Press: Woodbridge, 1992.

Rayner, Emma. 'AncientBiotics – A Medieval Remedy for Modern Day

Superbugs?'. University of Nottingham. Consulted at <http://www.nottingham.ac.uk/news/pressreleases/2015/march/ancientbiotics---a-medieval-remedy-for-modern-day-superbugs.aspx>. Accessed 27 June 2016.

Reid, Jennifer. '"Caro Verbum Factum Est": Incarnations of Word in Early English and Celtic Texts'. Unpublished Ph.D. Dissertation. University of Toronto, 2007.

—— 'The Lorica of Laidcenn: The Biblical Connections'. *Journal of Medieval Latin*. 2002, 12, 141–53.

Riddle, John. *Quid Pro Quo: Studies in the History of Drugs*. Variorum: Aldershot, 1992.

—— *Contraception and Abortion in the Ancient World to the Renaissance*. Harvard University Press: London and Cambridge, MA, 1992.

—— *Dioscorides on Pharmacy and Medicine*. University of Texas Press: Austin, 1985.

—— 'Pseudo-Dioscorides' *Ex herbis femininis* and Early Medieval Medical Botany'. *Journal of the History of Biology*. 1981, 14.1, 43–81.

—— 'Theory and Practice in Medieval Medicine'. *Viator*. 1974, 5, 157–84.

Risse, Guenter B. *Mending Bodies, Saving Souls: A History of Hospitals*. Oxford University Press: Oxford, 1999.

Rivard, Derek A. *Blessing the World: Ritual and Lay Piety of Medieval Religion*. Catholic University of America Press: Washington, D.C., 2009.

Robinson, J. Armitage. *The Times of Saint Dunstan: The Ford Lectures, delivered in the University of Oxford in the Michaelmas Term, 1922*. Clarendon Press: Oxford, 1923.

Rodrigues, Louis J. *Anglo-Saxon Verse Charms, Maxims and Heroic Legends*. Anglo-Saxon Books: Pinner, 1993.

Rowley, Sharon M. *The Old English Version of Bede's Historia Ecclesiastica*. D. S. Brewer: Cambridge, 2011.

Rubin, Stanley. 'The Anglo-Saxon Physician'. *Medicine in Early Medieval England: Four Papers*, ed. Marilyn Deegan and Donald Scragg. Centre for Anglo-Saxon Studies, University of Manchester: Manchester, 1989, pp. 7–15.

—— *Medieval English Medicine*. David & Charles: Newton Abbot, 1974.

Rumble, Alexander R. 'The Laity and the Monastic Reform in the Reign of Edgar'. *Edgar, King of the English, 959–975*, ed. Donald Scragg. Boydell Press: Woodbridge, 2008, pp. 242–51.

Rusche, Philip G. 'Dioscorides' *De materia medica* and Late Old English Herbal Glossaries'. *From Earth to Art: The Many Aspects of the Plant-World in Anglo-Saxon England: Proceedings of the First ASPNS Symposium, University of Glasgow, 5–7 April 2000*, ed. C. P. Biggam. Rodopi: New York, 2003, pp. 181–94.

Sabbah, Guy, Pierre-Paul Corsetti, and Klaus-Dietrich Fischer. *Bibliographie des textes médicaux latins: Antiquité et haut moyen age*. Université de Saint

Etienne: Saint Etienne, 1987.

Sacraments and Sacramentals, ed. Anscar J. Chupungco. Handbook for Liturgical Studies 4. Liturgical Press: Collegeville, MN, 1997.

Saunders, Corinne. *Magic and the Supernatural in Medieval English Romance*. D. S. Brewer: Cambridge, 2010.

Scribner, Robert W. *Popular Culture and Popular Movements in Reformation Germany*. Hambledon Press: London, 1987.

Searle, William George. *Onomasticon Anglo-Saxonicum: A List of Anglo-Saxon Proper Names From the Time of Beda to that of King John*. Cambridge University Press: Cambridge, 1897.

Sharpe, Richard. 'Churches and Communities in Early Medieval Ireland'. *Pastoral Care Before the Parish*, ed. John Blair and Richard Sharpe. Leicester University Press: Leicester, 1992, pp. 81–109.

Shaw, Philip. 'The Manuscript Texts of Against a Dwarf'. *Writing and Texts in Anglo-Saxon England*, ed. Alexander R. Rumble. D. S. Brewer: Cambridge, 2006, pp. 96–113.

Shippey, T. A. 'Light-elves, Dark-elves, and Others: Tolkien's Elvish Problem'. *Tolkien Studies*, 2004, 1, 1–15.

Sigerist, H. E. 'The Latin Medical Literature of the Early Middle Ages'. *Journal of the History of Medicine and Allied Sciences*, 1958, 13, 127–46.

Simek, Rudolf. 'Demons and Alfar'. *Conversions: Looking for Ideological Change in the Early Middle Ages*, ed. Leszek Slupecki and Rudolf Simek. Fassbaender: Vienna, 2013, pp. 321–42.

—— 'Elves and Exorcism: Runic and Other Lead Amulets in Medieval Popular Religion'. *Myths, Legends, and Heroes: Essays on Old Norse and Old English Literature in Honour of John McKinnell*, ed. Daniel Anlezark. University of Toronto Press: Toronto, Buffalo, and London, 2011, pp. 25–52.

Sims-Williams, Patrick. *Religion and Literature in Western England, 600–800*. Cambridge University Press: Cambridge, 1990.

—— 'Thought, Word and Deed: An Irish Triad'. *Ériu*, 1978, 29, 78–111.

Singer, Charles J. *From Magic to Science: Essays on the Scientific Twilight*. Ernest Benn: London, 1928. Reprinted, Dover: New York, 1958.

—— 'The Herbal in Antiquity and its Transmission to Later Ages'. *The Journal of Hellenic Studies*. 1927, 47.1, 1–52.

—— 'Early English Medicine and Magic'. *Proceedings of the British Academy*. 1920, 9, 341–74.

Siraisi, Nancy G. *Medieval & Early Renaissance Medicine: An Introduction to Knowledge and Practice*. University of Chicago Press: London, 1990.

Slover, Clark H. 'Glastonbury Abbey and the Fusing of English Literary Culture'. *Speculum*. 1935, 10.2, 147–60.

Stanley, E. O. 'Did the Anglo-Saxons Have a Social Conscience Like Us?'. *Anglia*. 2003, 121.2, 238–64.

—— *The Search for Anglo-Saxon Paganism*. D. S. Brewer: Cambridge, 1975.

Stannard, Jerry. 'The Herbal as a Medical Document'. *Herbs and Herbalism in the Middle Ages and Renaissance*, ed. Katherine E. Stannard and Richard Kay. Variorum: Aldershot, 1999, pp. 212–20.

—— 'The Theoretical Bases of Medieval Herbalism'. *Herbs and Herbalism in the Middle Ages and Renaissance*. Variorum: Aldershot, 1999, pp. 186–96.

—— 'Medieval Herbals and their Development'. *Herbs and Herbalism in the Middle Ages and Renaissance*. Variorum: Aldershot, 1999, pp. 23–33.

Stanton, Robert. *The Culture of Translation in Anglo-Saxon England*. D. S. Brewer: Cambridge, 2002.

Stevenson, Jane. 'Literacy in Ireland: The Evidence of the Patrick Dossier in the Book of Armagh'. *The Uses of Literacy in Early Medieval Europe*, ed. Rosamond McKitterick. Cambridge University Press: Cambridge, 1990, pp. 11–35.

Storms, Gordon. *Anglo-Saxon Magic*. Nijhoff: Hague, 1948.

Symes, Carol. 'Liturgical Texts and Performance Practices'. *Understanding Medieval Liturgy: Essays in Interpretation*, ed. Helen Gittos and Sarah Hamilton. Ashgate: Farnham, 2016, pp. 239–67.

Szarmach, Paul E. 'Augustine's *Soliloquia* in Old English'. *A Companion to Alfred the Great*, ed. Nicole Guenther Discenza and Paul E. Szarmach. Brill: Leiden and Boston, 2014, pp. 227–55.

Talbot, Charles. H. *Medicine in Medieval England*. Oldbourne: London, 1967.

—— 'Some Notes on Anglo-Saxon Medicine'. *Medical History*. 1965, 9, 156–69.

Temkin, Owsei. *Hippocrates in a World of Pagans and Christians*. John Hopkins University Press: Baltimore and London, 1991.

—— *Galenism: Rise and Decline of a Medical Philosophy*. Cornell University Press: London, 1973.

Thompson, Victoria. *Dying and Death in Later Anglo-Saxon England*. Boydell Press: Woodbridge, 2004.

Thornbury, Emily. 'Aldhelm's Rejection of the Muses and the Mechanics of Poetic Inspiration in Early Anglo-Saxon England'. *Anglo-Saxon England*. 2007, 36, 71–92.

Thorndike, Lynn. *The Place of Magic in the Intellectual History of Europe*. AMS Press: New York, 1967.

—— and Pearl Kibre. *A Catalogue of Incipits of Mediaeval Scientific Writings in Latin*. Medieval Academy: Cambridge, MA, 1963.

Thun, Nils. 'The Malignant Elves: Notes on Anglo-Saxon Magic and Germanic Myth'. *Studia Neophilologica*. 1969, 41.2, 378–96.

Van Arsdall, Anne. 'Rehabilitating Medieval Medicine'. *Misconceptions about the Middle Ages*, ed. Stephen Harris and Byron L. Grisby. Routledge Studies in Medieval Religion and Culture 7. Routledge: New York and London, 2008.

—— 'Challenging the "Eye of Newt" Image of Medieval Medicine'. *The*

Medieval Hospital and Medical Practice, ed. Barbara S. Bowers. Ashgate: Aldershot, 2007, pp. 195–208.

—— 'Medical Training in Anglo-Saxon England: An Evaluation of the Evidence'. *Form and Content of Instruction in Anglo-Saxon England in the Light of Contemporary Manuscript Evidence: Papers Presented at the International Conference, Udine, 6–8 April 2006*, ed. Patrizia Lendinara, Loredana Lazzari, and Maria Amalia D'Aronco. Brepols: Turnhout, 2007, pp. 415–34.

—— 'Reading Medieval Medical Texts with an Open Mind'. *Textual Healing: Essays in Medieval and Early Modern Medicine*, ed. Elizabeth Furdell. Brill: Leiden, 2005, pp. 9–30.

—— *Medieval Herbal Remedies: The Old English Herbarium and Anglo-Saxon Medicine*. Routledge: New York, 2002.

Vaughan-Sterling, Judith A. 'The Anglo-Saxon "Metrical Charms": Poetry as Ritual'. *JEGP*. 1983, 82, 186–200.

Versnel, H. S. 'The Poetics of the Magical Charm: An Essay in the Power of Words'. *Magic and Ritual in the Ancient World*, ed. Paul Mireki and Marvin Meyer. Brill: Leiden, Boston, and Cologne, 2002, pp. 105–58.

Voigts, Linda. 'Anglo-Saxon Plant Remedies and the Anglo-Saxons'. *Isis*. 1979, 70, 250–68.

—— 'The Significance of the Name "Apuleius" to the *Herbarium Apulei*'. *Bulletin of the History of Medicine*. 1978, 52, 214–27.

—— and Patricia Deery Kurtz. *Scientific and Medical Writings in Old and Middle English: An Electronic Reference*. University of Michigan Press: Ann Arbor, 2000. Consulted at <http://http://cctr1.umkc.edu/search>. Accessed 14 September 2015.

Voth, Christine Bobbitt. 'An Analysis of the Tenth-Century Anglo-Saxon Manuscript London, British Library, Royal 12. D. xvii'. Unpublished Ph.D. Dissertation. University of Cambridge, 2015.

Wallis, Faith. 'The Experience of the Book: Manuscripts, Texts, and the Role of Epistemology in Early Medieval Medicine'. *Knowledge and the Scholarly Medical Traditions*, ed. Don Bates. Cambridge University Press: Cambridge, 1995, pp. 101–26.

Waterhouse, Ruth. 'Tone in Alfred's Version of Augustine's Soliloquies'. *Studies in Earlier Old English Prose*, ed. Paul E. Szarmach. State University of New York Press: Albany, 1986, pp. 47–86.

Watkins, Francis *et al*. 'Antimicrobial Assays of Three Native British Plants Used in Anglo-Saxon Medicine for Wound Healing Formulations in 10th Century England'. *Journal of Ethnopharmacology*. 2012, 144, 408–15.

—— *et al*. 'Anglo-Saxon Pharmacopoeia Revisited: A Potential Treasure in Drug Discovery'. *Drug Discovery Today*. 2011, 16, 1069–75.

Weston, L. M. C. 'Women's Medicine, Women's Magic: The English Metrical Childbirth Charms'. *Modern Philology*. 1995, 92.3, 279–93.

Whitelock, Dorothy. 'The Prose of Alfred's Reign'. *Continuations and*

Beginnings, ed. E. G. Stanley. Nelson: London, 1966, pp. 67–103.

The Wiley-Blackwell Encyclopedia of Anglo-Saxon England, ed. Michael Lapidge, John Blair, Simon Keynes, and Donald Scragg. 2nd Edition. John Wiley & Sons: Chichester, 2014.

Woolf, R. E. 'The Devil in Old English Poetry'. *The Review of English Studies*. 1953, 13.4, 1–12.

Wormald, Patrick. 'Æthelwold and his Continental Counterparts: Contact, Comparison, Contrast'. *Bishop Æthelwold: His Career and Influence*, ed. Barbara Yorke. Boydell Press: Woodbridge, 1997, pp. 13–42.

Wright, Charles D. '*The Apocalypse of Thomas*: Some New Latin Texts and their Significance for the Old English Versions'. *Apocryphal Texts and Traditions in Anglo-Saxon England*, ed. Kathryn Powell and Donald Scragg. D. S. Brewer: Cambridge, 2003, pp. 27–64.

—— 'The Irish Tradition'. *A Companion to Anglo-Saxon Literature*, ed. Phillip Pulsiano and Elaine Treharne. Blackwell Publishers: Oxford, 2001, pp. 345–74.

—— *The Irish Tradition in Old English Literature*. Cambridge Studies in Anglo-Saxon England 6. Cambridge University Press: Cambridge, 1993.

Wright, Neil. 'The Sources of the Collectanea'. *Collectanea pseudo-Bedae*, ed. Martha Bayless and Michael Lapidge. Scriptores Latini Hiberniae. Dublin Institute for Advanced Studies: Dublin, 1998, pp. 25–34.

Yearl, Mary K. K. 'Medieval Monastic Customaries on *Minuti* and *Infirmi*'. *The Medieval Hospital and Medical Practice*, ed. Barbara S. Bowers. Ashgate: Aldershot, 2007, pp. 176–94.

Yorke, Barbara. 'Aldhelm's Irish and British Connections'. *Aldhelm and Sherborne: Essays to Celebrate the Founding of the Bishopric*, ed. Katherine Baker and Nicholas Brooks. Oxbow Books: Oxford, 2010, pp. 164–80.

Zavoti, Susan. 'Blame it on the Elves: Perception of Illness in Anglo-Saxon England'. *Medieval and Early Modern Literature, Science and Medicine*, ed. Rachel Falconer and Denis Renevey. Narr Verlag: Tübingen, 2013, pp. 67–78.

Zimmer, Heinrich. 'Keltische Studien. 13. Ein altirischer Zauberspruch aus der Vikingerzeit'. *Zeitschrift für vergleichende Sprachforschung*. 1895, 33, 144–45.

Index

Ad Glauconem de methodo medendi 13, 19–20, 55 n 80
Alcuin 148, 170
Aldhelm 89, 93, 129
Alexander of Tralles 18–19
   See also Latin Alexander
Alfred, King 45–47, 49
   See also Alfredian translations
Alfredian translations 45–46, 49, 141
   Bald's Leechbook as an Alfredian text 46–53, 55–56
   See also Bald's Leechbook
Amand Abbey 54
Anglo-Saxon Chronicle see Parker Chronicle
Antiphonary of Bangor 88, 91 n 112, 119
Arzneibuch see Lorsch *Arzneibuch*
Audite omnes amantes 119
Augustine of Hippo 77, 154, 158, 165, 167, 169
   De videndo deo 51
   Soliloquies, Old English translation 45–46, 49
      comparison with *Bald's Leechbook* 50–52
   See also Alfredian translations
Aurelius-Esculapius Complex 19–20, 38, 54
æcerbot 114
   See also metrical charms
ælf-adl 65, 67–68
   water-ælfadl 65–68, 85
   See also ælfe
ælf-cynne 65, 75
   See also ælfe
ælf-siden 61–62, 63, 64, 73, 75
   See also ælfe
ælf-sogoþa 59, 65–68, 75–76, 82, 83, 85, 86–92, 99
   See also ælf-adl, ælfe
ælf-þone 73–74
ælfe 58, 68, 72–73, 73–75
   association with internal pains 63
   association with skin disorders 66, 71 n 45

diseases in *Bald's Leechbook* 61–63, 83–84
diseases in the *Lacnunga* 63–64, 72–74
diseases in *Leechbook III* 64–68, 72–74, 83–84
relationship to demons 71, 74–78, 81–82, 86, 89–91
relationship to *mære* and *nihtgengan* 59–61
treatment with herbs 69–71, 76, 92
   See also ælf-adl, ælf-cynne, ælf-sogoþa, demons, *dweorh, leod-rune, mære, nihtgengan, ofscoten*
Ælfric, abbot of Eynsham 75, 77, 150, 157, 158
   attitude towards medicine 161, 164–70, 83–184, 186
   forbidden practices 168–70, 172–73, 176–84
Ælfric Bata 155
Æthelthryth, abbess of Ely 153
Æthelwold, bishop of Winchester 137, 147, 150–51

Bald see *Bald's Leechbook*, colophon
Bald's Leechbook 5
   authorship 24, 26–28, 44, 53–56
   colophon 23–24, 53–54, 57
   dialect 45, 47
   educational aims 50, 52–53
   Latin source material 19, 37–38, 54–55
   length 57
   location of composition 45, 47–49, 55, 150
   organisation 24–26, 130
   relationship between Books I and II 28–30, 42–44
   relationship with *Leechbook III* 23, 57–58, 69
   remedies involving *ælfe* 60, 82
   scriptorium 48
   translation skill 39–40, 42, 54–56
   translation styles 28–44, 49–53, 53–54

Index

See also Alfredian translations, Old English medical collections
Baldwin, abbot of Bury St Edmunds 21, 149
Bede 153, 162
  Ecclesiastical History, Old English translation 106, 127
beer 143–44
Benedictine reform movement 131, 137, 149–52, 172
Benedictine Rule 149–50
  Old English translation 150–51
Bernard of Clairvaux 153
Boethius
  Consolation of Philosophy, Old English translation 45, 49, 51–52, 136
  See also Alfredian translations
Book of Cerne 104, 116, 118, 124
  See also Insular Prayerbooks
Book of Nunnaminster 104, 118, 119
  See also Insular Prayerbooks
Bury St Edmunds 21, 149
Byrhtferth of Ramsey 89

Cambridge, Corpus Christi College, MS 41 59, 106–14, 194–98
  grammatica 118–26
  location of composition 126–28
  See also Journey Charm, Lacnunga
Canons of Edgar 178
Canons of Theodore see penitentials
Canterbury 16 n 48, 128, 150–52
Carolingian *renovatio* 148, 170
  See also Old English medical collections, Carolingian influence
Cassiodorus 149
cattle theft charms 108–11, 119, 194–96
  See also metrical charms
charms see *galdru*
Cild see *Bald's Leechbook*, colophon
Cockayne, Oswald
  editions 7–8, 9, 23, 57, 95, 132
Collectanea Pseudo-Bedeae 124
Consolation of Philosophy see Boethius
Curae herbarium 16–17, 132, 148
  See also Dioscorides
Danelaw 179–81
De medicamentis 13, 29, 31–32, 38, 96
demonic possession 76–78, 80, 81–84, 86, 88, 93
  See also demons, exorcism
demons 78

relationship to *ælfe* 71, 74–78, 81–82, 89–94
treatment with herbs 71, 76, 82, 92
  See also ælfe, demonic possession
deofol see demons
Dioscorides 15–17, 132, 149
  See also Curae herbarium, Liber medicinae ex herbis femininis
drycræft 6, 155, 168–69, 171–73, 177–84, 185
  in penitentials 174–78
  women 176–77
  See also galdru, Lacnunga, relationship with popular belief
Dunstan 127–28, 150
Durham Ritual 104
dweorh 73–74

elf shot see *ofscoten*
elves see *ælfe*
Exeter 106
exorcism 76–81
  Anglo-Saxon England 77, 79–81
  different types 79–80
  in the medical corpus 81–86, 83–84, 86–91, 112, 120

feondes costungum 63, 65, 67, 71, 75–76, 83, 87, 105
  See also demonic possession, demons
For Sudden Stabbing Pain see *Wið færstice*
Francia 13, 54, 148, 155

galdru 6, 11–12, 67, 155, 168–69, 171–74, 177–78, 182–84, 185
  in penitentials 174–78
Galen 18–19, 38
  See also Ad Glauconem de methodo medendi
Gelasian Sacramentary 104
gibberish charms 100–03, 121–22, 129, 182, 183
  See also galdru
Glastonbury 127–28
grammatica 114–16, 129
  See also Cambridge, Corpus Christi College, MS 41, Insular Prayerbooks, *Lacnunga*
Gregory the Great 158–59, 160, 165
  Dialogues, Old English translation 48, 158

230

Index

Pastoral Care, Old English
    translation 158–59
  See also Alfredian translations
Grendel 60

Harleian Prayerbook 105
  See also Insular Prayerbooks
Herbarium Complex 20, 38, 147–48
  Old English translations 34–37,
    131–34, 136
  *See also Medicina de Quadrupedibus,
    Old English Herbarium, Pseudo-
    Apuleius Herbal,*
herbs 155, 170
  exotic ingredients 143–44
  use in Old English medical corpus 3
  use in treating elf-diseases 69–71
  See also medical training, medicine
Hisperica Famina 118, 121
Historia adversum paganos see Orosius
Hrabanus Maurus 148, 170
humours 18

incubus 60
  See also mære
Insular Prayerbooks 91, 104–05, 114–18
Irish see Old English medical
  collections, Irish influence
Isidore of Seville 115–16, 171

Journey Charm 59, 113–14, 118, 126
  See also metrical charms
Judgement Day II 157, 162–63

Lacnunga 5
  date 95
  dialect 95, 104
  exotic languages 100–03
  grammatica 116–24, 128–29
  Latin text 97–100, 104–05
  manuscript context 104–07, 128–29
  organisation 95, 130
  relationship to CCCC 41 106–14,
    119–20, 128, 194–98
  relationship to the *Leechbook III* 69,
    71–74, 94
  relationship with popular
    belief 72–74, 94, 95–97, 129
  remedies involving *ælfe* 61, 63–64, 82
  translation style of Latin medical
    remedies 35–36
  See also Old English medical
    collections

Lanalet Pontifical 80, 82
Latin Alexander 19, 29 n 21, 37–42, 44,
    54–55, 188–91
  See also Alexander of Tralles
Leechbook III 5
  dialect 57
  diseases related to *ælfe* 61, 64–68,
    83–84, 86–94
  length 57–58
  organisation 57–58, 130
  relationship with *Bald's Leechbook* 23,
    57–58, 69, 71–72
  relationship to the *Lacnunga* 69,
    71–74, 94
  relationship with popular
    belief 58–59, 60–61, 91–94
  translator's skill 91–92
  See also Old English medical
    collections
leod-rune 61–62
  See also ælfe
Leofric Missal 88–91, 104
leprosy 21, 166
Liber de taxone 132–33
  See also Herbarium Complex
Liber Hymnorum 111
Liber medicinae ex animalibus 132–33,
    148
  See also Herbarium Complex
Liber medicinae ex herbis femininis 16–17,
    20, 132, 148, 149
  See also Dioscorides
Liber Tertius 13, 19, 20, 29, 37–42, 44,
    54–55, 187–88
Life of Guthlac 82
Life of St Cuthbert 82
liturgy see Old English medical
    collections, relationship to liturgy
London, BL, MS Cotton Otho B. xi 2,
    27, 33
London, BL, MS Cotton Tiberius
    B. v 151
London, BL, MS Cotton Vitellius
    C. iii 130, 135, 137, 148, 151
  See also Old English Pharmacopeia
London, BL, MS Harley 585 95, 126,
    130, 134–35, 151
  See also Lacnunga, Old English
    Pharmacopeia
London, BL, MS Harley 6258b 2, 130,
    137, 151
  See also Old English Pharmacopeia

Index

London, BL, MS Royal 12 D. xvii 23, 45, 47–48, 53, 57
   See also *Bald's Leechbook*, *Leechbook III*
Lord's Prayer II 157
lorica prayers 117, 119, 125
Lorica of Laidcenn 116–18, 119, 121
   See also *lorica* prayers
Lorsch *Arzneibuch* 148, 170
Lotharius, monk 54 n 78

Marcellus see *De medicamentis*
Maxims I 164
mære 58, 59–50
   See also *ælfe*, *nihtgengan*
medical training 156, 164
   in Francia 148–49, 164
Medicina de Quadrupedibus 6, 15,130–43
   date 135–36
   translation style 41, 133–34, 140
   See also Herbarium Complex, *Old English Pharmacopeia*
Medicina Plinii 15, 37, 54
   See also Pliny the Elder, *Physica Plinii*
medicine
   attitudes towards 153–61, 166–68, 185–86
   depiction in Old English literature 157–64
   practice of in Anglo-Saxon England 155–56, 161, 164
   See also Old English medical collections, medical training
menstruation 145–46
metrical charms 103, 109–10, 112–14
   See also cattle theft charms, *Nine Herbs Charm*, *Wið færstice*
Monastic communities
   ownership of medical texts 20–22, 55
   See also Benedictine reform movement
Montecassino Biblioteca della Badia, MS 97 147–48

Naturalis historia 14–15, 20, 21, 31–32, 54, 171
   See also Pliny the Elder
nightmare see *mære*
nihtgengan 58, 59–60
   See also *ælfe*, *mære*
Nine Herbs Charm 112–14, 121
   See also metrical charms
Nowell transcript see London, BL, MS Cotton Otho B. xi

ofscoten 62–64, 72–73
   See also *ælfe*, *Wið færstice*
Old English Handbook see penitentials
Old English Herbarium 6, 15, 55, 60
   date 134–37
   location of composition 147, 148, 150–52
   practicality 139–40, 143–44
   relationship to *Bald's Leechbook* 136
   relationship to *Medicina de Quadrupedibus* 130–31, 133–34, 140
   translation style 34–36, 133–34, 138–47
   women's remedies 145–46, 150
   See also Herbarium Complex, Old English medical collections, *Old English Pharmacopeia*
Old English medical collections
   Carolingian influence 13, 147–48
   efficacy 9–11
   Greek 8, 16 n 48, 86–87, 93, 100–01, 142, 182
   Irish influence 101–03, 110–14, 121–22, 126, 128–29, 173
   Latin medical source material 8–9, 13, 12–20, 130, 184–85
   medical texts in Anglo-Saxon libraries 20–22, 152, 186
   orthodoxy 11–12, 154, 169–70, 182–86
   relationship to liturgy 81, 85–86, 97–99
   use by practitioners 156
   See also *Bald's Leechbook*, *Lacnunga*, *Leechbook III*, *Medicina de Quadrupedibus*, medicine, *Old English Herbarium*, *Old English Pharmacopeia*
Old English Penitential see penitentials
Old English Pharmacopeia 6, 15, 95, 130–34
   See also Herbarium Complex
Oribasius 18–19
   See also *Synopsis* and *Europistes*
Origen 154
Orosius
   Historia adversum paganos, Old English translation 46, 48, 49, 50–52, 136
   See also Alfredian translations
Oxford, Bodleian Library, MS Hatton 76 130, 134, 137, 151
   See also *Old English Pharmacopeia*

Index

Parker Chronicle 47–48, 49
Passionarius see *Aurelius-Esculapius* Complex
penitentials 159–60, 163, 173–77, 183–84
Peterborough 152
Physica Plinii 15, 21, 29, 31–32, 37, 54, 96
 See also Medicina Plinii, Pliny the Elder
Pliny the Elder 14–15, 21, 171
 See also Medicina Plinii, *Physica Plinii*
Pseudo-Apuleius Herbal 13, 15, 17, 131–32, 138 n 23, 148
 See also Herbarium Complex
Pseudo-Egbert Confessional see penitentials
Pseudo-Egbert Penitential see penitentials

reform movement see Benedictine reform movement
Regula S. Benedicti see *Benedictine Rule*
Romano-Germanic Pontifical 85
Royal Prayerbook 91, 104–05, 116
 See also Insular Prayerbooks

Sacramentary of Ratoldus 88, 90
sator formula 108, 122–23

scriftboc see penitentials
sogoþa see *ælf-sogoþa*
Soliloquies see Augustine of Hippo
Solomon and Saturn 106, 124–26, 127, 157
St Gall monastery 55 n 80, 149–50
Stow Missal 88, 91 n 112, 120
St Patrick's Breastplate see *Lorica* prayers
surgery 3 n 4
Synopsis and *Europistes* 18–19, 37–38, 54–55, 55 n 80, 192–93

theft charms see cattle theft charms
tres linguae sacrae 97, 99–100, 116 n 69, 121

Virgilius Maro Grammaticus 122

Winchester 45, 47–48, 55, 150–52
wine 143–44
witchcraft see *drycræft*
Wið færstice 63–64, 72–73, 92, 112–14
 See also ælfe, metrical charms
Worcester 55, 151–52
Wulfstan, archbishop of York 172, 178–81, 183–84, 186

ANGLO-SAXON STUDIES

Volume 1: The Dramatic Liturgy of Anglo-Saxon England,
M. Bradford Bedingfield

Volume 2: The Art of the Anglo-Saxon Goldsmith: Fine Metalwork in Anglo-Saxon England: its Practice and Practitioners, *Elizabeth Coatsworth and Michael Pinder*

Volume 3: The Ruler Portraits of Anglo-Saxon England, *Catherine E. Karkov*

Volume 4: Dying and Death in Later Anglo-Saxon England, *Victoria Thompson*

Volume 5: Landscapes of Monastic Foundation: The Establishment of Religious Houses in East Anglia, c. 650–1200, *Tim Pestell*

Volume 6: Pastoral Care in Late Anglo-Saxon England, *edited by Francesca Tinti*

Volume 7: Episcopal Culture in Late Anglo-Saxon England,
Mary Frances Giandrea

Volume 8: Elves in Anglo-Saxon England: Matters of Belief, Health, Gender and Identity, *Alaric Hall*

Volume 9: Feasting the Dead: Food and Drink in Anglo-Saxon Burial Rituals,
Christina Lee

Volume 10: Anglo-Saxon Button Brooches: Typology, Genealogy, Chronology, *Seiichi Suzuki*

Volume 11: Wasperton: A Roman, British and Anglo-Saxon Community in Central England, *edited by Martin Carver with Catherine Hills and Jonathan Scheschkewitz*

Volume 12: A Companion to Bede, *George Hardin Brown*

Volume 13: Trees in Anglo-Saxon England: Literature, Lore and Landscape,
Della Hooke

Volume 14: The Homiletic Writings of Archbishop Wulfstan,
Joyce Tally Lionarons

Volume 15: The Archaeology of the East Anglian Conversion, *Richard Hoggett*

Volume 16: The Old English Version of Bede's *Historia Ecclesiastica*,
Sharon M. Rowley

Volume 17: Writing Power in Anglo-Saxon England: Texts, Hierarchies, Economies, *Catherine A. M. Clarke*

Volume 18: Cognitive Approaches to Old English Poetry, *Antonina Harbus*

Volume 19: Environment, Society and Landscape in Early Medieval England: Time and Topography, *Tom Williamson*

Volume 20: Honour, Exchange and Violence in *Beowulf*, *Peter S. Baker*

Volume 21: *John the Baptist's Prayer* or *The Descent into Hell* from the Exeter Book: Text, Translation and Critical Study, *M. R. Rambaran-Olm*

Volume 22: Food, Eating and Identity in Early Medieval England, *Allen J. Frantzen*

Volume 23: Capital and Corporal Punishment in Anglo-Saxon England, *edited by Jay Paul Gates and Nicole Marafioti*

Volume 24: The Dating of *Beowulf*: A Reassessment, *edited by Leonard Neidorf*

Volume 25: The Cruciform Brooch and Anglo-Saxon England, *Toby F. Martin*

Volume 26: Trees in the Religions of Early Medieval England, *Michael D. J. Bintley*

Volume 27: The Peterborough Version of the Anglo-Saxon Chronicle: Rewriting Post-Conquest History, *Malasree Home*

Volume 28: The Anglo-Saxon Chancery: The History, Language and Production of Anglo-Saxon Charters from Alfred to Edgar, *Ben Snook*

Volume 29: Representing Beasts in Early Medieval England and Scandinavia, *edited by Michael D. J. Bintley and Thomas J. T. Williams*

Volume 30: Direct Speech in *Beowulf* and Other Old English Narrative Poems, *Elise Louviot*

Volume 31: Old English Philology: Studies in Honour of R. D. Fulk, *edited by Leonard Neidorf, Rafael J. Pascual and Tom Shippey*

Volume 32: 'Charms', Liturgies, and Secret Rites in Early Medieval England, *Ciaran Arthur*

Volume 33: Old Age in Early Medieval England: A Cultural History, *Thijs Porck*

Volume 34: Priests and their Books in Late Anglo-Saxon England, *Gerald P. Dyson*

Volume 35: Burial, Landscape and Identity in Early Medieval Wessex, *Kate Mees*

Volume 36: The Sword in Early Medieval Northern Europe: Experience, Identity, Representation, *Sue Brunning*

Volume 37: The Chronology and Canon of Ælfric of Eynsham, *Aaron J. Kleist*

Volume 38: Medical Texts in Anglo-Saxon Literary Culture, *Emily Kesling*

Volume 39: The Dynastic Drama of *Beowulf, Francis Leneghan*

Volume 40: Old English Lexicology and Lexicography: Essays in Honor of Antonette diPaolo Healey, *edited by Maren Clegg Hyer, Haruko Momma and Samantha Zacher*

Volume 41: Debating with Demons: Pedagogy and Materiality in Early English Literature, *Christina M. Heckman*

Volume 42: Textual Identities in Early Medieval England: Essays in Honour of Katherine O'Brien O'Keeffe, *edited by Jacqueline Fay, Rebecca Stephenson and Renée R. Trilling*

Volume 43: Bishop Æthelwold, his Followers, and Saints' Cults in Early Medieval England: Power, Belief, and Religious Reform, *Alison Hudson*

Volume 44: Global Perspectives on Early Medieval England, *edited by Karen Louise Jolly and Britton Elliott Brooks*

Volume 45: Performance in *Beowulf* and other Old English Poems, *Steven J. A. Breeze*

Volume 46: Wealth and the Material World in the Old English Alfredian Corpus, *Amy Faulkner*

Volume 47: Law, Literature, and Social Regulation in Early Medieval England, *edited by Anya Adair and Andrew Rabin*

www.ingramcontent.com/pod-product-compliance
Lightning Source LLC
Chambersburg PA
CBHW070800230426
43665CB00017B/2431